Infections Associated with Indwelling Medical Devices

SECOND EDITION

Infections Associated with Indwelling Medical Devices

SECOND EDITION

Edited by

Alan L. Bisno

Miami Veterans Administration Medical Center
and Department of Medicine
University of Miami School of Medicine
Miami, Florida

and

Francis A. Waldvogel

Department of Medicine
Clinique Médicale Thérapeutique
University Hospital
Geneva, Switzerland

ASM PRESS
Washington, D.C.

Library of Congress Cataloging-in-Publication Data

Infections associated with indwelling medical devices/edited by Alan L. Bisno and
Francis A. Waldvogel.—2nd ed.
    p. cm.
  Includes index.
  ISBN 1-55581-077-2
  1. Implants, Artificial—Complications. 2. Prosthesis—Complications.
3. Infection—Etiology. I. Bisno, Alan L. II. Waldvogel, Francis A., 1938–
  [DNLM: 1. Implants, Artificial—adverse effects. 2. Prosthesis—adverse effects.
  3. Catheters, Indwelling—adverse effects. 4. Infection—etiology. WE 172 I427 1994]
  RD755.5.I54   1994
  617.9′5—dc20
  DNLM/DLC
  for Library of Congress   94-12592
                                                                                      CIP

Cover photos: Colonization of *n*-butyl-cyanoacrylate by a strain of *Staphylococcus
epidermidis* recovered from a patient with endocarditis. Reprinted with permission of
John Wiley & Sons, Inc. (**Olson, M. E., I. Ruseska, and J. W. Costerton.** 1988.
Colonization of *n*-butyl-2-cyanoacrylate tissue adhesive by *Staphylococcus epidermidis.
J. Biomed. Mater. Res.* **22:**485–495). Copyright 1988, John Wiley & Sons, Inc. Inset:
Radiograph of an infected total knee arthroplasty.

To the memory of our fathers,
Ralph Bisno and Paul Waldvogel

Contents

Contributors

Ann Sullivan Baker • Infectious Disease Service, Massachusetts Eye & Ear Infirmary, and Massachusetts General Hospital, Boston, Massachusetts 02114, and Harvard Medical School, Boston, Massachusetts 02115

Lucilla Baldassarri • Laboratorio di Ultrastrutture, Istituto Superiore di Sanitá, Viale Regina Elena 299, 00161 Rome, Italy

Alan L. Bisno • Department of Veterans Affairs Medical Center, 1201 Northwest 16th Street, Miami, Florida 33125

P. Joan Chesney • Department of Pediatrics, University of Tennessee, Memphis, and LeBonheur Children's Medical Center, 848 Adams Avenue, Memphis, Tennessee 38103

Gordon D. Christensen • Research Service (151), Harry S. Truman Memorial Veterans' Hospital, 800 Hospital Drive, Columbia, Missouri 65201

T. J. Foster • Microbiology Department, Moyne Institute, Trinity College, Dublin 2, Ireland

Gary W. Gibbons • Department of Surgery, Harvard Medical School, and Division of Vascular Surgery, New England Deaconess Hospital, Boston, Massachusetts 02215

David W. Haas • Department of Medicine, Vanderbilt University School of Medicine, 911 Oxford House, Nashville, Tennessee 37232-4751

Margaret T. Hessen • The Medical College of Pennsylvania, 3300 Henry Avenue, Philadelphia, Pennsylvania 19129

Waldemar G. Johanson, Jr. • Department of Medicine, MSB I-506, UMDNJ-New Jersey Medical School, 185 South Orange Avenue, Newark, New Jersey 09103

Allen B. Kaiser • Department of Medicine, Vanderbilt University School of Medicine, Nashville, Tennessee 37232-4751

Adolf W. Karchmer • Department of Medicine, Harvard Medical School, and Infectious Disease Section, New England Deaconess Hospital, 185 Pilgrim Road, Kennedy-6, Boston, Massachusetts 02215

Donald Kaye • Department of Medicine, The Medical College of Pennsylvania, 3300 Henry Avenue, Philadelphia, Pennsylvania 19129

Daniel P. Lew • Infectious Disease Division, University Hospital, CH-1211 Geneva 14, Switzerland

Dennis G. Maki • Section of Infectious Diseases, Department of Medicine, University of Wisconsin Medical School, and Infection Control Department, Center for Trauma and Life Support, University of Wisconsin Hospital and Clinics, Madison, Wisconsin 53792

D. McDevitt • Microbiology Department, Moyne Institute, Trinity College, Dublin 2, Ireland

Douglas R. Osmon • Orthopedic Infectious Diseases Focus Group, Division of Infectious Diseases, Mayo Clinic and Mayo Foundation, Rochester, Minnesota 55905

Richard A. Proctor • Department of Medical Microbiology and Immunology, 407 SMI, University of Wisconsin, Madison, Wisconsin 53706

Oliver D. Schein • Cornea Service and Dana Center for Preventive Ophthalmology, The Wilmer Eye Institute, Johns Hopkins University, Baltimore, Maryland 21287-9019

W. Andrew Simpson • Research Service (151), Harry S. Truman Memorial Veterans' Hospital, 800 Hospital Drive, Columbia, Missouri 65201

James M. Steckelberg • Division of Infectious Diseases, Orthopedic Infectious Diseases Focus Group, Mayo Clinic and Mayo Foundation, Rochester, Minnesota 55905

Linda Sternau • University of Miami School of Medicine, Miami, Florida

Parvathi Tiruviluamala • Division of Pulmonary Diseases, Department of Medicine, MSB I-506, UMDNJ-New Jersey Medical School, 185 South Orange Avenue, Newark, New Jersey 09103

Stephen I. Vas • Departments of Microbiology and Medicine, University of Toronto, Toronto, Ontario M5T 2S8, Canada

Pierre E. Vaudaux • Infectious Disease Division, University Hospital, CH-1211 Geneva 14, Switzerland

Francis A. Waldvogel • Department of Medicine, Clinique Médicale 2, University Hospital, CH-1211 Geneva 14, Switzerland

Introduction

Modern medical and surgical practice has increasingly come to rely upon indwelling devices of various kinds. Such devices may be utilized briefly or intermittently (e.g., intravenous catheters), for months to years (intrauterine devices), or permanently (prosthetic heart valves and hips). The number and variety of devices continue to increase. It has been estimated, for example, that some 140,000 hip prostheses and 115,000 other joint prostheses were inserted in the United States in 1987 alone.

Certainly, indwelling prosthetic devices have been instrumental in saving the lives of a large number of patients and have enhanced the quality of life for a great many more. As with all forms of therapeutic intervention, however, adverse side effects are to be anticipated. In practice, one of the most frequent and serious complications of the use of these devices has been the development of infections. That this should be true comes as no surprise to clinicians specializing in infectious diseases and to microbiologists, who have long recognized that the presence of an indwelling foreign body both predisposes a patient to and greatly complicates the eradication of bacterial and fungal infections.

The magnitude of the problems posed by infections of medical devices has grown pari passu with the proliferation of the devices themselves. It's an ill wind that blows no good, however, and one fortuitous result of these developments has been a renaissance of interest in both the basic scientific and clinical aspects of foreign body infections. On the basic level, scientists have begun to elucidate the nature of the host response to foreign bodies, to assess the effects which prosthetic materials themselves might have on host defenses, and to learn more about which microorganisms are most likely to cause infections and why. Studies of the last issue have been greatly facilitated by knowledge developed over the past 2 decades of ligand-receptor interactions between microorganisms, host cells, and prosthetic materials and of the role played by bacterial glycocalyces in facilitating microbial persistence on colonized surfaces. Finally, there has been heightened interest in those physiocochemical properties of synthetic materials which both permit and retard bacterial and fungal colonization.

Meanwhile, clinicians have become increasingly concerned with accurately describing the syndromes associated with these foreign body infections as well as their natural history. At times diagnosis may be obvious and at other times it may be agonizingly difficult. Likewise, in certain cases therapy may require astute choices of antimicrobial agents, while in others removal of the infected device is mandatory for cure. The latter course of action may have very serious implications should the infection be in a strategic location, such as on a heart valve or vascular graft.

In recognition of this developing field of scientific interest, the first edition of this book was published by the American Society for Microbiology in 1989. The intent of that volume was to define the state of the art at both the laboratory bench and the bedside. The second edition is intended to serve the same ends and to document advances in our knowledge that have occurred in the intervening years. All chapters included in the first edition have been revised and updated to reflect current data and concepts. The content has been amplified by new contributions on the molecular basis of adherence of staphylococci to biomaterials and on infections associated with cardiac pacemakers. The chapter on prosthetic joint infections includes a summary of Mayo Clinic data on the incidence of such infections, based on the more than 39,000 large joint implants with some 275,000 joint years of follow-up. Such data are critical to decision making regarding the necessity of "endocarditis-like" prophylaxis for prosthetic joint recipients undergoing invasive dental and surgical procedures. The thorny issues regarding necessity for and preferred types of prophylaxis at the time of prosthesis insertion are considered in individual chapters and in the succinct summary of the topic provided by Drs. Haas and Kaiser. We are indeed grateful to all our contributors for their thoughtful and comprehensive treatment of the complex issues relating to both the basic and clinical aspects of device-related infections. We trust that this book will serve as a useful reference for all those whose endeavors will ultimately lead to much more effective means of prevention and therapy of these "diseases of medical progress."

Alan L. Bisno
Francis A. Waldvogel

Infections Associated with Indwelling Medical Devices, 2nd ed.
Edited by Alan L. Bisno and Francis A. Waldvogel
© 1994 American Society for Microbiology, Washington, DC 20005

Chapter 1

Host Factors Predisposing to and Influencing Therapy of Foreign Body Infections

Pierre E. Vaudaux, Daniel P. Lew, and Francis A. Waldvogel

HOST RESPONSES TO IMPLANTED BIOMATERIALS

Materials implanted for many months or years must meet several criteria. First, they must have specific mechanical properties, to replace the functions of defective body tissues or organs (30). Second, they must be accepted and integrated by the host in a controlled and predictable way (30). No implanted artificial material can be considered totally inert in the body, as suggested by Hench and Wilson (44), who described four major categories of host responses: (i) the material releases some toxic compounds, leading to the death of surrounding tissue (2, 73); (ii) the material is nontoxic but is gradually resorbed and replaced by the surrounding tissue that is under repair; (iii) the material is nontoxic and biologically inactive but cannot be degraded by the host, which reacts by encapsulation. (several metallic and plastic biomaterial implants belong to this category); and (iv) the material is nontoxic but highly interactive with the surrounding tissues in forming chemical bonds with it, which stabilize the implant. Dense hydroxylapatite ceramics, bioactive glasses, bioactive glass-ceramics, and bioactive composites are examples of this last category of biomaterials (44).

The mechanisms subtending these variable host responses to the different categories of biomaterial implants are complex and still poorly

Pierre E. Vaudaux and Daniel P. Lew   •   Infectious Disease Division, University Hospital, CH-1211 Geneva 14, Switzerland.   **Francis A. Waldvogel**   •   Department of Medicine, Clinique Médicale 2, University Hospital, CH-1211 Geneva 14, Switzerland.

1

understood. An interesting situation is that of nontoxic and biologically inactive plastic or metallic biomaterials. Depending on the circumstances, some of these materials can elicit a chronic inflammatory response, also called foreign body reaction (16, 72, 73), which has the following characteristics: after an initial acute inflammatory reaction, a chronic granulomatous tissue reaction may persist, even after encapsulation has occurred (16, 72). The foreign body reaction seems to be induced by continuous chemical or mechanical stimuli arising from the biomaterial implants (16). Morphological analysis of this reaction reveals the presence of a large number of macrophages, which generally attempt to phagocytize the material (16). Usually, the foreign body is much larger than individual macrophages and is not easily degraded (16). Some of the macrophages then merge their cytoplasm to become multinucleated giant cells, also called foreign body giant cells (16). If the foreign body cannot be degraded by phagocytes, granulation tissue is formed to encapsulate the foreign body in order to isolate the implant from the rest of the body tissues (16). The foreign body reaction may be assessed in a semiquantitative way by the enumeration of inflammatory cells, namely, the polymorphonuclear leukocytes (PMN) and activated macrophages or giant cells found either at the surface of implanted biomaterials or in the inflammatory exudative fluid elicited by implants (16, 72, 73).

The contribution of phagocytic cells to the foreign body reaction may involve two closely related mechanisms. In the first, the neutrophils or macrophages phagocytize the smaller fragments of biodegraded or corroded metallic or plastic implants. These fragments cannot be degraded further, and they may persist intracellularly in the neutrophils or macrophages for a prolonged period of time or may be ingested by other phagocytes if cell death does occur. In the second reaction, also called "frustrated phagocytosis," phagocytic cells are confronted with foreign particles, such as nylon wool, glass, cotton, polysulfone fibers, or polystyrene or polypropylene materials, too large to be ingested (45, 57, 60, 123, 124). Phagocytes coming into contact with this nonphagocytizable foreign material become permanently activated, in a way similar to phagocytes containing the smaller fragments of nondegradable foreign particles; each kind of phagocyte may separately or in concert secrete or passively release several important inflammatory mediators (6, 73), including acidic or neutral hydrolases, activated complement components, tumor necrosis factor (TNF), interleukins, prostaglandins, plasminogen activator, and coagulation factors. The respective roles and relative importance of these secreted factors in the control and maintenance of acute and chronic phases of the inflammatory response to implants are not yet well defined (3, 6, 33).

Materials coming in contact with blood must fulfill additional requirements: they must not damage blood cells or encourage the formation of blood clots (30, 78). When blood meets foreign materials, there is an immediate reaction leading to some degree of protein and blood-cell deposition on the material (30, 78). If this process continues, clotting and thrombosis may result, leading to severe complications (30, 78). Thus, the development of thromboresistant materials is an absolute requirement for implanted durable cardiac prostheses, artificial heart valves, or blood vessels (30, 78). Besides interacting with fibrinogen, coagulation factors, and platelets, materials can also affect various other plasma proteins and cellular components (78). One example is complement activation (78, 120), which may cause adverse effects during extracorporeal circulation such as hemodialysis (18), cardiopulmonary bypass (9), and membrane plasmapheresis (78). An interesting global approach of blood interaction with biomaterials has been proposed by Murabayashi and Nosé (78). First, these authors stress the multiple interactions occurring between various host defense enzymatic systems, such as the coagulation, fibrinolytic, kallikrein-kinin, and complement systems, which may in turn interact with cellular components such as neutrophils, lymphocytes, macrophages, and platelets. Second, there is a systemic reaction resulting from the initially local blood-material interaction; this systemic reaction may ultimately modify the local interaction itself. Similar reactions to those documented in the blood-material interface may also be predicted to occur in extravascular compartments, when exudative fluid is produced in contact with the material.

Finally, host responses to biomaterial implants are not restricted to adverse humoral or cellular responses. One example of a contact surface advantageously modified by the host is the production of a pseudoneointima (30, 42, 78) on the surface of artificial vessels or blood pump devices. The pseudoneointima is a biological cellular approximation of a natural lining, which makes the foreign surface more compatible with the host and may eventually lead to endothelialization of the artificial materials (42). Another example of a complex host response to biomaterial implants is found with rigid and stress-resistant metallic bone implants (see review in reference 31). In contrast to normal bone, which is stimulated to grow by stress (7, 30, 66, 90), metallic implants, which are stronger than normal bones, do not transfer stress (30, 66). Such a stress "shielding" by the implant can lead to bone resorption and in turn to loosening of the implant. In the hope of increasing the life of bone implants, several investigators are now studying materials transferring stress from the implant to the nearby bone, thereby avoiding excessive bone loss.

All these examples illustrate the complexity of the multiple host interactions with biomaterials. Not only the composition, size, and mechanical and surface properties of the materials, but also their location within the human body, modulate the host responses.

Host Factors Involved in Staphylococcal Infections

On their surface staphylococci express specific receptors for interacting with host-derived adhesins (see reviews in reference 52 and chapter 2). Host adhesins include some of the major proteins and glycoproteins, components from plasma, platelets, connective tissue, and basement membranes. The most active host proteins interacting with *Staphylococcus aureus* in the fluid phase or promoting its in vitro attachment when in contact with surfaces are fibronectin (29, 48, 62–64, 76, 77, 82, 83, 85, 86, 89, 97, 106, 107, 109, 110, 114), fibrinogen and fibrin (10, 12, 21, 43, 48, 65, 100, 106, 107), collagen (50, 92, 96, 114, 117, 118), laminin (48, 68, 69, 114), vitronectin (11, 81), thrombospondin (47), bone sialoprotein (87), elastin (122), and a recently described extracellular matrix-binding protein with broad specificity (51). Fibronectin, which is a large multidomain glycoprotein, can be found either in soluble form in blood and other body fluids or in an insoluble form in connective tissues and on cell surfaces (54). Invasive strains of staphylococci have been reported to bind more fibronectin than commensal strains can (77, 82). Thus, fibronectin is one major target of *S. aureus* in traumatized tissues, blood clots, and abnormal heart valves, which have ample quantities of fibronectin exposed to circulating organisms (62, 77, 89, 98, 113). In these situations, fibrin also may contribute to *S. aureus* attachment and colonization either directly (43) or indirectly by incorporating fibronectin into the clots, a process stabilized by the cross-linking action of the coagulation factor XIII$_a$ (12, 76, 77, 85, 98, 100). In contrast to *S. aureus*, interaction of coagulase-negative strains of staphylococci with host-derived adhesins has not been well characterized at the molecular level, but at least we know that these interactions are weaker than those described with coagulase-positive staphylococci with the proteins described above (48, 118).

The production of pyogenic exudates or abscesses by *S. aureus* infections indicates a major role for neutrophils in the host defense against such infections. The crucial host defense contribution of neutrophils and mononuclear phagocytes against staphylococcal infections is further documented by clinical observations of patients suffering from phagocytic disorders (32, 84, 116).

Another important aspect of the host response to staphylococcal infection is the directed migration of the phagocytes toward an infectious focus, which acts as a stimulus (32, 34). Establishment of an inflammatory focus leads to the liberation of humoral mediators, which attract and modulate the cellular components of the inflammatory response (32, 34). This complex set of events involves activation or inactivation of several humoral pathways, which interact with the migrating phagocytes (32, 34). Neutrophils are not only migrating to infectious foci for phagocytic purposes but also acting as secretory cells; by releasing their granule contents of hydrolytic enzymes into the surrounding medium, they can selectively activate or inactivate the chemotactic factors (32, 34). In this way, inflammatory cells can control by themselves the extent of the inflammatory response. A further important effect mediated by the release of neutrophil hydrolases has been recently demonstrated: elastase, which is a major neutral protease of neutrophils, was shown to inactivate significantly the complement-derived opsonic activity of infected pleural effusions (67, 94). A major target of the elastolytic activity was the important complement factor C3, which underwent extensive degradation in the infected site (67, 94). Degradation of the most important group of staphylococcal opsonins by elastase may be an important factor contributing significantly to the persistence of infection, despite the presence of high concentrations of neutrophils in the infected exudates (119).

Host Factors Predisposing to Foreign Body Infections

Alterations in the host defense mechanisms in the vicinity of implanted foreign bodies have been frequently suggested, although they have rarely been confirmed by experimental data. Since the presence of a foreign body markedly increases the pathogenic potential of organisms of low virulence, such as *Staphylococcus epidermidis* (70), patients infected with such organisms in connection with a biomaterial implant(s) may be considered in some way immunocompromised patients. In one study, the humoral immune response to *S. epidermidis* during prosthetic joint infections was followed for extended periods of time but failed to demonstrate any significant rise in infection-specific antibodies (55).

Another major argument in favor of local defects in the host defense against staphylococcal foreign body infections was obtained by studies performed with experimentally infected animals. Many studies have shown that a bacterial inoculum that would be considered "subinfective" for a particular kind of experimental wound was sufficient to cause a severe clinical infection in the presence of foreign materials such as sutures, hemostats, soil, devitalized and crushed muscle tissue, gelatin, or oxidized cellulose (see review in reference 35). Particularly impressive were the differences obtained for minimal infective doses for *S. aureus;* in the presence of silk sutures, as few as 100 CFU produced a permanent infection, whereas 10^7 organisms were noninfective in the absence of foreign material (23, 56, 79). Although neutrophils accumulating around a foreign body appeared to be microscopically normal in these experiments (79), their functional status as well as the opsonizing capacity of the surrounding fluid could not be explored in these animal models. Thus, the model developed by these authors did not allow a quantitative evaluation of the microbiological, immunological, and cellular events preceding, or associated with, a foreign body infection.

EXPERIMENTAL STUDY OF HOST FACTORS PREDISPOSING TO FOREIGN BODY INFECTIONS

Development of a Tissue Cage Model in Guinea Pigs

To analyze the role of local host factors in foreign body infections, we developed an experimental model suitable for analysis of the various microbiological, immunological, and cellular events preceding, or associated with, a foreign body infection. Polymethylmethacrylate (PMMA) or polytetrafluoroethylene (Teflon) perforated cylinders (i.e., tissue cages) were implanted subcutaneously into guinea pigs under strict aseptic conditions and general anesthesia (127). An important characteristic of this and other types of subcutaneous implants with a dead space (5, 73) was the presence of a sterile inflammatory exudate that accumulated inside the tissue cages within the 2 to 4 weeks after their implantation (127). This tissue cage fluid (TCF) could be easily aspirated for analysis of its humoral and cellular components and also to exclude occasional spontaneous bacterial contamination (127).

The course of inflammatory reaction elicited by implantation has previously been described in detail (126). The presence of TCF allowed the injection of a well-defined volume of a bacterial suspension of S. aureus to produce infection. The induction of experimental foreign body infection was generally performed after 4 weeks of implantation, at which time the acute inflammatory reaction was complete (127). S. aureus Wood 46 was selected for this study for two main reasons: (i) this strain is devoid of staphylococcal protein A, which reacts in a nonspecific way with the Fc portion of immunoglobulin G subclasses 1, 2, and 4 (61), and (ii) this strain was shown to be primarily opsonized by complement activation through the alternative pathway, leading to C3b deposits on the bacterial surface.

The minimal infective dose of S. aureus Wood 46 was indeed very low in our model, as shown in other systems (56, 79, 91), since 10^2 CFU was sufficient to infect more than 95% of the tissue cages and inoculation of 10^3 CFU produced infections in all tissue cages tested (127). Other strains of *S. aureus*, including protein A producers and methicillin-resistant ones, and *S. epidermidis* are also highly infective in the tissue cage model.

In contrast, no infection could be produced by either subcutaneous or intraperitoneal injection of 10^8 CFU of *S. aureus* Wood 46 in the absence of tissue cages (127), thus confirming that this harmless strain showed an increased virulence only when associated with foreign implants. This increased virulence of *S. aureus* Wood 46 was not significantly influenced by the chemical, physical, or structural properties of the tissue cages (127), confirming previous findings with silk sutures (23, 56, 79). As shown in previous observations (23, 56, 79), there was an abundant influx of neutrophils into tissue cages after inoculation of *S. aureus* Wood 46, resulting in abscess formation (127). Despite this intense inflammatory response, formation of a spontaneous fistula with purulent discharge and subsequent spontaneous shedding of the foreign bodies occurs in most cases, followed by spontaneous wound healing. No signs of bacteremic spread can be demonstrated, and bacteriological cultures of other organs were uniformly negative (127).

A last characteristic of this tissue cage model is the response to parenteral antistaphylococcal antibiotics. Whereas vancomycin or rifampin prevented or eradicated tissue cage infections if treatment was initiated before or during the first 6 to 12 h after inoculation of 10^3 CFU of *S. aureus* Wood 46 (99), it was ineffective if initiated more than 12 h after inoculation (99). Such inefficacy of antibiotic therapy initiated after infection has developed is commonly observed in the clinical context of staphylococcal foreign body infections.

Phagocytic Defects in the Presence of Foreign Materials

Complement-mediated opsonic activity and total hemolytic complement levels were measured before infection, at various intervals after implantation of tissue cages, or during the course of experimental infection (127). Before the onset of infection, decreased levels of complement-mediated opsonins, reflecting a low amount of the C3 component of complement, were recorded in TCF (Fig. 1). However, such decreased levels of complement-mediated opsonins were not a rate-limiting factor favoring the development of experimental foreign body infection (127), since after in vitro preopsonization under optimal conditions, namely, in 10% guinea pig serum, 10^2 CFU of *S. aureus* Wood 46 injected into sterile tissue cages was still infective in the experimental model (127). The opsonic coating of *S. aureus* Wood 46 was tested after incubation of the microbial organism with TCF in vivo or in vitro. This opsonic coating

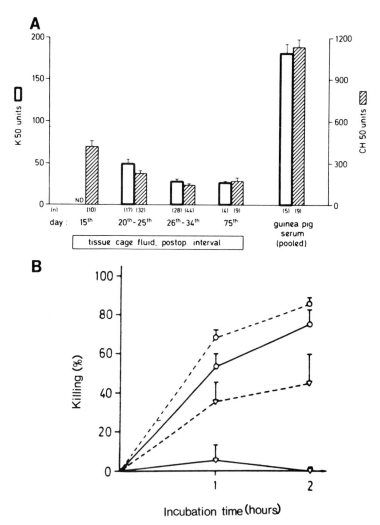

Figure 1. Local host defense during the early onset of experimental foreign body infections. (A) Opsonic activity and total hemolytic complement levels in tissue cage fluid at intervals after implantation and in pooled guinea pig serum. Data are means ± standard errors of the means (bars) of the reciprocal dilutions that gave either 50% killing of the bacteria in a phagocytic-bactericidal assay (K 50) or 50% hemolysis in a hemolytic system (CH 50). (Reprinted from reference 127 with permission.) (B) Bactericidal capacity of neutrophils obtained from sterile tissue cage fluid (▽) compared with peritoneal exudate neutrophils obtained after stimulation with glycogen (○). The phagocytic assay mixture contained, in a volume of 1 ml, 10^6 PMN, 10% pooled guinea pig serum, and either 2×10^6 cells of S. aureus Wood 46 (—) or 2×10^6 cells of S. faecalis (- -). (Reprinted from reference 125 with permission.)

was steady at 1 h after infection but decreased significantly later on during infections (127). Reduced opsonic coating of the bacteria either drawn directly from infected fluids or incubated in vitro with such fluids had already been observed in various clinical situations of purulent exudates: loss of complement-mediated opsonins, as well as proteolytic cleavage of C3, was found for pleural empyema (67, 94), infected cerebrospinal fluid (128), or bronchial secretions of cystic fibrosis patients (95).

In contrast to initially normal opsonic activity, the phagocytic-bactericidal activity of neutrophils drawn from the sterile TCF was markedly deficient (127) and considerably lower than activities observed with neutrophils from acute and chronic peritoneal exudates and from peripheral blood (127). In a further study, the phagocytic and metabolic functions of tissue cage neutrophils were analyzed in more detail (125). Whereas neutrophils derived from the sterile tissue cage fluid were unable to kill a catalase-positive organism such as *S. aureus* Wood 46, they still possessed some bactericidal activity against catalase-negative bacteria, such as *Streptococcus faecalis* (Fig. 1). These observations indicated that oxygen-dependent killing mechanisms were defective (125). Specific assays verified that superoxide production by tissue cage neutrophils was markedly reduced when compared with that of neutrophils from acute or chronic peritoneal exudates (125). Tissue cage neutrophils also showed evidence of previous degranulation events (125). The mechanisms leading to such an acquired granulocyte defect were further investigated in a simplified in vitro system (125). Peritoneal exudate neutrophils were incubated with Teflon fibers, leading to significant increases in hexose monophosphate shunt activity and exocytosis of secondary granules. Neutrophils eluted after such interaction showed defective bactericidal activity, oxidative metabolism, and granular enzyme content similar to those observed in tissue cage neutrophils (125). These observations gave additional support to the hypothesis that neutrophils could be damaged by contacting the foreign surface of tissue cages (125), in accordance with the concept of frustrated phagocytosis along nonphagocytizable surfaces, reported by other investigators (45, 57, 60, 123, 124) using different foreign materials. Finally, effective protection from foreign body infection was indeed obtained by injection of fresh neutrophils into tissue cages (125). Results of these protection experiments supported the view that the neutrophils' defects in the vicinity of tissue cages were responsible, at least in part, for the high susceptibility of foreign bodies to infection.

Besides their intrinsic defects, tissue cage neutrophils may also exhibit defective antibacterial responses because of selective defects in the levels of some cytokines in tissue cage fluid. Indirect evidence for this

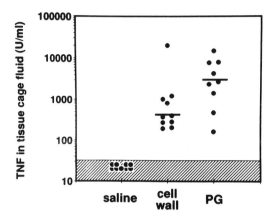

Figure 2. Tumor necrosis factor (TNF) concentrations in tissue cage fluid in guinea pigs (units per milliliter), measured 2 h after local injection of either 0.5 ml of saline, purified cell wall components, or purified peptidoglycan (PG). Bars indicate median values. (Reprinted from reference 103 with permission.)

hypothesis was found by recent observations showing that components inducing tumor necrosis factor (TNF) production could partly restore the local host defense against a bacterial challenge (103). Locally injected components derived from the cell wall of *S. aureus* Wood 46 (in particular, peptidoglycan) raised TNF levels in tissue cage fluid (Fig. 2) and prevented infection by the test strain (103). Furthermore, injection of the murine recombinant TNF into tissue cages could substitute for bacterial components in preventing experimental infection (103). This protective effect could be neutralized by anti-TNF antibodies (103).

To summarize the phagocytic defects observed in this animal model (125, 127), we can differentiate two sequential phases of defects during the course of experimental foreign body infections: (i) in the early phase (0 to 6 h), complement-mediated opsonic activity in TCF is adequate, whereas local neutrophil functions and local levels of the cytokine TNF are markedly deficient and (ii) in the second phase (6 to more than 48 h), complement-mediated opsonic activity is markedly reduced, whereas neutrophils freshly attracted into infected TCF exhibit normal activity. Thus, the full sequence of opsonophagocytic events cannot be performed under optimal conditions at any time of the infection.

Modulation of *S. aureus* Adhesion to Foreign Surfaces by Solid-Phase Host Factors

Development of an in vitro assay

A large number of studies have evaluated the characteristics of bacterial attachment either to normal or damaged host tissues or to artificial surfaces, reviewed elsewhere (19). However, most of the reported studies have evaluated bacterial attachment to surfaces in simplified in vitro systems, frequently in the absence of serum proteins in the incubation medium. We will focus on the argument that host proteins, whether surface bound or in the fluid phase, play an essential role in staphylococcal attachment to artificial human or animal implants.

As mentioned above, exposure of any biomaterial to blood results in the immediate formation of a conditioning layer of blood proteins and cells on its surface (4, 9, 17, 18, 27, 30, 42, 78, 120). These protein layers may influence the process of staphylococcal attachment in two different ways: (i) by masking nonspecifically any direct interaction between bacterial adhesive surface components and artificial surfaces (28, 49, 80, 93) and (ii) by increasing more specifically the attractive properties of biomaterials for staphylococci. The blood components and tissue proteins containing specific binding sites for staphylococci (see previous sections) are evidently ideal candidates for such a phenomenon, if they can be adsorbed in adequate amounts on the surface of biomaterials.

The best way to understand how different proteins either promote or prevent staphylococcal adhesion to indwelling devices seemed implied in the comparison between unimplanted and implanted foreign surfaces. We developed a modified in vitro assay to quantify staphylococcal adhesion to small-sized polymer surfaces, presented as either cover slips of 1 by 1 cm (109, 111) or 1-cm-long segments of polymeric tubing (106, 107). Several studies performed in our and other laboratories have demonstrated that the presence of whole plasma (49), serum (80, 109), or purified serum albumin (20, 48, 104, 109, 110, 112) prevented staphylococcal adhesion to a number of different unimplanted artificial surfaces, such as PMMA (48, 109, 110), Teflon (104), fluorinated polyethylene-propylene films (49), polyvinyl chloride (106, 112), and polyurethane tubing segments (106, 107). It was also observed with various metallic surfaces such as stainless steel, pure titanium, and titanium alloy (20). Inhibition of adhesion by either whole serum or purified serum albumin was observed with almost all coagulase-positive and -negative staphylococcal strains and species thus far tested, including laboratory and clinical bacteremic isolates (48, 101, 105). Thus, there are indeed plasma or serum components that can form protein layers by adsorption on various artificial surfaces and interfere nonspecifically with staphylococcal attachment. Since a major component of this inhibition is human serum albumin, many recent studies of bacterial adhesion on protein-coated surfaces have included this protein in the fluid phase of bacterial suspensions to reduce the contribution of nonspecific physicochemical forces to the process of staphylococcal attachment.

Role of fibronectin in staphylococcal adhesion to foreign implants

In contrast to unimplanted PMMA, cover slips implanted subcutaneously inside the tissue cages into guinea pigs and subsequently excised after 4 weeks showed entirely different characteristics toward S. aureus (109) or S. epidermidis (20) adhesion: (i) they allowed significant bacterial attachment, even in the presence of serum, albumin, or tissue cage fluid (20, 109); (ii) the new attachment characteristics of either PMMA (109) or metallic (20) cover slips, acquired during their implantation, were due to the presence of trypsin-sensitive adhesins on the surface of implants; and (iii) these acquired adhesins were likely to be host conditioned. Microscopic examination revealed that explanted PMMA cover slips were coated with fibers and cellular materials that stained intensely with antifibronectin antibodies (109). The presence of fibronectin was linked to the development of connective tissue (22, 44) on the surface of PMMA, as evidenced by the presence of numerous fibroblasts and collagen fibers. The specificity of the immunological staining of fibronectin deposited on PMMA was demonstrated using appropriate controls: neither sera depleted of antifibronectin antibodies nor antibodies directed against unrelated host proteins, such as fibrinogen and albumin (109), produced any fluorescent staining of the protein deposits of explanted PMMA cover slips (109).

To demonstrate that fibronectin deposited on PMMA cover slips during in vivo exposure was a major factor mediating the adhesion of S. aureus Wood 46, the potential binding sites of S. aureus were blocked by specific antibodies to fibronectin. Treatment of explanted cover slips with such antibodies (Fig. 3B) strongly reduced staphylococcal adhesion (20, 109). A similar inhibition was observed on unimplanted cover slips coated in vitro with purified fibronectin (Fig. 3A). Antibody-mediated inhibition of S. aureus adhesion could only be demonstrated by using strain Wood 46, which is devoid of protein A.

In vitro adsorption of fibronectin and other host proteins on artificial surfaces

To study in more detail the interaction of S. aureus and S. epidermidis with fibronectin and other host proteins selectively deposited on foreign surfaces, several investigators have used simplified in vitro bacterial adhesion assays. A common feature of these assays was the in vitro coating of artificial surfaces with individual blood or matrix protein or sometimes a mixture of them. A frequent limitation of many studies has been the empirical choice of protein concentrations used for coating the artificial

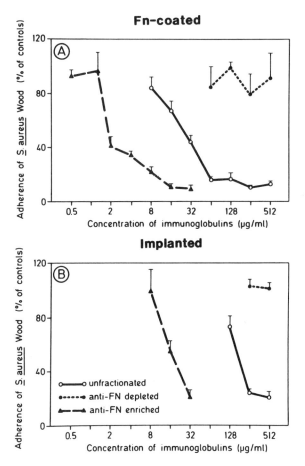

Figure 3. Inhibition of *S. aureus* adhesion by antifibronectin (anti-FN) antibodies. (A) Unimplanted cover slips coated in vitro with purified fibronectin. (B) PMMA cover slips excised from the guinea pigs after 4 weeks of subcutaneous implantation. Each cover slip was incubated with rabbit antifibronectin immunoglobulins, either unfractionated or selectively enriched for antifibronectin antibodies by affinity chromatography on fibronectin-Sepharose. Control incubations were performed with immunoglobulins selectively depleted of antifibronectin antibodies by affinity chromatography on fibronectin-Sepharose. (Reprinted from reference 109 with permission.)

surfaces. To compare in vitro assays with in vivo conditions, it is important to estimate the amount of host protein(s) adsorbed on unimplanted artificial surfaces in relation to the amounts deposited in vivo. Another interest of quantitating protein adsorption is the possibility of comparing the relative affinities of the different proteins for each artificial surface and determining their monolayer concentrations. Quantitative adsorption of most proteins can be easily determined either by using radiolabeled preparations of these macromolecules or by appropriate immunoassays. In various studies performed with purified fibronectin radiolabeled with either ^{125}I or ^{3}H, we found that protein adsorption on PMMA (110), Teflon (104), polyvinyl chloride tissue culture plates (112), or polyurethane (107) was dose dependent and saturable. Similar data were also obtained with cover slips of various metallic compositions (20, 102). Quantitative dose-dependent and saturable adsorption on artificial surfaces was also observed with either radiolabeled fibrinogen (106) or thrombospondin (47).

Promotion of *S. aureus* adhesion (20, 47, 107, 110, 112) by either surface-bound fibronectin, fibrinogen, or thrombospondin was dose dependent, being a linear function of both the quantity in solution and the quantity adsorbed on each type of artificial surfaces at intermediate protein concentrations. However, a significant difference was observed between thrombospondin and fibronectin or fibrinogen, in terms of quantitative dose-response. Whereas a minimal amount of 500 ng of thrombospondin per cover slip was required for significant promotion of *S. aureus* Cowan 1 adhesion (47), tenfold lower quantities of adsorbed fibrinogen or fibronectin, such as 20 ng/cm^2, were sufficient to promote equivalent bacterial adhesion. In three recent studies, we found that fibrinogen and fibronectin were reliably adsorbed on either PMMA cover slips (74, 101) or polyurethane catheter segments (107) from solutions containing submicrogram amounts of each protein per ml. In contrast to fibrinogen, which could be directly adsorbed on native polymer surfaces from such highly diluted protein solutions (74, 107), precoating of the materials with gelatin was required for fibronectin (101, 107). This precoating step significantly improved the wettability of the different polymer surfaces. Of interest was the observation that optimal adhesion of *S. aureus* was promoted by levels of fibrinogen or fibronectin much lower than those leading to a monolayer coating of the surfaces (74, 101, 107).

Fibronectin adsorption onto PMMA was also studied with purified radiolabeled fibronectin in complex protein mixtures such as human serum, after sequential depletion of endogenous plasma fibronectin and serum reconstitution. Under these conditions, fibronectin adsorption on PMMA cover slips was inhibited by 98%, compared with that occurring in the absence of serum proteins (110). Not only fibronectin but also thrombospondin (47) was prevented from adsorbing on PMMA cover slips by the presence of serum. Other studies have confirmed the decreased affinity of fibronectin for various hydrophobic surfaces in the presence of serum proteins (38, 39, 58).

The quantity of fibronectin adsorbed on PMMA in the presence of serum proteins was indeed too low to promote a significant adhesion of *S. aureus* Wood 46 to PMMA cover slips. These observations allowed explanation of why native PMMA or Teflon cover slips preincubated with 10% whole serum, containing approximately 30 μg/ml of fibronectin, were unable to promote subsequent adhesion of either *S. aureus* Wood 46 (104, 109, 110) or other strains of *S. aureus* or *S. epidermidis* (48, 105).

Precoating of either PMMA (110) or Teflon (104) with gelatin or heat-denatured collagen restored the ability of the foreign material to adsorb fibronectin from the mixture of serum proteins. Both denatured collagen and gelatin can interact with the specific collagen-binding site (75) of fibronectin by a specific domain (54, 59) containing the mammalian collagenase cleavage site. The quantity of fibronectin adsorbed on either PMMA (110) or Teflon (104) in the presence of serum proteins was at least 25% of the quantity adsorbed in the absence of serum proteins. Interestingly, equivalent amounts of fibronectin had a much higher adhesion-promoting activity on *S. aureus* Wood 46 when adsorbed from serum mixtures on collagen-precoated PMMA (110) or Teflon (104) than when adsorbed on native cover slips. These data suggest a potential role for collagen as a cofactor contributing to *S. aureus* adhesion onto fibronectin-coated surfaces. Collagen-fibronectin interactions could favor conformational changes in the fibronectin molecules, such as exposure of a maximal number of binding sites to *S. aureus.*

In a previous section, we briefly mentioned the contribution of other host proteins, such as collagen, laminin, vitronectin, bone sialoproteins, and even multifunctional adhesins, to staphylococcal adhesion (see also chapter 2). A detailed description of the binding conditions of each of these potential adhesins is outside the scope of this chapter. With regard to indwelling devices, the quantity of these different adhesins needs to be accurately estimated to evaluate how each of them might contribute to bacterial attachment onto indwelling devices. A combined approach of bacterial adhesion studies using significant numbers of clinical isolates and of experimental models of bacterial colonization or infection of indwelling devices is needed to assess the specific contribution of each adhesin to implant colonization by *S. aureus* and *S. epidermidis.*

The following summarizes the characteristics of host-mediated staphylococcal adhesion to artificial surfaces measured under in vitro and in vivo conditions. (i) Fibronectin is by far the best-characterized protein adhesin interacting with both coagulase-positive and -negative staphylococci in vitro and in vivo. (ii) Except for fibrin (or fibrinogen), which has been either visualized by electron microscopy or quantified by immunoassay, the presence and contribution of additional blood or matrix adhesins to bacterial adhesion and colonization of indwelling devices still need to be fully assessed. (iii) Serum considerably limits adsorption of fibronectin and thrombospondin onto freshly implanted plastic materials. (iv) The presence of collagen on the surface of biomaterial implants may circumvent the serum-mediated inhibition of fibronectin adsorption. (v) Biomaterials implanted in the subcutaneous space are progressively colonized by cellular and fibrillar connective tissue components, and fibroblasts may contribute by their own protein synthesis machinery to the deposition of fibronectin on the extracellular matrix coating the artificial material. This cellular form of fibronectin is closely related to the plasma form of fibronectin (53, 54) and can be deposited on artificial surfaces despite the presence of serum components (39). (vi) The presence of fibrin clots on the surface of blood-exposed biomaterials may also contribute to fibronectin deposition covalently cross-linked by factor XIII$_a$.

Clinical Relevance of Staphylococcal Adhesion

The clinical significance of in vitro bacterial adhesion could be documented using two approaches: (i) the testing of adhesion characteristics of a significant number of clinical isolates relevant to a particular type of indwelling device infection and (ii) the study of adhesion-promoting properties of devices retrieved from patients, using isolates with well-defined affinities for major adhesins.

In the first approach (48), we tested the adhesion properties of 27 bacteremic isolates of either *S. aureus* or coagulase-negative staphylococci responsible for intravascular catheter infections in hospitalized patients. Adhesion of all clinical isolates was promoted by the fibronectin coating of PMMA cover slips. In contrast, the same polymer surfaces coated in vitro with fibrinogen selectively promoted adhesion of *S. aureus* clinical isolates but not of coagulase-negative staphylococci, except for a few of them. Finally, in vitro coating with laminin promoted staphylococcal adhesion to a much lower extent.

In the second prospective approach, we studied the role in staphylococcal adhesion played by fibrinogen or fibrin and fibronectin deposited on 187 peripheral or central catheters removed from hospitalized patients (106). Compared with uninserted catheters, which allowed only minimal bacterial adhesion in the albumin-containing medium (used for blocking nonspecific adhesion), inserted catheters promoted significant adhesion of five *S. aureus* and five *S. epidermidis* isolates from patients with intravenous-device infections. Comparison of results obtained with three laboratory strains with well-defined affinities for fibrinogen or fibronectin again suggested a role for in vivo-deposited fibronectin in promoting adhesion of coagulase-negative staphylococci. In contrast, the much higher adhesion of *S. aureus* clinical isolates was suggested to be promoted by fibrinogen/fibrin, by fibronectin, or by the concerted action of both adhesins.

To further define the respective role of fibrinogen/fibrin and fibronectin in adhesion of *S. aureus* to central venous catheters, we assayed in parallel, on adjacent segments of previously inserted cannulas, the amount, chemical integrity, and biological activity of plasma proteins adsorbed on their surface (107). Comparison of polyurethane with polyvinyl chloride and Hickman cannulas removed from patients showed that the first category of intravenous lines promoted a significantly lower adhesion of *S. aureus* than the other types of cannulas (Fig. 4). When the group of inserted polyurethane catheters was compared with the same materials in vitro coated with either native fibrinogen or fibronectin, bacterial adhesion to ex vivo cannulas was equivalent to that promoted by very low amounts of in vitro-added proteins, namely, less than 70 and 25 ng of fibrinogen and fibronectin per segment, respectively (Fig. 4). Comparison for all three groups of inserted catheters of their biological activity with their immunologically assayed contents of fibrinogen/fibrin and fibronectin indicated an extensive loss of biological activity for the former, but not the latter, protein. Amounts of fibronectin recovered from ex vivo cannulas were equivalent to those determined to significantly promote *S. aureus* adhesion once coated in vitro onto each type of catheter. Finally, the extent of *S. aureus* adhesion promoted by inserted cannulas was significantly correlated with their content of immunologically assayed fibronectin (107).

To further analyze the selective inactivation of fibrinogen/fibrin, sodium dodecyl sulfate-polyacrylamide gel electrophoresis (SDS-PAGE) and immunoblots of cannula-associated proteins were performed. Figure 5 shows that proteins extracted from cannulas by SDS-Laemmli buffer represented only a few major bands, compared with proteins present in whole plasma. This indicated an expected selective protein adsorption process from plasma to inserted cannulas (Fig. 5A). Immunoblots of the same extracts stained with specific antibodies to fibrinogen/fibrin and plasminogen (Fig. 5B) or to fibronectin (not shown) indicated that these proteins were the major protein components recovered from inserted cannulas. Besides identifying native proteins, immunoblots also revealed the presence of proteolytic fragments of fibrinogen/fibrin (Fig. 5B) and fibronectin in cannula-extracted proteins. These fragments were related to the presence and activity of plasmin(ogen), whose content was significant among cannula-adsorbed proteins. In vitro studies dem-

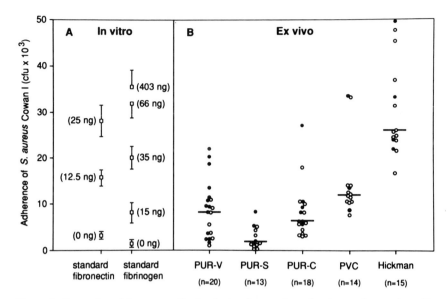

Figure 4. Promotion of *S. aureus* adhesion by in vitro coating of uninserted cannulas with native fibrinogen or fibronectin (A) or by ex vivo protein coating of cannulas previously inserted in 80 patients (B). Strain Cowan 1 was selected as representative of six bacteremic isolates of *S. aureus*. Cannulas significantly contaminated with blood after the rinsing procedure (●) or uncontaminated with blood (○) are indicated. Three brands of polyurethane (PUR) cannulas, previously inserted in patients, were compared with ex vivo polyvinyl chloride (PVC) and Hickman cannulas (PUR-V, Vialon; PUR-S, Seldiflex; PUR-C, Cavafix; see reference 107 for details). Duplicate 1-cm-long segments were assayed. Bars: median values of each group. Comments: *S. aureus* adhesion to ex vivo cannulas (B) correlates with their content of immunoassayed fibronectin and is equivalent to that promoted by low amounts of native in vitro-added fibronectin (A). In contrast, *S. aureus* adhesion to ex vivo cannulas (B) is unrelated to their content of immunoassayed fibrin or fibrinogen, which shows biological and chemical evidence (see text for details) of extensive inactivation by the fibrinolytic process. (Reprinted from reference 107 with permission.)

onstrated that whereas fibrinogen-promoting activity of *S. aureus* adhesion was extensively inactivated by plasmin cleavage, this was not the case with fibronectin, whose fragments could still promote bacterial adhesion (107). These data led us to conclude that intact fibronectin or its active fragments, although present in much lower amounts than fibrinogen/fibrin, was the critical determinant of *S. aureus* adhesion to intravascular lines chronically inserted in patients. These observations are concordant with the demonstration that with cannulas exposed to blood for a much shorter period of time in a canine model of arteriovenous shunt, *S. aureus* adhesion to such cannula segments (108) was essentially promoted by fibrinogen (see chapter 2).

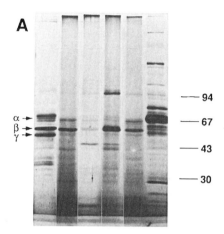

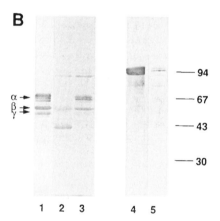

Figure 5. Analysis of SDS-extracted proteins from inserted cannulas by SDS-PAGE (A) and identification of either fibrinogen/fibrin or plasmin(ogen) by immunoblots with specific antibodies (B). (A) Protein extracts from four different cannulas (lanes 2 to 5) were electrophoresed in parallel with 100 ng of purified fibrinogen (lane 1) and 1,000-fold-diluted plasma (lane 6) in a 5 to 15% PAGE gradient and silver stained. (B) Two of these protein extracts were further probed by immunoblot with antifibrinogen antibodies (lanes 2 and 3) in parallel with purified fibrinogen (lane 1). The first extract (lane 2) shows mainly beta-chains, but not alpha- and gamma-chains, whereas the second extract (lane 3) shows both alpha- and beta-chains. Immunoblots show one additional band of 95 kDa in both extracts, representing cross-linked dimers of gamma-chains, plus a major proteolytic fragment of 40 to 43 kDa in one extract (lane 2). Immunoblots with antiplasminogen antibodies also show the presence of plasminogen in one cannula protein extract (lane 5) run in parallel with purified plasminogen (lane 4). (Lerch, P., J. J. Morgenthaler, D. Pittet, and P. E. Vaudaux, unpublished data.)

Role of host factors on phagocytic killing of *S. aureus* attached to foreign surfaces

The susceptibility to phagocytosis of *S. aureus* attached to PMMA cover slips was studied in two different ways. In the first study (111), we compared the susceptibility to phagocytic killing of *S. aureus* Wood 46 attached to a single side of uncoated PMMA cover slips, either spontaneously or artificially by centrifugation. After exposure to guinea pig peritoneal exudate neutrophils, both attached bacteria and phagocytes were removed from the cover slips using a harmless two-step procedure (111).

When the viability of resuspended bacteria was estimated by CFU counts, extensive killing of those attached artificially by centrifugation and immediately exposed to neutrophils was observed. In contrast, bacteria adhering spontaneously to cover slips for a prolonged period of time and incubated with phagocytes in similar conditions were more resistant to the killing action of phagocytes (111). The mode of bacterial attachment to the polymer surfaces was therefore a critical determinant of bacterial susceptibility or resistance to phagocytosis.

A more recent study was performed to evaluate the promotion of neutrophil bactericidal activity by extracellular matrix proteins against *S. aureus* attached to PMMA cover slips (46). Compared with uncoated surfaces, the bactericidal activity of human neutrophils adherent to fibronectin, fibrinogen, laminin, vitronectin, or type IV collagen was markedly enhanced. These matrix proteins appeared to enhance intracellular bactericidal activity of adherent neutrophils by integrin recognition of arginine-glycine-aspartic acid-serine (RGDS)-containing ligands (46). These results indicate a role for extracellular matrix proteins in the enhancement of host defense against pyogenic infections. Precise analysis of the composition and quantity of the different extracellular matrix proteins before and during infection needs to be further studied, to understand in closer detail how the contact of foreign bodies with neutrophils may eventually disturb their phagocytic and bactericidal functions.

Host factors influencing antibiotic susceptibility of *S. aureus* in a chronic model of infection

Persistence of staphylococcal foreign body infections despite the use of appropriate antibiotics is a major clinical problem. Several experimental studies have shown that bacteria either grown in vitro as adherent biofilms or recovered from infected prosthetic devices have decreased susceptibility to antimicrobial killing (1, 24–26, 36, 37, 40, 41, 91, 115, 121). To explore host and microbial factors hampering antibiotic efficacy in the vicinity of implants, three different but related approaches were taken.

(i) In vivo approach. A novel animal model of localized chronic foreign body infection was developed in rats to explore the in vivo activity of various bactericidal antibiotics (71). Four weeks after surgery, subcutaneously implanted tissue cages (with enclosed PMMA cover slips) were injected with 10^5 CFU of methicillin-susceptible or -resistant *S. aureus*, yielding stable counts (10^6 CFU/ml of TCF) at 2 weeks and later (14, 71). After 3 weeks of persistent infection, treatment with various antibiotics was given for 7 days. Concentrations of antibiotics in TCF continuously exceeded their MBCs for the test strains, whose batch cultures in Mueller-Hinton broth showed an elimination rate of 3 $\log_{10}$ CFU within 2 to 6 h. In vivo, a much lower decrease in viable counts of *S. aureus*, ranging from 0.5–2 $\log_{10}$ CFU per ml of tissue cage fluid, was obtained by intensive 7-day therapy with a number of beta-lactams, glycopeptides, and quinolones (8, 13, 14, 71, 88). Despite the fact that combined regimens of antibiotics (13, 14, 71) and longer durations (13) led to significant improvements of microbial elimination in vivo, the very poor efficacy of 7-day therapies with single agents clearly indicated a drastic loss of susceptibility to antibiotic killing for *S. aureus* chronically infecting tissue cages.

(ii) **Ex vivo approach.** After 3 weeks of tissue cage infection, suspensions of either methicillin-susceptible or -resistant strains of *S. aureus* were recovered from the foreign body surface and TCF (14). These ex vivo bacteria showed markedly less susceptibility to the in vitro killing effects of antistaphylococcal antibiotics than did bacteria of the same strains grown in batch cultures under conventional conditions (14).

(iii) **In vitro approach.** An artificial system of in vitro bacterial colonization was also developed by growing *S. aureus* on fibronectin-coated surfaces (15). At selected time points during growth, surface-bound organisms were exposed to bactericidal concentrations of four antistaphylococcal antibiotics. Whereas at 2 h organisms actively growing on surfaces were still optimally killed by all antibiotics, bacteria entering the stationary phase expressed markedly altered susceptibilities to each antimicrobial agent (15). Results from this in vitro study further suggest the occurrence of significant physiological and biochemical changes underlying decreased antibiotic susceptibilities of biomaterial-attached organisms (1, 24–26, 36, 37, 40, 41, 91, 115, 121). Overall, these data support the notion that in vivo conditions prevailing around implants may confer to *S. aureus* a broad-spectrum tolerance to most bactericidal antibiotics.

CONCLUDING REMARKS

Experimental models of foreign body infections and related in vitro models allowed exploration of major host factors predisposing to staphylococcal infections. Important defects in cytokine levels and in the phagocytic and bactericidal functions of local neutrophils were documented in the vicinity of subcutaneously implanted tissue cages challenged by *S. aureus* or *S. epidermidis*. Furthermore, such implanted tissue cages or cover slips were found to be progressively colonized by host-derived humoral and cellular elements. The extracellular matrix protein fibronectin was shown to play a significant role in promoting initial staphylococcal attachment to subcutaneously located polymer and metallic surfaces, thus eventually leading to microbial colonization and infection of indwelling devices. Finally, numerous in vivo and in vitro observations suggest that the host environment of indwelling devices may drastically alter metabolic properties of *S. aureus* or *S. epidermidis* infecting the implants, thus decreasing their susceptibility to bactericidal antibiotics.

Further progress in reducing the incidence or severity of foreign body infections will require the continuation of experimental studies; each category of implanted biomaterial needs to be more precisely analyzed in terms of composition of adsorbed host proteins and cell populations. The nature of adsorbed proteins will define which of them may preferentially promote bacterial attachment and colonization. The composition of the cell population in the vicinity of implants may critically influence the intensity and efficacy of the host immunological and phagocytic response to any bacterial challenge.

A number of approaches may be considered for reducing host susceptibility to foreign body infections. One of them is the development of new biomedical materials showing an improved compatibility with the host defense mechanisms or/and reducing adsorption of the most active host proteins promoting bacterial adhesion.

Besides having improved surface properties, biomedical materials might become protected from bacterial challenges by fluid-phase agents interfering with microbial adhesin or enhancing the phagocytic host defenses. Promising agents in this respect might be immunoglobulins raised against staphylococcal adhesins and blocking their activity (see details in chapter 2) or selective inducers of cytokine(s) improving the phagocytic clearance of microbial invaders. Finally, a better understanding of the tolerance of microorganisms toward antibiotics may offer new, effective treatment strategies in the future.

Notwithstanding the expected improvements in biocompatibility of indwelling devices, which should increase their resistance to colonization and reduce their susceptibility to pyogenic infections, we can still insist that strictly aseptic procedures during insertion or further handling of artificial implants will continue to be required to prevent their colonization and infection by pyogenic organisms.

Acknowledgments. This work was supported by grants 3.829.0.-87 and 32.30161.90 from the Swiss National Research Foundation.

Our gratitude extends to all previous or actual colleagues of the Division des Maladies Infectieuses and other collaborating institutions having contributed to this work. We especially thank M. Bento for expert technical assistance.

REFERENCES

1. **Anwar, H., M. K. Dasgupta, and J. W. Costerton.** 1990. Testing the susceptibility of bacteria in biofilms to antibacterial agents. *Antimicrob. Agents Chemother.* **34:**2043–2046.

2. **Autian, J.** 1977. Toxicological evaluation of biomaterials: primary acute toxicity screening program. *Artif. Organs* **1:**53–60.

3. **Baggiolini, M.** 1982. Proteinases and acid hydrolases of neutrophils and macrophages and the mechanisms of their release. *Adv. Inflammation Res.* **3:**313–327.

4. **Baier, R. E.** 1977. The organization of blood components near interfaces. *Ann. N. Y. Acad. Sci.* **283:**17–36.

5. **Bergan, T.** 1981. Pharmacokinetics of tissue penetration of antibiotics. *Rev. Infect. Dis.* **3:**45–66.

6. **Beutler, B., and A. Cerami.** 1987. Cachectin: more than a tumor necrosis factor. *N. Engl. J. Med.* **316:**379–385.

7. **Boyde, A., and S. Jones.** 1985. Bone modeling in the implantation bed. *J. Biomed. Mater. Res.* **19:**199–224.

8. **Cagni, A., C. Chuard, P. Vaudaux, F. A. Waldvogel, and D. P. Lew.** 1993. Comparative efficacy of sparfloxacin, temafloxacin, and ciprofloxacin in the therapy of experimental foreign body infection due to *Staphylococcus aureus. Program Abstr. 33rd Intersci. Conf. Antimicrob. Agents Chemother.,* abstr. 1160.

9. **Chenoweth, D. E., S. W. Cooper, T. E. Hugli, R. W. Stewart, E. H. Blackstone, and J. W. Kinklin.** 1981. Complement activation during cardiopulmonary bypass: evidence for generation of C3a and C5a anaphylotoxins. *N. Engl. J. Med.* **304:**497–508.

10. **Cheung, A. L., and V. A. Fischetti.** 1990. The role of fibrinogen in staphylococcal adherence to cathers in vitro. *J. Infect. Dis.* **161:**1177–1186.

11. **Chhatwal, G. S., G. Preissner, Müller-Berghaus, and H. Blobel.** 1987. Specific binding of the human S protein (vitronectin) to streptococci, *Staphylococcus aureus,* and *Escherichia coli. Infect. Immun.* **55:**1878–1883.

12. **Chhatwal, G. S., P. Valentin Weigand, and K. N. Timmis.** 1990. Bacterial infection of wounds: fibronectin-mediated adherence group A and C streptococci to fibrin thrombi in vitro. *Infect. Immun.* **58:**3015–3019.

13. **Chuard, C., M. Herrmann, P. Vandaux, F. A. Waldvogel, and D. P. Lew.** 1991. Successful therapy of experimental chronic foreign-body infection due to methicillin-resistant *Staphylococcus aureus* by antimicrobial combinations. *Antimicrob. Agents Chemother.* **35:**2611–2616.

14. **Chuard, C., E. C. Lucet, P. Rohner, M. Herrmann, R. Auckenthaler, F. A. Waldvogel, and D. P. Lew.** 1991. Resistance of *Staphylococcus aureus* recovered from infected foreign body in vivo to killing by antimicrobials. *J. Infect. Dis.* **163:**1369–1373.

15. **Chuard, C., P. Vaudaux, F. A. Waldvogel, and D. P. Lew.** 1993. Susceptibility of *Staphylococcus aureus* growing on fibronectin-coated surfaces to bactericidal antibiotics. *Antimicrob. Agents Chemother.* **37:**625–632.

16. **Coleman, D. L., R. N. King, and J. D. Andrade.** 1974. The foreign body reaction: a chronic inflammatory response. *J. Biomed. Mater. Res.* **8:**199–211.

17. **Cottonaro, C. N., H. V. Rookh, G. Shimica, and D. R. Sperling.** 1981. Quantitation and characterization of competitive protein binding to polymers. *Trans. Am. Soc. Artif. Intern. Organs* **27:**391–395.

18. **Craddock, P. R., J. Fehr, A. P. Dalmasso, K. L. Bringham, and H. S. Jacobs.** 1977. Hemodialysis leukopenia: pulmonary vascular leukostasis resulting from complement activation by dialyzer cellophane membranes. *J. Clin. Invest.* **59:**879–888.

19. **Dankert, J., A. H. Hogt, and J. Feijen.** 1986. Biomedical polymers: bacterial adhesion, colonization and infection. *Crit. Rev. Biocompat.* **2:**219–301.

20. **Delmi, M., P. Vaudaux, D. P. Lew, and H. Vasey.** Role of fibronectin on staphylococcal adhesion to metallic surfaces used as models of orthopaedic devices. *J. Orthop. Res.*, in press.
21. **Doolittle, R. F.** 1984. Fibrinogen and fibrin. *Annu. Rev. Biochem.* **53:**195–229.
22. **Dvorak, H. F.** 1986. Tumors: wounds that do not heal. Similarities between tumor stroma generation and wound healing. *N. Engl. J. Med.* **315:**1650–1659.
23. **Elek, S. D., and P. E. Conen.** 1957. The virulence of *Staphylococcus pyogenes* for man: a study of the problems of wound infection. *Br. J. Exp. Pathol.* **38:**573–586.
24. **Evans, D. J., D. G. Allison, M. R. Brown, and P. Gilbert.** 1991. Susceptibility of *Pseudomonas aeruginosa* and *Escherichia coli* biofilms towards ciprofloxacin: effect of specific growth rate. *J. Antimicrob. Chemother.* **27:**177–184.
25. **Evans, D. J., M. R. Brown, D. G. Allison, and P. Gilbert.** 1990. Susceptibility of bacterial biofilms to tobramycin: role of specific growth rate and phase in the division cycle. *J. Antimicrob. Chemother.* **25:**585–591.
26. **Evans, R. C., and C. J. Holmes.** 1987. Effect of vancomycin hydrochloride on *Staphylococcus epidermidis* biofilm associated with silicone elastomer. *Antimicrob. Agents Chemother.* **31:**889–894.
27. **Feijen, J., T. Beugeling, A. Bantjes, and C. T. H. Smit Sibinga.** 1979. Biomaterials and interfacial phenomena. *Adv. Cardiovasc. Phys.* **3:**100–134.
28. **Fletcher, M.** 1976. The effects of proteins on bacterial attachment to polysterene. *J. Gen. Microbiol.* **94:**400–404.
29. **Fröman, G., L. M. Switalski, P. Speziale, and M. Höök.** 1987. Isolation and characterization of a fibronectin receptor from *Staphylococcus aureus*. *J. Biol. Chem.* **262:**6564–6571.
30. **Fuller, R. A., and J. J. Rosen.** 1986. Materials for medicine. *Sci. Am.* **255:**118–125.
31. **Galante, J. O., J. Lemons, M. Spector, P. D. Wilson, Jr., and T. M. Wright.** 1991. The biologic effects of implant materials. *J. Orthop. Res.* **9:**760–775.
32. **Gallin, J. I.** 1981. Abnormal phagocyte chemotaxis: pathophysiology, clinical manifestations, and management of patients. *Rev. Infect. Dis.* **3:**1196–1220.
33. **Gallin, J. I.** 1984. Neutrophil specific granules: a fuse that ignites the inflammatory response. *Clin. Res.* **32:**320–328.
34. **Gallin, J. I., D. G. Wright, H. L. Malech, J. M. Davis, M. S. Klempner, and C. H. Kirkpatrick.** 1980. Disorders of phagocyte chemotaxis [clinical conference]. *Ann. Intern. Med.* **92:**520–538.
35. **Georgiade, N. G., E. H. King, W. A. Harris, J. H. Tenery, and B. A. Schlech.** 1975. Effect of three proteinaceous foreign materials on infected and subinfected wound models. *Surgery* **77:**569–576.
36. **Gilbert, P., D. G. Allison, D. J. Evans, P. S. Handley, and M. R. Brown.** 1989. Growth rate control of adherent bacterial populations. *Appl. Environ. Microbiol.* **55:**1308–1311.
37. **Gilbert, P., P. J. Collier, and M. R. Brown.** 1990. Influence of growth rate on susceptibility to antimicrobial agents: biofilms, cell cycle, dormancy, and stringent response. *Antimicrob. Agents Chemother.* **34:**1865–1868.
38. **Grinnell, F., and M. K. Feld.** 1981. Adsorption characteristics of plasma fibronectin in relationship to biological activity. *J. Biomed. Mater. Res.* **15:**363–381.
39. **Grinnell, F., and M. K. Feld.** 1982. Fibronectin adsorption on hydrophilic and hydrophobic surfaces detected by antibody binding and analysed during cell adhesion in serum-containing medium. *J. Biol. Chem.* **257:**4888–4893.
40. **Gristina, A. G., C. D. Hobgood, L. X. Webb, and Q. N. Myrvik.** 1987. Adhesive colonization of biomaterials and antibiotic resistance. *Biomaterials* **8:**423–426.

41. **Gristina, A. G., R. A. Jennings, P. T. Naylor, Q. N. Myrvik, and L. X. Webb.** 1989. Comparative in vitro antibiotic resistance of surface-colonizing coagulase-negative staphylococci. *Antimicrob. Agents Chemother.* **33:**813–816.

42. **Harasaki, H., R. Kiraly, and Y. Nose.** 1978. Endotheliziation in blood pumps. *Trans. Am. Soc. Artif. Intern. Organs* **24:**415–425.

43. **Hawiger, J., S. Timmons, D. Strong, B. A. Cottrell, M. Riley, and R. F. Doolittle.** 1982. Identification of a region of human fibrinogen interacting with staphylococcal clumping factor. *Biochem. J.* **21:**1407–1413.

44. **Hench, L. L., and J. Wilson.** 1984. Surface-active biomaterials. *Science* **226:**630–636.

45. **Henson, P. M.** 1971. The immunologic release of constituents from neutrophil leukocytes. I. The role of antibody and complement on nonphagocytosable surfaces or phagocytosable particles. *J. Immunol.* **107:**1535–1546.

46. **Herrmann, M., M. E. E. Jaconi, C. Dahlgren, F. A. Waldvogel, O. Stendahl, and D. P. Lew.** 1990. Neutrophil bactericidal activity against *Staphylococcus aureus* adherent on biological surfaces. *J. Clin. Invest.* **86:**942–951.

47. **Herrmann, M., S. J. Suchard, L. A. Boxer, F. A. Waldvogel, and D. P. Lew.** 1991. Thrombospondin binds to *Staphylococcus aureus* and promotes staphylococcal adherence to surfaces. *Infect. Immun.* **59:**279–288.

48. **Herrmann, M., P. Vaudaux, D. Pittet, R. Auckenthaler, D. P. Lew, F. Schumacher-Perdreau, G. Peters, and F. A. Waldvogel.** 1988. Fibronectin, fibrinogen and laminin act as mediators of adherence of clinical staphylococcal isolates to foreign material. *J. Infect. Dis.* **158:**693–701.

49. **Hogt, A., J. Dankert, and J. Feijen.** 1985. Adhesion of *Staphylococcus epidermidis* and *Staphylococcus saprophyticus* to a hydrophobic material. *J. Gen. Microbiol.* **131:**2485–2591.

50. **Holderbaum, D., T. Spech, A. Ehrhart, T. Keys, and G. S. Hall.** 1987. Collagen binding in clinical isolates of *Staphylococcus aureus*. *J. Clin. Microbiol.* **25:**2258–2261.

51. **Homonylo McGavin, M., D. Krajewska-Pietrasik, C. Rydén, and M. Höök.** 1993. Identification of a *Staphylococcus aureus* extracellular matrix-binding protein with broad specificity. *Infect. Immun.* **61:**2479–2485.

52. **Höök, M., L. M. Switalski, T. Wadström, and M. Lindberg.** 1989. Interactions of pathogenic microorganisms with fibronectin, p. 295–308. *In* D. F. Mosher (ed.), *Fibronectin.* Academic Press, Inc., San Diego.

53. **Hynes, R. O.** 1986. Fibronectins. *Sci. Am.* **254:**32–41.

54. **Hynes, R. O., and K. M. Yamada.** 1982. Fibronectins: multifunctional modular glycoproteins. *J. Cell Biol.* **95:**369–377.

55. **Inman, R. D., K. V. Gallegos, B. D. Brause, P. D. Redecha, and C. L. Christian.** 1984. Clinical and microbial features of prosthetic joint infection. *Am. J. Med.* **77:**47–53.

56. **James, R. C., and C. J. MacLeod.** 1961. Induction of staphylococcal infections in mice with small inocula introduced on sutures. *Br. J. Exp. Pathol.* **42:**266–277.

57. **Johnston, R. B., and J. E. Lehmeyer.** 1976. Elaboration of toxic oxygen by-product by neutrophils in a model of immune complex disease. *J. Clin. Invest.* **57:**836–841.

58. **Klebe, R. J., K. L. Bentley, and R. C. Schoen.** 1981. Adhesive substrates for fibronectin. *J. Cell. Physiol.* **109:**481–488.

59. **Kleinman, H. K., E. B. McGoodwin, G. R. Martin, R. J. Klebe, P. P. Fietzek, and D. E. Wooley.** 1978. Localization of the binding site for cell attachment in the alpha(I) chain of collagen. *J. Biol. Chem.* **253:**5642–5646.

60. **Klock, J. C., and D. F. Bainton.** 1976. Degranulation and abnormal bactericidal function of granulocytes procured by reversible adhesion to nylon wool. *Blood* **48:**149–161.

61. **Kronvall, G., and R. C. Williams, Jr.** 1969. Differences in anti-protein A activity among IgG subgroups. *J. Immunol.* **103**:828–833.
62. **Kuusela, P.** 1978. Fibronectin binds to *Staphylococcus aureus. Nature* (London) **276**: 718–720.
63. **Kuusela, P., T. Vartio, M. Vuento, and E. B. Myhre.** 1984. Binding sites for streptococci and staphylococci in fibronectin. *Infect. Immun.* **45**:433–436.
64. **Kupyers, J. M., and R. A. Proctor.** 1989. A fibronectin low-binding mutant of *Staphylococcus aureus* shows reduced adherence to traumatized heart valves. *Infect. Immun.* **57**:2306–2312.
65. **Lämmler, C., J. C. De Freitas, G. S. Chatwal, and H. Blobel.** 1985. Interactions of immunoglobulin G, fibrinogen and fibronectin with *Staphylococcus hyicus* and *Staphylococcus intermedius. Zentralbl. Bakteriol. Mikrobiol. Hyg. (A.)* **260**:232–237.
66. **Langlais, F.** 1985. Les nouveaux biomatériaux en orthopédie. *Presse Med.* **14**: 1424–1428.
67. **Lew, D. P., R. Zubler, P. Vaudaux, J. J. Farquet, F. A. Waldvogel, and P. H. Lambert.** 1979. Decreased heat-labile opsonic activity and complement levels associated with evidence of C3 breakdown products in infected pleural effusions. *J. Clin. Invest.* **63**:326–334.
68. **Lopes, J. D., M. Dos Reis, and R. R. Brentani.** 1985. Presence of laminin receptors in *Staphylococcus aureus. Science* **229**:275–277.
69. **Lopes, J. D., M. Dos Reis, and R. R. Brentani.** 1985. Presence of laminin receptors in *Staphylococcus aureus. Science* **229**:275–277.
70. **Lowy, F. D., and S. M. Hammer.** 1983. *Staphylococcus epidermidis* infections. *Ann. Intern. Med.* **99**:834–839.
71. **Lucet, J. C., M. Herrmann, P. Rohner, R. Auckenthaler, F. A. Waldvogel, and D. P. Lew.** 1990. Treatment of experimental foreign body infection caused by methicillin-resistant *Staphylococcus aureus. Antimicrob. Agents Chemother.* **34**:2312–2317.
72. **Marchant, R. E., and J. M. Anderson.** 1986. In vivo biocompatibility studies. VII. Inflammatory response to polyethylene and to a cytotoxic polyvinylchloride. *J. Biomed. Mater. Res.* **20**:37–50.
73. **Marchant, R. E., A. Hiltner, C. Hamlin, A. Rabinovitch, R. Slobodkin, and J. M. Anderson.** 1986. In vivo biocompatibility studies. I. The cage implant system and a biodegradable hydrogel. *J. Biomed. Mater. Res.* **17**:301–325.
74. **McDevitt, D., P. Vaudaux, and T. J. Foster.** 1992. Genetic evidence that bound coagulase of *Staphylococcus aureus* is not clumping factor. *Infect. Immun.* **60**:1514–1523.
75. **McDonald, J. A., T. J. Broekelmann, D. G. Kelley, and B. Villiger.** 1981. Gelatin-binding domain-specific anti-human plasma fibronectin Fab inhibits fibronectin-mediated gelatin binding but not cell spreading. *J. Biol. Chem.* **256**:5583–5587.
76. **Mosher, D. F., and R. A. Proctor.** 1980. Binding and factor XIII-mediated cross-linking of a 27-kilodalton fragment of fibronectin to *Staphylococcus aureus. Science* **209**: 927–929.
77. **Mosher, D. F., R. A. Proctor, and J. E. Grossman.** 1981. Fibronectin: role in inflammation, p. 187–206. *In* G. Weissmann (ed.), *Advances in Inflammation Research.* Raven Press, New York.
78. **Murabayashi, S., and Y. Nosé.** 1986. Biocompatibility: bioengineering aspects. *Artif. Organs* **10**:114–121.
79. **Noble, W. C.** 1965. The production of subcutaneous staphylococcal skin lesions in mice. *Br. J. Exp. Pathol.* **46**:254–262.
80. **Pascual, A., A. Fleer, N. A. C. Westerdaal, and J. Verhoef.** 1986. Modulation of adherence of coagulase-negative staphylococci to Teflon catheters in vitro. *Eur. J. Clin. Microbiol.* **5**:518–522.

81. **Paulsson, M., and T. Wadström.** 1990. Vitronectin and type-I collagen binding by *Staphylococcus aureus* and coagulase-negative staphylocci. *FEMS Microbiol. Immunol.* **2:**55–62.

82. **Proctor, R. A., G. Christman, and D. F. Mosher.** 1984. Fibronectin-induced agglutination of *Staphylococcus aureus* correlates with invasiveness. *J. Lab. Clin. Med.* **104:** 455–469.

83. **Proctor, R. A., D. F. Mosher, and P. J. Olbrantz.** 1982. Fibronectin binding to *Staphylococcus aureus. J. Biol. Chem.* **257:**14788–14794.

84. **Quie, P. G.** 1975. Pathology of bactericidal power of neutrophils. *Semin. Hematol.* **12:** 143–160.

85. **Raja, R. H., G. Raucci, and M. Höök.** 1990. Peptide analogs to a fibronectin receptor inhibit attachment of *Staphylococcus aureus* to fibronectin-containing substrates. *Infect. Immun.* **58:**2593–2598.

86. **Ryden, C., K. Rubin, P. Speziale, M. Höök, M. Lindberg, and T. Wadström.** 1983. Fibronectin receptors from *Staphylococcus aureus. J. Biol. Chem.* **258:**3396–3401.

87. **Ryden, C., A. I. Yacoub, I. Maxe, D. Heinegard, A. Oldberg, A. Franzen, A. Ljungh, and K. Rubin.** 1989. Specific binding of bone sialoprotein to *Staphylococcus aureus* isolated from patients with osteomyelitis. *Eur. J. Biochem.* **184:**331–336.

88. **Schaad, H., C. Chuard, P. Vaudaux, F. A. Waldvogel, and D. P. Lew.** 1993. *Program Abstr. 33rd Intersci. Conf. Antimicrob. Agents Chemother.*, abstr. 122.

89. **Scheld, W. M., R. W. Strunk, G. Balion, and R. A. Colderone.** 1985. Microbial adhesion to fibronectin in vitro correlates with production of endocarditis in rabbits. *Proc. Soc. Exp. Biol. Med.* **180:**474–482.

90. **Sela, J., and I. Bab.** 1985. The mechanism of primary mineralization in the reaction of bone to injury and administration of implant. *J. Biomed. Mater. Res.* **19:**225–231.

91. **Sheth, N. K., T. R. Franson, and P. G. Sohnle.** 1985. Influence of bacterial adherence to intravascular catheters on in vitro antibiotic susceptibility. *Lancet* **ii:**1266–1268.

92. **Speziale, P., G. Raucci, L. Visai, L. M. Switalski, R. Timpl, and M. Höök.** 1986. Binding of collagen to *Staphylococcus aureus* Cowan 1. *J. Bacteriol.* **167:**77–81.

93. **Stinson, M. W., D. C. Jincks, and J. M. Merrick.** 1981. Adherence of *Streptococcus mutans* and *Streptococcus sanguis* to salivary components bound to glass. *Infect. Immun.* **32:**583–591.

94. **Suter, S., U. E. Nydegger, L. Roux, and F. A. Waldvogel.** 1981. Cleavage of C3 by neutral proteases from granulocytes in pleural empyema. *J. Infect. Dis.* **144:**499–508.

95. **Suter, S., U. B. Schaad, L. Roux, U. E. Nydegger, and F. A. Waldvogel.** 1984. Granulocyte neutral proteases and Pseudomonas elastase as possible causes of airway damage in patients with cystic fibrosis. *J. Infect. Dis.* **149:**523–531.

96. **Switalski, L. M., J. M. Patti, W. Butcher, A. G. Gristina, P. Speziale, and M. Höök.** 1993. A collagen receptor on *Staphylococcus aureus* strains isolated from patients with septic arthritis mediates adhesion to cartilage. *Mol. Microbiol.* **7:**99–107.

97. **Switalski, L. M., C. Rydén, K. Rubin, A. Ljungh, M. Höök, and T. Wadström.** 1983. Binding of fibronectin to *Staphylococcus* strains. *Infect. Immun.* **42:**628–633.

98. **Toy, P. T. C., L.-W. Lai, T. Drake, and M. A. Sande.** 1985. Effect of fibronectin on adherence of *Staphylococcus aureus* to fibrin thrombi in vitro. *Infect. Immun.* **48:**83–86.

99. **Tshefu, K., W. Zimmerli, and F. A. Waldvogel.** 1983. Short-term administration of rifampin in the prevention or eradication of infection due to foreign bodies. *Rev. Infect. Dis.* **5**(Suppl.)**:**S474–S480.

100. **Valentin Weigand, P., K. N. Timmis, and G. S. Chhatwal.** 1993. Role of fibronectin in staphylococcal colonisation of fibrin thrombi and plastic surfaces. *J. Med. Microbiol.* **38:**90–95.

101. **Vaudaux, P.** Interaction of *Staphylococcus aureus* with implanted artificial surfaces used as biomaterials. *In* R. Möllby and J. I. Flock (ed.), *Proceedings of the VIIth International Symposium on Staphylococci and Staphylococcal Infections,* in press.

102. **Vaudaux, P., X. Clivaz, R. Emch, P. Descouts, and D. P. Lew.** 1990. Heterogeneity of antigenic and proadhesive activity of fibronectin adsorbed on various metallic or polymeric surfaces, p. 31–36. *In* G. Heimke, U. Soltösz, and A. J. C. Lee (ed.), *Clinical Implant Materials.* Elsevier Science Publishers, B. V., Amsterdam.

103. **Vaudaux, P., G. E. Grau, E. Huggler, F. Schumacher Perdreau, F. Fiedler, F. A. Waldvogel, and D. P. Lew.** 1992. Contribution of tumor necrosis factor to host defense against staphylococci in a guinea pig model of foreign body infections. *J. Infect. Dis.* **166:**58–64.

104. **Vaudaux, P., P. Lerch, M. I. Velazco, U. E. Nydegger, and F. A. Waldvogel.** 1986. Role of fibronectin in the susceptibility of biomaterial implants to bacterial infections. *Adv. Biomater.* **6:**355–360.

105. **Vaudaux, P., D. P. Lew, and F. A. Waldvogel.** 1987. Host-dependent pathogenic factors in foreign body infection: a comparison between *Staphylococcus epidermidis* and *Staphylococcus aureus,* p. 183–193. *In* G. Pulverer, P. G. Quie, and G. Peters (ed.), *Pathogenicity and Clinical Significance of Coagulase-Negative Staphylococci.* Gustav-Fischer-Verlag, Stuttgart.

106. **Vaudaux, P., D. Pittet, A. Haeberli, E. Huggler, U. E. Nydegger, D. P. Lew, and F. A. Waldvogel.** 1989. Host factors selectively increase staphylococcal adherence on inserted catheters: a role for fibronectin and fibrinogen/fibrin. *J. Infect. Dis.* **160:** 865–875.

107. **Vaudaux, P., D. Pittet, A. Haeberli, P. G. Lerch, J. J. Morgenthaler, R. A. Proctor, F. A. Waldvogel, and D. P. Lew.** 1993. Fibronectin is more active than fibrin or fibrinogen in promoting *Staphylococcus aureus* adherence to inserted intravascular catheters. *J. Infect. Dis.* **167:**633–641.

108. **Vaudaux, P., R. A. Proctor, D. McDevitt, T. Foster, D. P. Lew, H. Wabers, and S. Cooper.** 1991. *Program Abstr. 31st Intersci. Conf. Antimicrob. Agents Chemother.,* abstr. 1067.

109. **Vaudaux, P., R. Suzuki, F. A. Waldvogel, J. J. Morgenthaler, and U. E. Nydegger.** 1984. Foreign body infection: role of fibronectin as a ligand for the adherence of *Staphylococcus aureus. J. Infect. Dis.* **150:**546–553.

110. **Vaudaux, P., F. A. Waldvogel, J. J. Morgenthaler, and U. E. Nydegger.** 1984. Adsorption of fibronectin onto polymethylmethacrylate and promotion of *Staphylococcus aureus* adherence. *Infect. Immun.* **45:**768–774.

111. **Vaudaux, P., G. Zulian, E. Huggler, and F. A. Waldvogel.** 1985. Attachment of *Staphylococcus aureus* to polymethylmethacrylate increases its resistance to phagocytosis in foreign body infection. *Infect. Immun.* **50:**472–477.

112. **Velazco, M. I., and F. A. Waldvogel.** 1987. Monosaccharide inhibition of *Staphylococcus aureus* adherence to human solid-phase fibronectin. *J. Infect. Dis.* **155:**1069–1072.

113. **Vercellotti, G. M., D. Lussenhop, P. K. Peterson, L. T. Furcht, J. B. McCarthy, H. S. Jacob, and C. F. Moldow.** 1984. Bacterial adherence to fibronectin and endothelial cells: a possible mechanism for bacterial tissue tropism. *J. Lab. Clin. Med.* **103:**34–43.

114. **Vercellotti, G. M., J. B. McCarthy, P. Lindholm, P. K. Peterson, H. S. Jacob, and L. T. Furcht.** 1985. Extracellular matrix proteins (fibronectin, laminin, and type IV collagen) bind and aggregate bacteria. *Am. J. Pathol.* **120:**13–31.

115. **Vergeres, P., and J. Blaser.** 1992. Amikacin, ceftazidime, and flucloxacillin against suspended and adherent *Pseudomonas aeruginosa* and *Staphylococcus epidermidis* in an in vitro model of infection. *J. Infect. Dis.* **165:**281–289.

116. **Verhoef, J., and H. A. Verbrugh.** 1981. Host determinants in staphylococcal disease. *Annu. Rev. Med.* **32:**107–122.

117. **Voytek, A., A. G. Gristina, E. Barth, Q. Myrvik, L. Switalski, M. Höök, and P. Speziale.** 1988. Staphylococcal adhesion to collagen in intra-articular sepsis. *Biomaterials* **9:**107–110.

118. **Wadström, T., P. Speziale, Rozgonyi, A. Ljungh, I. Maxe, and C. Ryden.** 1987. Interactions of coagulase-negative staphylococci with fibronectin and collagen, as possible first step of tissue colonization in wounds and other tissue trauma, p. 83–91. *In* G. Pulverer, P. G. Quie, and G. Peters (ed.), *Pathogenicity and Clinical Significance of Coagulase-Negative Staphylococci.* Gustav Fischer Verlag, Stuttgart.

119. **Waldvogel, F. A., P. Vaudaux, D. P. Lew, A. Zwahlen, S. Suter, and U. E. Nydegger.** 1982. Deficient phagocytosis secondary to breakdown of opsonic factors in infected exudates, p. 603–610. *In* F. Rossi and P. Patriarca (ed.), *Biochemistry and Function of Phagocytes.* Plenum Publishing Corp., New York.

120. **Wegmüller, E., M. D. Kazatchkine, and U. E. Nydegger.** 1983. Complement activation during extracorporeal blood bypass. *Plasma Ther. Transfus. Technol.* **4:**361–371.

121. **Widmer, A. F., R. Frei, Z. Rajacic, and W. Zimmerli.** 1990. Correlation between in vivo and in vitro efficacy of antimicrobial agents against foreign body infections. *J. Infect. Dis.* **162:**96–102.

122. **Woo Park, P., D. D. Roberts, L. E. Grosso, W. C. Parks, J. Rosenbloom, W. R. Abrams, and R. P. Mecham.** 1991. Binding of elastin to *Staphylococcus aureus. J. Biol. Chem.* **266:**23399–23406.

123. **Wright, D. G., and J. I. Gallin.** 1979. Secretory responses of human neutrophils: exocytosis of specific (secondary) granules by human neutrophils during adherence in vitro and during exudation in vivo. *J. Immunol.* **123:**258–294.

124. **Yanai, M., and P. G. Quie.** 1981. Chemiluminescence by polymorphonuclear leukocytes adhering to surfaces. *Infect. Immun.* **123:**285–294.

125. **Zimmerli, W., D. P. Lew, and F. A. Waldvogel.** 1984. Pathogenesis of foreign body infection. Evidence for a local granulocyte defect. *J. Clin. Invest.* **73:**1191–1200.

126. **Zimmerli, W., and F. A. Waldvogel.** 1986. Models of foreign-body infections, p. 295–317. *In* O. Zak and M. A. Sande (ed.), *Experimental Models in Antimicrobial Chemotherapy,* vol. 1. Academic Press, Inc. (London), Ltd., London.

127. **Zimmerli, W., F. A. Waldvogel, P. Vaudaux, and U. E. Nydegger.** 1982. Pathogenesis of foreign body infection: description and characteristics of an animal model. *J. Infect. Dis.* **146:**487–497.

128. **Zwahlen, A., U. E. Nydegger, P. Vaudaux, P. H. Lambert, and F. A. Waldvogel.** 1982. Complement-mediated opsonic activity in normal and infected human cerebrospinal fluid: early response during bacterial meningitis. *J. Infect. Dis.* **145:**635–646.

Infections Associated with Indwelling Medical Devices, 2nd ed.
Edited by Alan L. Bisno and Francis A. Waldvogel
© 1994 American Society for Microbiology, Washington, DC 20005

Chapter 2

Molecular Basis of Adherence of Staphylococci to Biomaterials

T. J. Foster and D. McDevitt

Staphylococcus aureus is an important cause of infections associated with indwelling medical devices. The ability of the bacteria to adhere to biomaterial surfaces that have become coated with host plasma and matrix proteins such as fibrinogen and fibronectin is a major determinant for initiating a foreign body infection. In addition, the ability of bacteria to stick directly to plastic surfaces could play a role in biomaterial-related infection, but this is more likely to occur as a result of contamination prior to implanting.

In gram-negative bacteria, many important adhesins are associated with fimbriae that recognize sugar residues on glycoproteins or glycolipids on the surface of mammalian cells. In contrast, the major adhesins of *S. aureus* are monomeric cell surface-associated proteins that recognize host matrix proteins by direct protein-protein interactions.

Adhesion of *S. aureus* to biomaterial surfaces coated with fibrinogen and fibronectin is determined by protein adhesins located on the bacterial cell surface. The fibronectin-binding protein (FnBP) of *S. aureus* has been studied in considerable detail while the fibrinogen adhesin (clumping factor) has only recently been identified. The ligand-binding domain(s) of the adhesin is defined using truncated protein fragments and synthetic peptides in binding and inhibition studies. The role of the putative adhesin can be defined by isolating site-specific adhesin-defective mutants that can be compared with the parental strain in in vitro adhesion experiments and in animal models for foreign body infection.

T. J. Foster and D. McDevitt • Microbiology Department, Moyne Institute, Trinity College, Dublin 2, Ireland.

These complementary experimental approaches are being applied to the analysis of both fibronectin- and fibrinogen-binding proteins of *S. aureus.*

In contrast, there is relatively little information about the mechanisms of attachment of *Staphylococcus epidermidis.* This organism is the major cause of device-related infections, yet paradoxically much less is known about its adhesion mechanisms. The nature of the fibronectin adhesin is not known, and most research has focused on a surface polysaccharide that promotes adhesion to uncoated plastic.

BACTERIAL BINDING SITES ON FIBRONECTIN

Fibronectin is a dimeric glycopeptide that is composed of a series of repeats (Fig. 1) (42, 44). The N-terminal 27-kDa peptide formed by plasmin degradation (44) can bind to the bacterial cell surface with the same kinetics as native fibronectin (K_d, 1.8 nM) (2), and it can also promote attachment of *S. aureus* to coated surfaces. The five type I modules at the N terminus of fibronectin (modules 1 to 5) are implicated in the binding reaction with *S. aureus.* Site-directed mutagenesis of a recombinant truncated fibronectin gene expressed by a mammalian cell line in culture showed that each of the five type I modules is important in the binding reaction (52). Single amino acid substitutions in any of these modules reduced the affinity by about 50%, whereas deletion of any of the modules completely eliminated binding of the truncated fibronectin to bacteria.

A second binding domain (2, 29) with a K_d of 10 nM has been located in a single type III heparin-binding module, number 14 (Fig. 1). This domain may only be exposed in fibronectin that has taken on a fibrillar conformation when associated with surfaces. This could explain the observation that the C-terminal fragment in solution failed to bind to bacte-

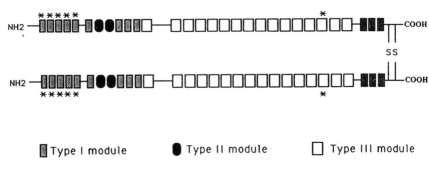

Figure 1. Structure of fibronectin (44). The binding sites for *S. aureus* are indicated (*).

rial cells, but when coated onto plastic surfaces, it promoted bacterial attachment. This apparently weak interaction might contribute synergistically with N-terminal type I sites to the binding of *S. aureus* cells to fibrillar fibronectin.

INTERACTIONS OF *S. AUREUS* WITH FIBRONECTIN

It has been known for some time that fibronectin can bind to receptors on the surface of *S. aureus* cells (28). In addition, *S. aureus* can also bind to fibronectin-coated surfaces. It is attractive to think that the same adhesin is responsible for both interactions.

A high-molecular-weight protein that can bind fibronectin was purified from extracts of the bacterial cell wall by affinity methods (11). Initially the molecular weight of the protein was underestimated (47), probably because of degradation. Molecular analysis of the genetic locus encoding the fibronectin-binding protein of *S. aureus* 8325-4 revealed two related *fnb* genes located 682 bp apart and showed that both could express a functional fibronectin-binding protein when cloned in *Escherichia coli* (23, 51). The availability of the DNA sequence facilitated the comparison of the primary structures of the two proteins (Fig. 2). It is interesting

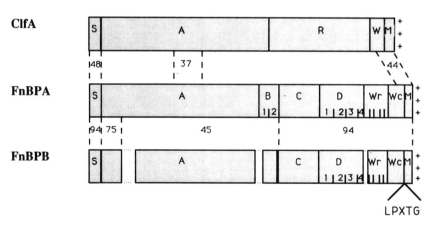

Figure 2. Comparison of the structures of the fibrinogen-binding protein (clumping factor, ClfA) of strain Newman and the fibronectin-binding proteins (FnBPA and FnBPB) of *S. aureus* 8325-4. The numbers between the vertical dashed lines indicate the percentage of amino acid identity between two proteins. In ClfA, a region between residues 272 and 349 is 37% identical and 41% identical with part of region A of FbpA and FbpB, respectively (35). S, signal sequence; R, repeat region; D, fibronectin-binding repeat domains; Wr, proline-rich wall-spanning region; W, wall-spanning region; M, membrane-spanning region; +, positive-charged residues. LPXTG, Leu-Pro-X-Thr-Gly motif.

to note that not all strains of *S. aureus* carry two *fnb* genes. Southern blotting has revealed that several phage group I and phage group II strains have a single *fnb* gene (13).

The fibronectin-binding proteins (FnBPs) have many features that are characteristic of wall-associated proteins of gram-positive bacteria (9, 26, 50). The functions of these regions have been inferred primarily from studies with protein A expressed by *S. aureus*. The primary translation products have a signal sequence that presumably specifies the cotranslational secretion of the FnBP across the plasma membrane. Several positively charged residues at the extreme C terminus are thought to act as a stop translation signal and could be located on the cytoplasmic side of the plasma membrane. This region also comprises a hydrophobic domain, which presumably spans the plasma membrane and may act as an anchor, and a conserved motif, Leu-Pro-X-Thr-Gly (LPXTG) (9). The latter is required for the accurate sorting and location of the protein in the cell wall. Situated N terminal to the membrane anchor region is the putative wall-spanning region. In FnBPs this comprises a constant region, Wc, and a repeated region, Wr, which has many proline and glycine residues (23, 51). The proline- and glycine-rich region may allow the protein to take up an extended structure with many turns, which could allow the protein to span the highly cross-linked peptidoglycan layer. Some cell wall-associated proteins such as protein A and FnBPs appear to be covalently linked to peptidoglycan. The intact protein can only be released by lysostaphin, which cleaves between glycine residues in the interpeptide bridge in peptidoglycan. In contrast, a muramidase which cleaves between *N*-acetylmuramic acid and *N*-acetylglucosamine releases proteins of higher molecular weight due to covalently attached peptidoglycan fragments. It is attractive to think that the LPXTG is cleaved proteolytically and a peptide bond is formed with the glycine in nascent peptidoglycan before final cross-linking occurs (9, 49, 50).

A repeated region located just upstream from the wall-spanning region contains the fibronectin-binding sites. Synthetic peptides representing each of the individual D repeats partially blocked binding of soluble fibronectin to bacterial cells, with D3 being the strongest (45). This could be explained because D3 carries two copies of the Glu-Glu-Asp-Thr (EEDT) motif implicated in the reaction with fibronectin. The strongest reaction occurred with the complete D1-D4 region expressed as a recombinant fusion protein. Recent studies with FnBPB revealed another fibronectin-binding domain located in region C, possibly at an EEDT sequence (23).

Studies with synthetic peptides based on fibronectin-binding repeat D3 showed that residues 15 to 36 comprised the minimum unit required for the blocking activity (37). Chemical modification of glutamate and aspartate residues led to the hypothesis that the EEDT motif present in each repeat was of crucial importance in the interaction with fibronectin.

By comparing the amino acid sequences of ligand-binding domains of staphylococcal and streptococcal FnBPs, a core fibronectin-binding sequence has been resolved: Glu-Asp-Thr/Ser-(X9, 10)-Gly-Gly-(X3, 4) Ile/Val-Asp-Phe. (32, 37, 38, 57). The validity of this motif in fibronectin binding was tested by adherence blocking experiments using a series of synthetic peptides with variant residues at core positions. Contrary to the original hypothesis, the Glu-Asp-Ser (EDT) motif seen in the staphylococcal FnBPs was shown not to be required for binding activity, whereas the conserved Gly-Gly dipeptide and the Ile/Val-Asp-Phe sequence together with additional acidic residues were required (38). The importance of these residues in the adherence of staphylococcal cells to fibronectin-coated surfaces could be confirmed by isolating site-directed mutants of *S. aureus* expressing FnBPs with specific changes in these regions.

Blocking studies with recombinant and synthetic peptides representing the D repeat region indicate that the FnBPs determine the ability of *S. aureus* to adhere to fibronectin-coated surfaces as well as to soluble fibronectin (45). This has been confirmed by our recent studies with site-specific mutants defective in FnBPs (14). The *fnbA* and *fnbB* genes of *S. aureus* 8325-4 were inactivated by cloning into the center of the genes DNA fragments expressing antibiotic resistance. The mutated genes were introduced into the chromosome in place of the wild-type genes by homologous recombination (allelic replacement). The single mutants had slightly reduced adherence to fibronectin-coated polymethylmeth-acrylate (PMMA) coverslips, while the double mutant was completely deficient. This shows that both *fnbA* and *fnbB* genes are required to promote adherence of *S. aureus* 8325-4 to fibronectin-coated surfaces (14).

The *fbpA fbpB* double mutant was also defective in adherence to ex vivo coverslips removed from subcutaneous chambers implanted in guinea pigs, a foreign body model (10). This indicates that the FnBPs contribute to adherence to biomaterial that has been coated with host proteins in vivo. This could be confirmed using ex vivo human catheters, for which degraded but functional fibronectin is the major determinant of staphylococcal adherence (62, 63).

As yet the only in vivo experiments with a fibronectin-binding-defective mutant are those reported by Kuypers and Proctor (30) with a derivative of the phage group I strain 879RF isolated by transposon Tn*918* mutagenesis. The low-fibronectin-binding mutant had a markedly reduced ability to adhere to traumatized rat heart valves, indicating that fibronectin binding is important in vivo. This observation takes on increased significance now that we have shown by Southern hybridization and DNA sequencing that the Tn*918* insertion is located 45 bp 5' to the single *fnb* gene in strain 879RF, where it presumably blocks transcription from the promoter lying upstream (13).

ADHERENCE TO FIBRONECTIN OF COAGULASE-NEGATIVE STAPHYLOCOCCI

The adherence of *S. epidermidis* to biomaterial is enhanced by bound fibronectin, but the number of adherent bacteria is significantly lower than for *S. aureus* strains under the same conditions (19, 62). Thus, *S. epidermidis* binds to fibronectin-coated biomaterial but less avidly than *S. aureus*. *S. epidermidis* also recognizes the 29-kDa N-terminal fibronectin fragment that contains the primary *S. aureus* binding domain (60). However, nothing is known about the molecular basis of *S. epidermidis* binding to fibronectin. It is perhaps reasonable to speculate that an FnBP similar to those found in *S. aureus* and streptococci is involved. Hybridization and PCR experiments using DNA probes and primers derived from the fibronectin-binding consensus might be profitable, as might adherence blocking experiments with synthetic peptides based on the binding motifs of known FnBPs.

ROLE OF POLYSACCHARIDES IN STAPHYLOCOCCAL ADHESION TO BIOMATERIAL

It has been postulated that the fibronectin-binding determinant of *S. aureus* is capsular polysaccharide, at least in strains that express serotype 8 polysaccharide (22, 61). Evidence cited to support this contention is as follows: (i) a macromolecular polysaccharide complex with fibronectin-binding activity has been purified from *S. aureus*, (ii) electron microscopic analysis of gold-labelled cells indicated that fibronectin attached to the bacteria at the extremity of the glycocalyx rather than close to the cell wall, and (iii) antibody to serotype 8 capsular polysaccharide inhibited binding of fibronectin to bacterial cells. An alternative explanation for the last observation is that the antibody caused steric blocking of fibronectin binding. Also, the fibronectin-binding activity of the polysaccharide could have been due to FnBP present in the complex.

There are several reports implicating surface polysaccharides in adhesion of *S. epidermidis* to naked plastic surfaces and in biofilm formation (34, 39, 46). Attachment of bacteria directly to plastic surfaces could be important in the contamination of biomaterial prior to implantation and also in infection via the exposed surfaces of indwelling catheters. A polysaccharide adhesin (PS/A) is required for adherence of S. *epidermidis* to naked plastic (39), and another possibly distinct polysaccharide appears to be involved in cell-cell adherence in biofilm formation (34). Another group has found evidence that a high-molecular-weight surface protein promotes binding of (at least one strain of) S. *epidermidis* to plastic (58). A monoclonal antibody to the surface protein blocked adherence.

The importance of the polysaccharide adhesin PS/A is supported by genetic manipulation (39) and by immunization experiments (27). Mutants defective in the polysaccharide adhesin PS/A were isolated by transposon insertion mutagenesis. These were defective in adherence to plastic surfaces in vitro and were less virulent in a foreign body infection model involving interaction of plastic material with bacterial cells prior to implantation. In addition, active and passive immunization of rabbits with PS/A reduced bacteremia and prevented experimental endocarditis (56). PS/A could form the basis of a vaccine to combat nosocomial infection caused by S. *epidermidis*.

Formation of a biofilm is a characteristic of staphylococcal infections associated with indwelling medical devices. The extracellular polysaccharide-containing material associated with aggregates of bacterial cells in the biofilm is called the glycocalyx. Slime is a term reserved for exopolymers that accumulate in broth culture supernatants. This material is predominantly teichoic acid (12). The polysaccharides previously identified in slime actually come from the growth medium (12). Slime formation in vitro does not correlate with adherence.

ADHESION OF *S. AUREUS* TO FIBRINOGEN

It has been known for many years that S. *aureus* cells form macroscopic clumps when a suspension is mixed with plasma. The clumping reaction is due to the avid binding of the dimeric plasma protein fibrinogen (Fig. 3) to the clumping factor located on the bacterial cell surface. Blocking experiments with proteolytic fragments of fibrinogen and with synthetic peptides showed that the S. *aureus* binding site is in the C terminus of the γ chain (15, 54).

Initially it was thought that the clumping factor is a cell-bound form of coagulase. However, Duthie demonstrated that coagulase and the clumping factor are independent entities (6). Coagulase is a predominantly extracellular protein that binds stoichiometrically with prothrombin to activate the proteolytic function characteristic of thrombin (16, 24,

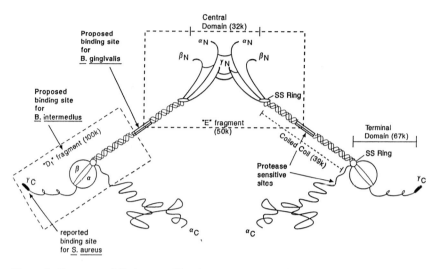

Figure 3. Structure of fibrinogen. This figure was first published in Lantz et al. (31) and is adapted from Doolittle (5). The dimeric molecule is composed of three polypeptide chains, α (66,000), β (54,000), and γ (48,000). The amino-terminal ends are held together by disulfide bridges. Protease treatment generates a number of fragments including D and E, which are indicated.

25). Thus, staphylothrombin converts fibrinogen to fibrin, resulting in the formation of a plasma clot.

Recently it was shown that coagulase could also bind directly to fibrinogen (1). In contrast to the reaction with prothrombin, which occurs at the N terminus of coagulase (24, 25, 43), the interaction with fibrinogen is with the C terminus (36). In addition, when cell wall extracts were probed by fibrinogen affinity blotting, the major activity was shown to be due to a cell-bound form of coagulase (1). It was postulated that bound coagulase was, after all, the clumping factor. However, a deletion mutant in the chromosomal *coa* gene isolated by allelic replacement retained the clumping phenotype but lost the plasma-clotting activity and the fibrinogen-binding proteins in the cell wall (36). Conversely, a clumping-factor-deficient transposon insertion mutant retained the plasma-clotting phenotype and the wall-bound fibrinogen-binding activity of coagulase (36). Thus, although coagulase binds to fibrinogen, the fibrinogen-binding region cannot be exposed on the bacterial cell surface and cannot be responsible for clumping.

There have been several reports describing the purification of the clumping factor (e.g., references 3, 59). However, the proteins obtained were not characterized further. We have exploited transposon mutagenesis to identify the genetic locus encoding clumping factor (35). Several independent transposon Tn917 mutants defective in clumping factor were isolated. Southern blotting showed that each transposon insertion was located in the same region of the chromosome. The locus containing the Tn917 insertion sites was cloned from a wild-type strain. It expressed a ca. 130-kDa fibrinogen-binding protein in E. coli. A similar-sized protein was seen in affinity blots of cell wall extracts of S. aureus strains harboring the clumping factor gene clfA on a multicopy plasmid. Subsequently, the 130-kDa ClfA protein expressed by a single copy of the gene was detected when the signal was amplified. The cloned clfA gene also restored the fibrinogen-binding defect of the clfA mutants.

Sequence analysis of the clfA gene predicted a protein of 896 residues after removal of the signal sequence. This protein has significant amino acid similarities with the N and C termini of the FnBPs of S. aureus (Fig. 2). The protein also has features characteristic of wall-associated proteins in the C terminus (LPXTG motif, hydrophobic region, positively charged residues) but lacks the extensive proline repeats of the FnBPs. Instead, ClfA has a remarkable dipeptide repeat comprising 154 alternating serine and aspartate residues. It is postulated that this is a novel structure for extending a protein through peptidoglycan and for exposing an adhesin on the bacterial cell surface. Experiments are under way to identify the fibrinogen-binding region by expressing recombinant truncated variants of ClfA and testing fibrinogen-binding activity in affinity blots and blocking activity in adherence experiments.

The availability of site-specific mutants defective in ClfA as well as derivatives carrying a complementing single copy of clfA has permitted the correlation of the clumping reaction with the ability of bacteria to adhere to plastic surfaces coated with fibrinogen (35). Indeed, all the evidence points to these phenotypes being specified by the same fibrinogen-binding determinant. The ClfA⁻ mutant was defective in adherence to coverslips coated in vitro with fibrinogen and to catheters that had been exposed for short periods (10 to 60 min) to canine blood in an arteriovenous shunt (10, 64). In this model, bacterial adherence is determined exclusively by fibrinogen-binding activity, while the presence of fibronectin binding does not contribute significantly. This suggests that fibrinogen is the most important determinant of adherence of S. aureus to newly implanted biomaterials.

ADHERENCE TO OTHER HOST MATRIX PROTEINS

S. aureus can bind specifically to several host tissue and matrix proteins other than fibronectin and fibrinogen described above, viz., collagen (20, 53), bone sialoprotein (48), vitronectin (41), laminin (4, 33), and elastin (65). Only the collagen adhesin associated with strains isolated from osteomyelitis and septic arthritis infections has been characterized at the molecular level (40, 55). A 135-kDa protein was purified from the cell surface, and the gene has been cloned and sequenced. The collagen receptor is strongly implicated in binding of bacteria to cartilage in the pathogenesis of septic arthritis.

The interaction of *S. aureus* with thrombospondin (18) may be of relevance to foreign body infections. Thrombospondin is the major platelet protein and is released from activated platelets that lodge on the surface of newly implanted biomaterial as part of the inflammatory response. Platelets are also directly implicated in catheter infections (17). Platelets bound to plastic surfaces promoted attachment of *S. aureus* cells. This process was enhanced by plasma and in particular by fibrinogen/fibrin, perhaps acting as a bridge between the immobilized platelet and the bacterial cell.

Another protein that could contribute to adherence to biomaterial is the recently described broad-specificity protein which interacts with fibrinogen, fibronectin, thrombospondin, vitronectin, and collagen in affinity (ligand) blotting experiments (21). In contrast to the FnBPs and ClfA, in which direct protein-protein interactions are involved, this protein probably recognizes carbohydrate residues on host glycoproteins.

SUMMARY AND FUTURE PROSPECTS

There is growing evidence that many of the biologically important interactions between staphylococci and host plasma and matrix proteins are conferred by protein adhesins exposed on the surface of the bacterial cell. However, until recent experiments with site-specific mutants, formal proof that these binding proteins were responsible for bacterial adherence to coated biomaterial surfaces was lacking. It now requires animal infection experiments to establish if these proteins are virulence factors and thus to fulfill molecular Koch's postulates (7).

One of the goals of research into staphylococcal adhesins is to investigate the possibility of intervening to prevent foreign body or wound infections. Agents that block bacterial adherence to biomaterial in vivo might be useful prophylactically in at-risk patients. Alternatively, a vaccine prepared from the capsular polysaccharide of *S. aureus* which stimulated the formation of opsonic antibodies (8) might be useful in combatting human nosocomial infection.

Acknowledgments. We thank Marilyn Lantz for permitting the use of the diagram of fibrinogen shown in Fig. 3.

Research performed in our laboratory is funded by the Wellcome Trust, London, U.K., and by the Health Research Board of Ireland.

REFERENCES

1. **Boden, M. K., and J.-I. Flock.** 1989. Fibrinogen-binding protein/clumping factor from *Staphylococcus aureus. Infect. Immun.* **57**:2358–2363.
2. **Bozzini, S., L. Visai, P. Pignatti, T. E. Petersen, and P. Speziale.** 1992. Multiple binding sites in fibronectin and the staphylococcal fibronectin receptor. *Eur. J. Biochem.* **207**:327–333.
3. **Chhatwal, G. S., G. Albohn, and H. Blobel.** 1987. Interaction between fibronectin and purified staphylococcal clumping factor. *FEMS Microbiol. Lett.* **44**:147–151.
4. **Chhatwal, G. S., K. T. Preissner, G. Muller-Berghaus, and H. Blobel.** 1987. Specific binding of the human S protein (vitronectin) to streptococci, *Staphylococcus aureus,* and *Escherichia coli. Infect. Immun.* **55**:1878–1883.
5. **Doolittle, R. F.** 1984. Fibrinogen and fibrin. *Annu. Rev. Biochem.* **53**:195–229.
6. **Duthie, E. S.** 1954. Evidence for two forms of staphylococcal coagulase. *J. Gen. Microbiol.* **10**:427–436.
7. **Falkow, S.** 1988. Molecular Koch's postulates applied to microbial pathogenicity. *Rev. Infect. Dis.* **10**:S274–S276.
8. **Fattom, A., J. Shiloach, D. Bryla, D. Fitzgerald, I. Pastan, W. W. Karakawa, J. B. Robbins, and R. Schneerson.** 1992. Comparative immunogenicity of conjugates composed of *Staphylococcus aureus* type 8 capsular polysaccharide bound to carrier proteins by adipic acid dihydrazide or N-succinimidyl-3-(2-pyridyldithio)propionate. *Infect. Immun.* **60**:584–589.
9. **Fischetti, V. A., V. Pancholi, and O. Schneewind.** 1990. Conservation of a hexapeptide sequence in the anchor region of surface proteins from gram-positive cocci. *Mol. Microbiol.* **4**:1603–1605.
10. **Francois, P., P. Vaudaux, C. Greene, D. McDevitt, and T. J. Foster.** Unpublished data.
11. **Froman, G., L. M. Switalski, P. Speziale, and M. Hook.** 1987. Isolation and characterization of a fibronectin receptor from *Staphylococcus aureus. J. Biol. Chem.* **262**:6564–6571.
12. **Hussain, M., M. H. Wilcox, and P. J. White.** 1993. The slime of coagulase-negative staphylococci: biochemistry and relation to adherence. *FEMS Microbiol. Rev.* **104**:191–208.
13. **Greene, C., D. McDevitt, and T. J. Foster.** Unpublished data.
14. **Greene, C., D. McDevitt, T. J. Foster, P. Francois, and P. Vaudaux.** Unpublished data.
15. **Hawiger, J., S. Timmons, D. D. Strong, B. A. Cottrell, B. A., M. Riley, and R. F. Doolittle.** 1982. Identification of a region of human fibrinogen interacting with staphylococcal clumping factor. *Biochemistry* **21**:1407–1413.
16. **Hemker, H. C., B. M. Bas, and A. D. Muller.** 1975. Activation of a proenzyme by stoichiometric reaction with another protein. The reaction between prothrombin and staphylocoagulase. *Biochim. Biophys. Acta* **379**:180–188.
17. **Herrmann, M., Q. J. Lai, R. M. Albrecht, D. F. Mosher, and R. A. Proctor.** 1992. Adhesion of *Staphylococcus aureus* to surface-bound platelets: role of fibrinogen/fibrin and platelet integrins. *J. Infect. Dis.* **167**:312–322.
18. **Herrmann, M., S. J. Suchard, L. A. Boxer, F. A. Waldvogel, and P. D. Lew.** 1991. Thrombospondin binds to *Staphylococcus aureus* and promotes staphylococcal adherence to surfaces. *Infect. Immun.* **59**:279–288.

19. **Herrmann, M., P. E. Vaudaux, D. Pittet, R. Auckenthaler, D. P. Lew, F. Schumacher-Perdreau, G. Peters, and F. A. Waldvogel.** 1988. Fibronectin, fibrinogen, and laminin act as mediators of adherence of clinical staphylococcal isolates to foreign material. *J. Infect. Dis.* **158:**693–701.

20. **Holderbaum, D., T. Spech, L. A. Ehrhart, T. Keys, and G. S. Hall.** 1987. Collagen binding in clinical isolates of *Staphylococcus aureus*. *J. Clin. Microbiol.* **25:**2258–2261.

21. **Homonylo McGavin, M., D. Krajewska-Pietrasik, C. Ryden, and M. Hook.** 1993. Identification of a *Staphylococcus aureus* extracellular matrix-binding protein with broad specificity. *Infect. Immun.* **61:**2479–2485.

22. **Huycke, M. M., J. M. Kuypers, and R. A. Proctor.** 1988. Characterization of a fibronectin (FN) binding exopolysaccharide from *Staphylococcus aureus*. *Clin. Res.* **36:**458A.

23. **Jonsson, K., C. Signas, H.-P. Muller, and M. Lindberg.** 1991. Two different genes encode fibronectin binding proteins in *Staphylococcus aureus*. The complete nucleotide sequence and characterization of the second gene. *Eur. J. Biochem.* **202:**1041–1048.

24. **Kawabata, S., T. Miyata, T. Morita, T. Miyata, S. Inagawa, and H. Igarashi.** 1986. The amino acid sequence of the procoagulant- and prothrombin-binding domain isolated from staphylocoagulase. *J. Biol. Chem.* **261:**527–531.

25. **Kawabata, S., T. Morita, S. Inagawa, and H. Igarashi.** 1985. Enzymatic properties of staphylothrombin, an active molecular complex fomed between staphylocoagulase and human prothrombin. *J. Biochem.* **98:**1603–1614.

26. **Kehoe, M. A.** 1994. Cell-wall-associated proteins in gram-positive bacteria, p. 217–261. *In* J.-M. Ghuysen and R. Hakenbeck (ed.), *New Comprehensive Biochemistry 1994. Bacterial Cell Wall.* Elsevier Science Publishing, Amsterdam.

27. **Kojima, Y., M. Tojo, D. A. Goldman, T. Tosteson, and G. B. Pier.** 1990. Antibody to the capsular polysaccharide/adhesin protects rabbits against catheter-related bacteremia due to coagulase-negative staphylococci. *J. Infect. Dis.* **162:**435–441.

28. **Kuusela, P.** 1978. Fibronectin binds to *Staphylococcus aureus. Nature* (London) **276:** 718–720.

29. **Kuusela, P., T. Varti, M. Vuento, and E. B. Myhre.** 1985. Attachment of staphylococci and streptococci on fibronectin, fibronectin fragments, and fibrinogen bound to a solid phase. *Infect. Immun.* **50:**77–81.

30. **Kuypers, J. M., and R. A. Proctor.** 1989. Reduced adherence to traumatized rat heart valves by a low-fibronectin-binding mutant of *Staphylococcus aureus. Infect. Immun.* **57:** 2306–2312.

31. **Lantz, M. S., R. D. Allen, P. Bounelis, L. M. Switalski, and M. Hook.** 1990. *Bacteroides gingivalis* and *Bacteroides intermedius* recognize different sites on human fibrinogen. *J. Bacteriol.* **172:**716–726.

32. **Lindgren, P.-E., M. J. McGavin, C. Signas, B. Guss, S. Gurusiddappa, M. Hook, and M. Lindberg.** 1993. Two different genes coding for fibronectin-binding proteins from *Streptococcus dysgalactiae.* The complete nucleotide sequences and characterization of the binding domains. *Eur. J. Biochem.* **214:**819–827.

33. **Lopes, J. D., M. dos Reis, and R. R. Brentani.** 1985. Presence of laminin receptors in *Staphylococcus aureus. Science* **229:**275–277.

34. **Mack, D., N. Siemssen, and R. Laufs.** 1992. Parallel induction by glucose of adherence and a polysaccharide antigen specific for plastic-adherent *Staphylococcus epidermidis:* evidence for functional relation to intercellular adhesion. *Infect. Immun.* **60:**2048–2057.

35. **McDevitt, D., P. Francois, P. Vaudaux, and T. J. Foster.** 1994. Molecular characterization of the fibrinogen receptor (clumping factor) of *Staphylococcus aureus. Mol. Microbiol.* **11:**237–248.

36. **McDevitt, D., P. Vaudaux, and T. J. Foster.** 1992. Genetic evidence that bound coagulase of *Staphylococcus aureus* is not clumping factor. *Infect. Immun.* **60:**1514–1523.

37. McGavin, M. J., S. Gurusiddappa, P. E. Lindgren, M. Lindberg, G. Raucci, and M. Hook. 1993. Fibronectin receptors from *Streptococcus dysgalactiae* and *Staphylococcus aureus*. Involvement of conserved residues in ligand binding. *J. Biol. Chem.* **268:** 23946–23953.

38. McGavin, M. J., G. Raucci, S. Gurusiddappa, and M. Hook. 1991. Fibronectin binding determinants of the *Staphylococcus aureus* fibronectin receptor. *J. Biol. Chem.* **266:** 8343–8347.

39. Muller, E., J. Hubner, N. Gutierrez, S. Takeda, D. A. Goldman, and G. B. Pier. 1993. Isolation and characterization of transposon mutants of *Staphylococcus epidermidis* deficient in capsular polysaccharide/adhesin and slime. *Infect. Immun.* **61:**551–558.

40. Patti, J. M., H. Jonsson, B. Guss, L. M. Switalski, K, Wiberg, M. Lindberg, and M. Hook. 1992. Molecular characterization and expression of a gene encoding *Staphylococcus aureus* collagen adhesin. *J. Biol. Chem.* **267:**4766–4772.

41. Paulsson, M., O. D. Liang, F. Ascencio, and T. Wadstrom. 1992. Vitronectin-binding surface proteins of *Staphylococcus aureus*. *Zentralbl. Bakteriol.* **277:**54–64.

42. Petersen, T. E., H. C. Thogersen, K. Skorstengaard, K. Vibe-Pedersen, P. Sahl, L. Sottrup-Jensen, and S. Magnusson. 1983. Partial primary structure of bovine plasma fibronectin: three types of internal homology. *Proc. Natl. Acad. Sci. USA* **80:**137–141.

43. Phonimdaeng, P., M. O'Reilly, P. Nowlan, A. J. Bramley, and T. J. Foster. 1990. The coagulase of *Staphylococcus aureus* 8325-4. Sequence analysis and virulence of site-specific coagulase-deficient mutants. *Mol. Microbiol.* **4:**393–404.

44. Proctor, R. A. 1987. Fibronectin: a brief overview of its structure, function and physiology. *Rev. Infect. Dis.* **9**(Suppl. 4):S317–S321.

45. Raja, R. H., G. Raucci, and M. Hook. 1990. Peptide analogs to a fibronectin receptor inhibit attachment of *Staphylococcus aureus* to fibronectin-coated substrates. *Infect. Immun.* **58:**2593–2598.

46. Rupp, M. E., and G. L. Archer. 1992. Hemagglutination and adherence to plastic by *Staphylococcus epidermidis*. *Infect. Immun.* **60:**4322–4327.

47. Ryden, C., K. Rubin, P. Speziale, M. Hook, M. Lindberg, and T. Wadstrom. 1982. Fibronectin receptors from *Staphylococcus aureus*. *J. Biol. Chem.* **258:**3396–3401.

48. Ryden, C., A. I. Yacoub, I. Maxe, D. Heinegard, A. Oldberg, A. Franzen, A. Ljungh, and K. Rubin. 1989. Specific binding of bone sialoprotein to *Staphylococcus aureus* isolated from patients with osteomyelitis. *Eur. J. Biochem.* **184:**331–336.

49. Schneewind, O., D. Mihaylova-Petkov, and P. Model. 1993. Cell wall sorting signals in surface proteins of gram-positive bacteria. *EMBO J.* **12:**4803–4811.

50. Schneewind, O., P. Model, and V. A. Fischetti. 1992. Sorting of protein A to the staphylococcal cell wall. *Cell* **70:**267–281.

51. Signas, C., G. Raucci, K. Jonsson, P.-E. Lindgren, G. M. Anantharamaiah, M. Hook, and M. Lindberg. 1989. Nucleotide sequence of the gene for a fibronectin-binding protein from *Staphylococcus aureus:* use of this peptide sequence in the synthesis of biologically active peptides. *Proc. Natl. Acad. Sci. USA* **86:**699–703.

52. Sottile, J., J. Schwarzbauer, J. Selegue, and D. F. Mosher. 1991. Five type I modules of fibronectin form a functional unit that binds to fibroblasts and to *Staphylococcus aureus*. *J. Biol. Chem.* **266:**12840–12843.

53. Speziale, P., G. Raucci, L. Visai, L. M. Switalski, R. Timpl, and M. Hook. 1986. Binding of collagen to *Staphylococcus aureus* Cowan 1. *J. Bacteriol.* **167:**77–81.

54. Strong, D. D., A. P. Laudano, J. Hawiger, and R. F. Doolittle. 1982. Isolation, characterization, and synthesis of peptides from human fibrinogen that block the staphylococcal clumping reaction and construction of a synthetic clumping particle. *Biochemistry* **21:**1414–1420.

55. Switalski, L. M., J. M. Patti, W. Butcher, A. G. Gristina, P. Speziale, and M. Hook. 1993. A collagen receptor on *Staphylococcus aureus* strains isolated from patients with septic arthritis mediates adhesion to cartilage. *Mol. Microbiol.* **7:**99–107.

56. Takeda, S., G. B. Pier, Y. Kojima, M. Tojo, E. Muller, T. Tosteson, and D. A. Goldman. 1991. Protection against endocarditis due to *Staphylococcus epidermidis* by immunization with capsular polysaccharide/adhesin. *Circulation* **84:**2539–2546.

57. Talay, S. R., P. Valentin-Weigand, P. G. Jerlstrom, K. N. Timmis, and G. S. Chhatwal. 1992. Fibronectin-binding protein of *Streptococcus pyogenes:* sequence of the binding domain involved in adherence of streptococci to epithelial cells. *Infect. Immun.* **60:** 3877–3844.

58. Timmerman, C. P., A. Fleer, J. M. Besnier, L. de Graaf, F. Cremers, and J. Verhoef. 1991. Characterization of a proteinaceous adhesin of *Staphylococcus epidermidis* which mediates attachment to polystyrene. *Infect. Immun.* **59:**4187–4192.

59. Usui, Y. 1986. Biochemical properties of fibrinogen binding protein (clumping factor) of the staphylococcal cell surface. *Zentralbl. Bakteriol. Hyg. A* **262:**287–297.

60. Valentin-Weigand, P., K. N. Timmis, and G. S. Chhatwal. 1993. Role of fibronectin in staphylococcal colonisation of fibrin thrombi and plastic surfaces. *J. Med. Microbiol.* **38:**90–95.

61. Vann, J. M., R. J. Hamill, R. M. Albrecht, D. F. Mosher, and R. A. Proctor. 1989. Immunoelectron microscopic localization of fibronectin in adherence of *Staphylococcus aureus* to cultured bovine endothelial cells. *J. Infect. Dis.* **160:**538–542.

62. Vaudaux, P., D. Pittet, A. Haeberli, E. Huggler, U. E. Nydegger, D. P. Lew, and F. A. Waldvogel. 1989. Host factors selectively increase staphylococcal adherence on inserted catheters: a role for fibronectin and fibrinogen or fibrin. *J. Infect. Dis.* **160:** 865–875.

63. Vaudaux, P., D. Pittet, A. Haeberli, P. G. Lerch, J.-J. Morgenthaler, R. A. Proctor, F. A. Waldvogel, and D. P. Lew. 1993. Fibronectin is more active than fibrin or fibrinogen in promoting *Staphylococcus aureus* adherence to inserted intravascular devices. *J. Infect. Dis.* **167:**633–641.

64. Vaudaux, P., R. A. Proctor, D. McDevitt, T. Foster, D. P. Lew, H. Wabers, and S. Cooper. 1991. Use of adherence-defective mutants of *Staphylococcus aureus* (SA) to identify adherence-promoting proteins deposited from perfusing blood in a canine shunt model. *Program Abstr. 31st Intersci. Conf. Antimicrob. Agents Chemother.,* abstr. 1068.

65. Woo Park, P., D. D. Roberts, L. E. Grosso, W. C. Parks, J. Rosenbloom, J., W. R. Abrams, and R. P. Mecham. 1991. Binding of elastin to *Staphylococcus aureus. J. Biol. Chem.* **266:**23399–23406.

Infections Associated with Indwelling Medical Devices, 2nd ed.
Edited by Alan L. Bisno and Francis A. Waldvogel
© 1994 American Society for Microbiology, Washington, DC 20005

Chapter 3

Colonization of Medical Devices by Coagulase-Negative Staphylococci

Gordon D. Christensen, Lucilla Baldassarri, and W. Andrew Simpson

PARADOX OF THE COAGULASE-NEGATIVE STAPHYLOCOCCI

The coagulase-negative staphylococci, particularly *Staphylococcus epidermidis*, cause more infections of medical devices than any other category of microorganisms. These gram-positive bacteria are the leading cause of infections of intravascular catheters (14, 77, 127), cerebrospinal fluid (CSF) shunts (56, 105), prosthetic valves (42, 57, 79, 94), orthopedic devices (49, 72, 74), artificial pacemakers (3, 17, 121), chronic ambulatory peritoneal dialysis (CAPD) catheters (5, 58, 100, 143), vascular grafts (8), and the total artificial heart (59).

This capacity to cause disease is surprising. Normally the coagulase-negative staphylococci (CoagNS) live in balanced harmony on our skin, forming the major component of the cutaneous microflora (80). Outside the setting of an infected medical device, these organisms virtually never

Gordon D. Christensen • Departments of Internal Medicine, Molecular Microbiology and Immunology, and Veterinary Microbiology, University of Missouri, and Harry S. Truman Memorial Veterans' Hospital, Research Service (151), 800 Hospital Drive, Columbia, Missouri 65201. **Lucilla Baldassarri** • Laboratorio di Ultrastrutture, Istituto Superiore di Sanitá, Viale Regina Elena 299, 00161 Rome, Italy. **W. Andrew Simpson** • Departments of Internal Medicine and Molecular Microbiology and Immunology, University of Missouri, and Harry S. Truman Memorial Veterans' Hospital, Research Service (151), 800 Hospital Drive, Columbia, Missouri 65201.

cause infections (91). In contrast, the coagulase-positive staphylococci (e.g., *Staphylococcus aureus*) are well known for their capacity to invade and infect healthy tissues, even though these organisms are also a common component of the cutaneous microflora. For many years, clinicians regarded the CoagNS as the prototypic avirulent microbe (91) while they viewed the coagulase-positive staphylococci as the prototypic bacterial pathogen. Only since the 1980s have physicians come to regard the isolation of CoagNS from sterile body sites as representing something more than a contaminated laboratory specimen (18, 91). Now they recognize that in the appropriate clinical setting, specifically when there is a possible infection of a medical device, the CoagNS can cause severe disease and even death (25, 91).

Considering the variety of materials used in constructing medical devices and the variety of anatomical locations selected for implanting them, it is difficult to understand why under almost all situations one particular group of avirulent organisms should emerge as the primary microorganism to cause medical device infections or, for that matter, why the number of medical device infections due to CoagNS should be so much greater than the number of infections caused by the more virulent coagulase-positive staphylococci (19, 27).

This pathologic paradox has been the subject of extensive investigation for more than a decade. An attractive explanation for this infectious tropism is the proposition that pathogenic strains of CoagNS have an unusual capacity to attach to and colonize medical devices. This proposition gained impetus from the discovery that many pathogenic strains of CoagNS colonize medical devices—or, more properly, "smooth" surfaces—in vitro by forming a tenacious bacterial film known as "slime." Although the production of slime is one likely explanation for this disease tropism, we now know that the colonization of medical devices in vivo is a complex multistep process. This chapter reviews our current understanding of mechanisms leading to the colonization of smooth surfaces by CoagNS.

FACTORS GOVERNING THE INITIAL ATTACHMENT OF CoagNS TO SURFACES

It is now evident that the colonization of inanimate surfaces by CoagNS, whether in vivo or in vitro, takes place through a series of sequential stages in which each stage in this process is dependent upon a different set of factors. We have diagrammed this sequence in Fig. 1 and demonstrated it in Fig. 2, which is a series of electron micrographs

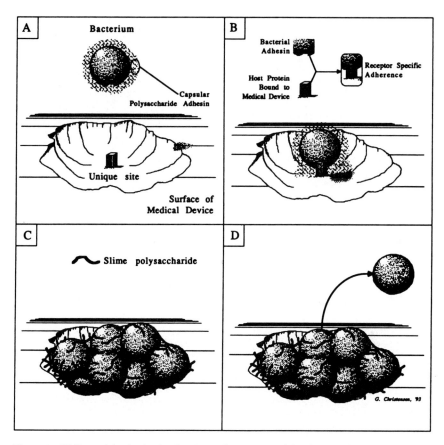

Figure 1. (A) Bacterial colonization begins with exposure of the device to bacteria. By virtue of mass effect, a certain proportion of the bacteria in the bathing solution will associate with the surface of the device. This association will always take place, even with surfaces that are designed to repel bacterial attachment. (B) Resulting bacterial attachment to the surface. This initial attachment is promoted by the unavoidable presence of "unique sites" on the surface of the device. These unique sites include local variations in surface hydrophobicity, surface irregularities (demonstrated in the three panels as a surface crater), and the presence of host proteins adsorbed onto the surface of the device. (C) The rare *S. epidermidis* cells that attach to the surface at unique sites can proceed to successfully colonize the surface by producing slime. The slime stabilizes the cell-to-cell and cell-to-surface associations, allowing the bacteria to accumulate on the medical device. (D) Final stage in surface colonization. By virtue of phase variation or phenotypic modulation, daughter cells that are not bound to the colony by slime emerge from the microcolony. These cells are then free to drift to new sites to repeat the colonization process.

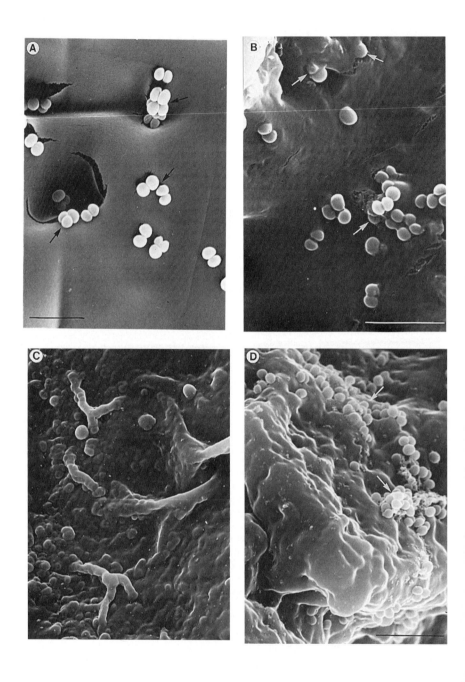

obtained by Olson, Ruseska, and Costerton portraying the colonization of n-butyl-2-cyanoacrylate (106).

The first stage of colonization, exposure, is almost an understatement but may actually be all-important in determining the spectrum of infecting microbes. As suggested by Maki (personal communication), the predominance of CoagNS over *S. aureus* in causing medical device infections could simply reflect opportunity, since the numerical density of CoagNS on the skin far exceeds that of *S. aureus* (80). Exposure is also an obvious explanation for finding clusters of medical device infections due to exceptionally virulent strains of bacteria carried on the skin (or mucous membranes) of health care workers (2). Exposure could also explain the atypical finding of a predominance of members of the family *Enterobacteriaceae* over CoagNS in causing infections of vascular grafts placed in the groin (8) as well as the observation that the spectrum of medical device pathogens in general parallels the spectrum of skin saprophytes.

According to the laws of mass action, following exposure to a suspension of microbial cells, some proportion of these cells will always come into contact with the medical device; the actual number of cells that come in contact with the device, however, is dependent upon the particular mix of forces acting upon the surfaces of both the device and the cells. While these forces may promote or discourage this initial contact, it should be remembered that given a high enough concentration of cells in suspension, some proportion of these cells will always come into contact with the surface.

The forces acting at this initial stage of colonization include active forces such as chemotaxis, passive forces such as gravity and the flow of fluids over the surface, and nonspecific forces resulting from the physicochemical characteristics of both the bacterial surface and the smooth

---

Figure 2. This series of microphotographs by Olson, Ruseska, and Costerton (106) (republished with permission of John Wiley & Sons, Inc. Copyright 1988, John Wiley & Sons.) illustrates the process diagrammed in Fig. 1. The microphotographs demonstrate the colonization of n-butyl-cyanoacrylate by a strain of *S. epidermidis* recovered from a patient with endocarditis. (A) After 2 h of exposure. The cells have collected in surface pits and have formed small microcolonies. (B) After 4 h of exposure. The surface texture of the plastic has noticeably changed, and the cells have developed "foot processes." These changes are due to condensation of a newly formed thin covering sheet of polysaccharide-rich extracellular material ("glycocalyx"). (C) After 8 h of exposure. The surface of the plastic is totally obscured by a thick mat of bacteria, known as "slime," which consists of individual cells buried in the amorphous extracellular material. (D) After 24 h of exposure. Nonadherent daughter cells, representing spontaneous phenotypic variants, have emerged from the slime and are now free to break away and drift to new colonization sites.

surface. These nonspecific forces include van der Waals' forces, electrostatic forces, surface tension, and surface hydrophobicity (reviewed in references 19 and 28). This stage of colonization is of prime interest to investigators because many of the forces that apply to the medical device can be modified by design engineering and material fabrication with the intent of minimizing attachment and, consequently, infection. For example, we now know that materials with rough surfaces are more likely to be colonized than those with smooth surfaces, because bacteria tend to collect in the microscopic pits as they flow over the surface (89).

Investigations into the physicochemical characteristics governing initial attachment have focused primarily upon understanding the bacterial surface, since this is the one variable not under control of the medical device engineers. The prominent factor at this stage appears to be bacterial surface hydrophobicity. Hogt and coworkers have convincingly demonstrated that hydrophobic CoagNS are more likely to colonize medical devices in vitro than hydrophilic strains (66, 107), a finding confirmed by other investigators (50) as well as our laboratory (125) (but not by all investigators [84]). Consistent with this observation was the recent analysis of a collection of clinical isolates by Martin and coworkers (97). These investigators reported that finding a strain with a high surface hydrophobicity was a reliable predictor of clinical pathogenicity.

Upon contact, bodily fluids immediately coat all surfaces, including medical devices, with a layer of host materials—primarily serum proteins and platelets—in a process known as surface conditioning. This layer of bound host materials, known as the biofilm, distinguishes the colonization of a medical device in vivo from colonization in vitro. Once bound to the surface, these host materials can serve as the "signal" or "target" for receptor-specific bacterial binding via an adhesin-mediated attachment (reviewed in references 19 and 28). As discussed in chapter 1, targeted binding to bound host proteins and platelets is a critical factor in the colonization of medical devices by S. aureus. For example, surface structures on S. aureus specifically recognize and bind fibronectin (51, 87). Fibronectin is adsorbed onto the conditioned surfaces of implanted foreign bodies (139), where it can serve as a specific target for the binding of S. aureus to the device (86, 99, 139, 140). Such fibronectin-specific binding has been demonstrated for both in vitro (123) and in vivo (137, 138) colonization of intravascular catheters by S. aureus. Surface deposits of fibrinogen and fibrin can also serve as specific targets for the attachment of S. aureus to smooth surfaces (86), including intravascular catheters (15, 137). Receptor-specific binding has also been observed for the host proteins collagen (67, 111, 132), vitronectin (16, 111), spreading factor (54), sialoprotein (124), laminin (90), and thrombospondin (65).

Serum proteins may also function as ligands to bind *S. aureus* to platelets deposited on a surface, such as an intravascular catheter (64).

Several investigators (123, 137) have demonstrated the attachment of CoagNS to intravascular catheters by a similar fibronectin-specific binding process; however, the binding avidity appears markedly less than that exhibited by *S. aureus*. In contrast, while using different experimental conditions, Pier's laboratory could not confirm that in vivo or in vitro coating of intravascular catheters with fibronectin enhanced the attachment of CoagNS to the device (102). Unlike *S. aureus*, the CoagNS do not bind fibrinogen (102, 137), and fibrinogen does not appear to be an immediate receptor for the attachment of CoagNS to surfaces (102, 137). Under more complex experimental conditions, Chugh and coworkers have reported that *S. epidermidis* does bind to fibrin-platelet clots via lipoteichoic acid (LTA) (32), and Wang and coworkers have found that platelets deposited on a hydrophobic plastic surface promote subsequent attachment of CoagNS (142). So far most studies examining the role of host proteins as specific surface receptors for the CoagNS have been inconclusive (reviewed in reference 27); however, this hypothesis continues to attract attention, such as the recently published report from Wadstrom's laboratory that demonstrated the interaction of CoagNS with a variety of host proteins including fibronectin, laminin, vitronectin, and collagen (110). Of concern is the perplexing but persistent observation that pretreatment of smooth surfaces with serum and plasma inhibits the attachment of most strains of CoagNS in vitro (50, 84, 102, 142), which further demonstrates the complexity of this issue.

Recently Timmerman and associates have reported a novel mechanism for the attachment of *S. epidermidis* to polystyrene (135). Using an immunogold label and electron microscopy, they were able to demonstrate proteinaceous pili-like structures that appeared to mediate the attachment of the test organism to polystyrene (135). Although pili are not usually associated with staphylococci, similar evidence of pili-mediated attachment of *Staphylococcus saprophyticus* (126) has also been reported. Pili-mediated attachment is usually due to a specific lectin incorporated into the pilus structure. Therefore it is possible that a lectin-based mechanism exists for *S. epidermidis* to attach to glycosylated proteins adsorbed onto the surface of intravascular catheters. This mechanism of adherence may be similar to the observations made by Rupp and Archer, who have found an association between intravascular catheter-associated sepsis and the binding of CoagNS to red blood cells (122). This binding could indicate the existence of a coagulase-negative staphylococcal surface lectin, perhaps even a pili-borne lectin, that recognizes a specific glycosylated protein adsorbed to the surface of the catheter, which is also on the surface of red blood cells (122).

Pier's laboratory has provided the most comprehensive description of an adhesin for the CoagNS. Beginning with the *S. epidermidis* sensu stricto strain RP62A (ATCC 35984), chosen because it was a strong producer of slime (21), they prepared bacterial extracts that were then used to pretreat silastic catheters. By concentrating upon the fractions that inhibited bacterial attachment within 2 h, they eventually identified and isolated a particular component that inhibited adherence (136). The material was extensively purified, including passage over a concanavalin A-Sepharose column to remove a mannan-rich contaminant (136); the purified product, referred to as "capsular polysaccharide/adhesin" (PS/A), was a large polysaccharide (>500,000 kDa) rich in galactose and glucosamine (136). In a rabbit model of intravascular catheter-induced endocarditis, active immunization with PS/A and passive immunization with polyclonal and monoclonal antibody to PS/A provided partial protection against endocarditis and bacteremia (81, 133).

Although PS/A was discovered in a search for the molecular identity of slime, PS/A and slime appear to be mutually independent phenomena. According to Pier's laboratory, only 57% of PS/A positive strains produce slime, while 17% of PS/A negative strains produce slime (103). The mechanism by which PS/A promotes colonization is not known. It appears that PS/A is important in mediating the initial attachment of CoagNS to surfaces, while the production of slime appears to be important in the subsequent accumulation of bacteria on surfaces (23).

The remainder of this chapter concerns the last stages of surface colonization, the accumulation of bacteria on a surface and the subsequent release of bacteria from the surface, which are stages dependent upon the production of slime.

ASSOCIATION OF SLIME PRODUCTION WITH CLINICAL INFECTIONS

In the early 1960s, the staphylococcal taxonomist Baird-Parker (6) parenthetically noted the production of "mucoid" material by many strains of CoagNS. In another publication, Jones and colleagues (76) specifically referred to this material as "slime" and associated its production with the presence of pyruvate in the media. It was not until a report by Bayston and Penny in 1972 (10) that any pathogenic significance was ascribed to slime. Bayston and Penny found that CoagNS isolated from children with cerebrospinal fluid shunt infections formed adherent "mucoid" deposits on the shunts in vitro (10), prompting them to speculate that this "mucoid" material was important to the pathogenesis of shunt infections (10). Unfortunately this perceptive report did not receive much attention for the next 10 years. Meanwhile, in the late 1970s and early 1980s, investigators worldwide began to recognize the CoagNS as increasingly common pathogens, particularly in the setting of nosocomial sepsis due to intravascular catheters (98, 118, 131).

Much of the work regarding slime was performed by investigators at the University of Tennessee (including authors of this chapter) who were among the first to report an increase in intravascular catheter associated sepsis due to CoagNS (25). In the course of conducting these clinical investigations, our group collected a large number of pathogenic and nonpathogenic strains of CoagNS from patients at the City of Memphis Hospital (26). In subsequent studies, this collection—which included the soon to be intensively studied strains RP12 (ATCC 35983), RP62A, and SP2 (ATCC 35982)—became a tool for exploring the pathogenesis of medical device infections. These investigations led to the recognition that in liquid media (particularly Trypticase soy broth), some of these strains of CoagNS covered the walls of the culture tube with a thick viscid layer of bacteria (29) referred to as "slime." (The unfortunate term "slime" was introduced by Jones and colleagues [76], who were the first to describe this phenomenon. This term also avoids confusion that might arise from the term "mucoid" material [used in the earlier parenthetical comment by Baird-Parker {6} and the later report by Bayston and Penny {10}], since mucoid material suggests both an animal origin and a specific chemical material, i.e., "mucopolysaccharide.")

We demonstrated the presence of slime by a simple procedure known as the tube test, which consisted of emptying the contents of the culture tube and staining the residual adherent film of bacteria (Fig. 3). Applying this test to our collection of CoagNS, we found that 63% of the pathogenic strains produced slime, and only 37% of the nonpathogenic strains produced slime ($P < 0.05$) (25, 29). In later studies we upgraded this qualitative test into a quantitative assay (known as the plate test) by substituting microtiter wells for culture tubes and by measuring the optical density of the stained adherent bacterial film with an automatic spectrophotometer (31) (Fig. 3). With this quantitative assay, strains associated with intravascular catheter sepsis produced significantly thicker bacterial films than blood culture contaminants ($P < 0.01$) or skin strains ($P < 0.05$) (31). Similar observations were made by our group in collaboration with Younger and Barrett in a pediatric population with infected cerebrospinal fluid (CSF) shunts (31, 144) and in collaboration with Baddour in an adult population with infected chronic ambulatory peritoneal

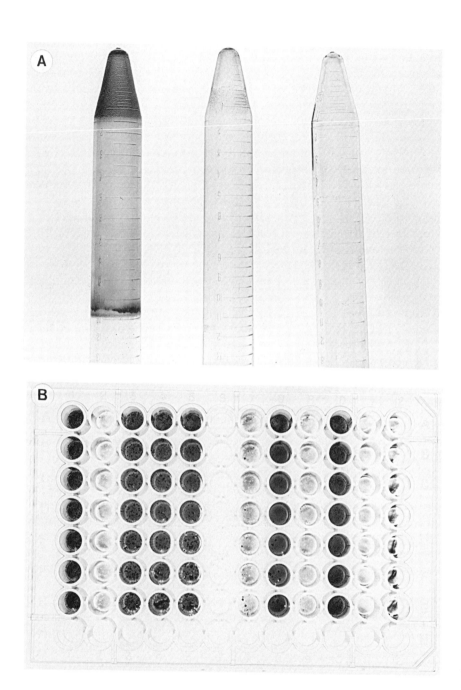

Table 1. Association of slime production with pathogenic strains of CoagNS

Investigator (reference)	% of bacteria producing slime[a]		P	Assay	Clinical collection
	Pathogens	Contaminant			
Memphis group					
Christensen (29)	63	37	<0.05	Tube test	Bacteremia
Christensen (31)	(0.602)	(0.295)	<0.01	Plate test	Repeat of (29)
Younger (144)	88	61	<0.01	Plate test	CSF shunt
Baddour (5)	(0.627)	(0.320)	<0.025	Plate test	CAPD catheter
Ishak (73)	93	23	0.0003	Tube test	Bacteremia
Martin (97)	77	56	0.036	Tube test	Bacteremia
Fidalgo (48)	77	43	<0.01	Tube test	Bacteremia
Kotilainen (82)	53	29	<0.001	Tube test	Septicemia
Hall (63)	75	58	0.027	Tube test	Bacteremia
Davenport (33)	79	54	0.003	Tube test	Miscellaneous
Dunne (44)	47	18	0.014	Tube test	Miscellaneous
Deighton (34)	Not noted	Not noted	<0.005	Plate test	Miscellaneous
Beaman (11)	89	29	Not done	Tube test	CAPD catheter
Kaebnick (78)	87	33	<0.01	Tube test	Vascular graft
Dobbins (41)	100	Not done	Not done	Tube test	Orthopedic

[a] The numbers in parentheses refer to the optical density of the adherent bacterial film when the assay was performed by the microtiter plate method.

dialysis (CAPD) catheters (5). Subsequently, a variety of independent investigators worldwide have performed analogous studies, which are summarized in Table 1. The recurrent finding by all of these groups is the repetitive epidemiologic association between slime production and CoagNS isolated from medical device infections.

Table 1 includes a particularly noteworthy study by Dobbins and colleagues (41) in which they found that 75% of electively explanted

Figure 3. (A) Tube test. On the left is a positive tube, on the right is a negative tube, and in the middle is an indeterminate result. (From reference 29, with permission.) (B) Plate test. Individual microtiter plate wells are covered with a bacterial film. The optical density of the film (read in an automatic spectrophotometer) is an index of the thickness of the bacterial film or "slime production." (From reference 31, with permission.)

orthopedic appliances were asymptomatically colonized with gram-positive coccoid bacteria. Not all of these organisms were viable, but with the exception of one diphtheroid isolate, all of the strains that could be propagated proved to be slime-producing CoagNS. Additional noncomparative clinical studies that support the association between slime production and clinical virulence included those of Skoutelis and coworkers (129), who reported 83% of intravascular catheter pathogens produced slime; Ponce de Leon and coworkers (117), who reported 66% of bacteremic isolates produced slime; Righter (120), who reported that 72% of septicemic strains of CoagNS arising from vascular access sites produced slime (while only 41% of all septicemia strains produced slime); and Etienne and coworkers (45), who reported 53% of endocarditis strains produced slime.

Slime production may have therapeutic implications. In separate clinical studies, both Younger et al. (144) and Davenport et al. (33) observed a link between the production of slime and the persistence of infection. In patients with CSF shunt infections, Diaz-Mitoma and coworkers (40) also found a significant ($P < 0.025$) association between antibiotic failure and slime production. Likewise, in patients with CAPD peritonitis, Deighton and colleagues observed an association between therapeutic failure and slime ($P < 0.003$) (36), as did Kristinsson and colleagues ($P = 0.02$) (85) and Beaman and colleagues (11).

The reader should know, however, that in a few cases investigators have not found an epidemiologic association between the production of slime and the production of disease by pathogenic isolates of CoagNS. For example, neither Diaz-Mitoma et al. (40) nor Kristinsson et al. (85) were able to demonstrate a simple epidemiologic association between clinical isolates of CoagNS and the production of slime (nevertheless, as already mentioned both of these groups found an association between slime and persistence of infection). For reasons that are not clear, the literature concerning CAPD isolates is particularly confusing. West and coworkers, for example, could not find an association between slime production by CAPD isolates and clinical complications, but they did find that 83% of the peritonitis strains produced slime (143) (there was no comparison group for calculating the significance of this observation). Using a small collection of 14 CAPD pathogens and both the tube test and a quantitative assay, Alexander and Rimland (1) failed to show any association between virulence and slime, but this failure may simply have been due to the small size of the study. In an informal report, Freeman and Falkiner (53) also failed to find a link between slime production and CAPD isolates; however, like previously quoted studies, they found an association ($P < 0.05$) between the production of slime and severity of infection (53). As far as we know, only the studies by Needham and Stempsey (104) (miscellaneous pathogens), Alexander and Rimland (1) (CAPD), and Beard-Pegler and coworkers (12) (CAPD) have failed to find any statistical association between disease and the production of slime by infecting strains of CoagNS.

A major problem in interpreting this literature is that there are no standard assays for measuring slime production, yet technical factors greatly influence the observed presence of slime. The formation of slime is dependent upon environmental factors such as the medium (29, 34, 69, 71, 93), the presence of carbohydrates (29, 34, 69, 76) or iron (35), CO_2 content (39, 71), and oxygenation (9). The tube test is variable (31, 34) and highly subjective (31), and it produces different results from the plate test (9, 31, 34). The demonstration of slime depends upon both the fixative (7) and the age of the culture (7). The importance of these technical concerns was nicely demonstrated by Deighton et al. While using the tube test in an early 1988 study (37) and in a later 1990 study (34), they failed to find an epidemiologic association between slime production and clinical isolates of CoagNS. When Deighton and Balkau applied the quantitative plate test to the 1990 collection, however, they successfully found this association (34).

The most noteworthy technical problem is that for at least some—if not all—strains of CoagNS, the production of slime is subject to phase variation (20, 21, 38) (Fig. 4). This means that slime production is a heterogeneous phenomenon in which there is unequal expression of slime by individual daughter cells from the same strain. As a consequence, the clinical detection of slime can vary from isolate to isolate of an infecting strain of CoagNS (38). The actual incidence of slime-producing cells in a slime-positive culture may be quite low; in the laboratory, we have demonstrated that as few as 1 slime-producing cell per 16,000 slime-nonproducing cells results in a culture that will grossly produce slime (20). Finally, because they are adhesive, slime-positive daughter cells may be difficult to recover from an infected device (41), whereas the nonadherent slime-negative daughter cells may be easily recovered. For these reasons, at the present time we cannot conclude that the failure to detect slime in vitro necessarily rules out either the in vivo or in vitro production of slime.

These problems have not dampened investigators' enthusiasm for this line of research because they can see slime—or what appears to be slime—on infected medical devices. When intravascular catheters (14, 52, 96, 108, 113, 119, 134) and cardiac pacemakers (95, 115) infected with CoagNS are removed from patients and examined with a scanning electron microscope, the devices are universally found to be colonized

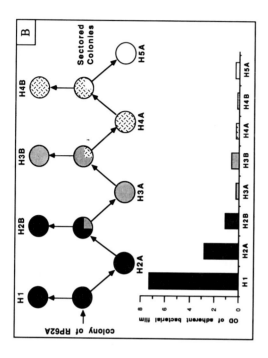

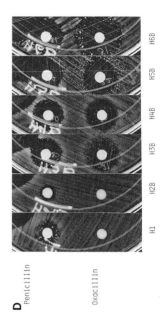

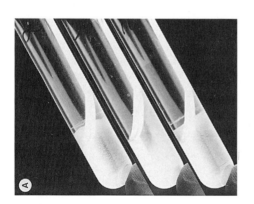

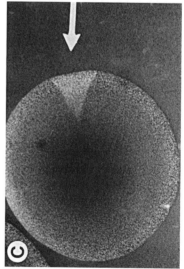

with a layer of bacteria embedded in an unknown amorphous extracellular material. The microscopic appearance of these in vivo colonized devices is identical to the appearance of intravascular catheters (29, 49, 89, 114) and cardiac pacemakers (115) colonized by CoagNS in vitro (Fig. 5). To be sure, the two phenomena cannot be identical, since the laboratory-colonized devices do not include host-derived materials; we do not even know the chemical composition and derivation of either the in vivo or in vitro material that forms the bacterial film. Nevertheless, considering the many clinical reports of an association between slime production and pathogenic strains of CoagNS as well as the similarity in appearance between the in vivo and in vitro colonized devices, one can make a persuasive argument that slime production is a critical factor in the pathogenesis of medical device infections.

Persuasive is not conclusive. Slime production has neither been conclusively demonstrated to be a virulence factor nor even been defined

---

Figure 4. (A) The three test tubes demonstrate phase variation of slime production. The top tube contained a broth culture of the slime-producing strain RP62A; the adherent bacterial film ("slime") was revealed by tipping the broth away from the walls of the tube. The middle tube contained a broth culture of a variant strain, RP62A-NA, which was directly derived from RP62A. This strain has lost the capacity to produce slime, which was evident from the diffuse growth of bacteria in the broth and the clean walls when the tube was tipped. The bottom tube contained a broth culture of the variant strain, RP62A-NAR, which was directly derived from the variant RP62A-NA. RP62A-NAR has recovered the capacity to produce slime, which was evident by tipping the tube. (From reference 21, with permission.) Panels B and D summarize the key experiments demonstrating phase variation of slime production and the associated change in β-lactam resistance. (B) The change in slime production is shown as we selected a sequential series of "sectored" colonies of RP62A on Memphis agar. A sector is a pie-shaped section of the colony with a color that is different from the rest of the colony, illustrated in this diagram as different shades of grey (panel C). Sectors signal the spontaneous emergence of new bacterial phenotypes. The top of panel B illustrates the selection process in which a sectored colony was first identified, followed by isolating the new phenotype, and then repeated by screening the new phenotype for even newer forms. Beginning with H1, a specific colony of RP62A, the serially selected phenotypes were identified as H2A and -B, H3A and -B, H4A and -B, and H5A. The bottom of panel B is a graph of the slime production by each clone, demonstrating that slime production was lost as the colonies were serially selected. (From reference 22, with permission.) The process was determined to be fully reversible; new clones emerged at a rate of 1.1×10^{-5} (20). (D) The simultaneous change in susceptibility to β-lactam antibiotics as the colonial variants of RP62A were selected in panel B. (From reference 20, with permission.) This experiment demonstrated linkage between the colonial morphology, slime production, and susceptibility to β-lactam antibiotics. In later experiments, virulence in two different animal models of medical device infection (20, 24) was also found to vary between the different clones, suggesting that for RP62A, multiple factors were subject to global regulation. The authors' suggestion as to how this might occur are diagrammed in Fig. 6.

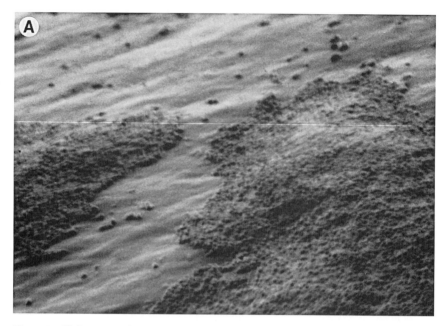

Figure 5. (A) Scanning electron micrograph of an intravascular catheter incubated in vitro with a slime-producing strain (RP12) of *S. epidermidis*. The microphotograph shows the surface of the device with accreted microcolonies of staphylococci. (From reference 29, with permission.) (B) Transmission electron micrograph of the same strain in panel A, RP12, showing a highly organized thick layer of extracellular material covering the bacterial cell. The extracellular material stains with Alcian blue, indicating that the material is a polysaccharide.

in terms of composition and function. There is ample evidence for the role of other factors in pathogenesis, and slime production may only be a marker of virulence rather than a virulence factor per se. Continuing studies have focused upon demonstrating the pathogenic importance of slime in animal models of infection, purification and analysis of slime, and determination of the role of slime in microbial pathogenesis.

ASSOCIATION OF SLIME PRODUCTION WITH DISEASE IN ANIMAL MODELS OF INFECTION

Our laboratory performed the first animal experiments to examine the role of slime in medical device infections. We inserted short sections of intravascular catheters under the skin of mice, injected the implanted catheters with either a slime-positive (RP12) or -negative (SP2) strain of

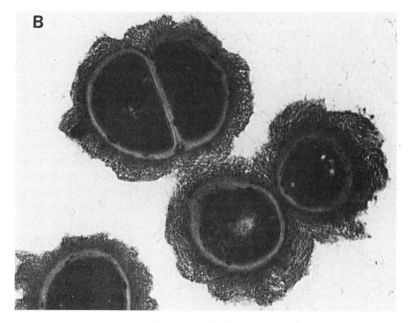

Figure 5. *Continued.*

CoagNS, and followed after a period of time by sacrificing the animals and counting the frequency of infected catheters (30). These experiments confirmed the clinical observation that a foreign body was a necessary prerequisite for CoagNS virulence (30). Since RP12 proved more virulent than SP2, the findings also supported the proposed pathogenic role of slime production; however, in follow-up collaborative studies with Baddour, using a rat model of intravascular catheter-associated endocarditis (4), we found this conclusion to be in error. The problem was that we had compared the virulence of unrelated strains of bacteria, which at a later date we found to be different species of staphylococci (RP12 was an *S. epidermidis* ss strain, while SP2 was a *Staphylococcus hominis* strain). In subsequent work with the endocarditis model, we discovered that this species assignment was an overriding factor in comparisons of virulence between unrelated strains of CoagNS. This observation has been confirmed by other investigators in both clinical studies (40, 97) and in animal models of infection (61, 88). In follow-up studies we tried to overcome this problem (with inconclusive results) by comparing mutants and phase variants of a single strain of *S. epidermidis* ss (20, 21, 24).

For similar reasons, Patrick and coworkers have also had problems demonstrating the pathogenic role of slime. Comparing the virulence of a small number of unrelated strains in the mouse foreign body infection model, these investigators failed to find a correlation between slime and virulence (109). They did note, however, that slime production increased the density of bacteria on the surface of the infected catheters (109). Gunn reported the best experimental evidence in support of a pathogenic role of slime when he compared the virulence of unrelated strains in an infant mouse weight-retardation model. The large number of strains used in this study allowed Gunn to reliably correlate virulence with slime production despite the limitation of comparing unrelated bacteria (61). Using the electron microscope (but without controls), Lambe and co-workers (88) and Gallimore and coworkers (55) reported visual data supporting the role of slime in experimental foreign body infections by CoagNS. In a variation of the mouse foreign body infection model, Lambe found that all infected catheters were coated with a biofilm, which these authors referred to as the glycocalyx (88). With a mouse model of intraperitoneal catheter infection, Gallimore found the bacteria bound to the catheters in a biofilm while the corresponding peritoneal fluid was sterile (55).

Recent observations have raised questions regarding the interpretation of animal experiments as well as clinical studies concerning slime production. Until now, investigators have understandably assumed a cause-and-effect relationship when correlating a laboratory-observed phenotype (i.e., slime production) with virulence. In the case of *S. epidermidis*, however, such a relationship does not necessarily exist. For example, using the slime-producing strain RP62A, we isolated a slime-negative variant that was found to be avirulent in both the mouse model of foreign body infection (24) and the rat model of catheter-induced endocarditis (20). Although these findings appeared to prove the proposition that slime is a virulence factor, they were only consistent with this hypothesis. The weakness in these types of studies stems from the observation that the phase variant was a pleiotropic variant. In other words, the variant demonstrated changes in multiple phenotypic features; specifically, for RP62A, the expression of slime (and virulence) was correlated with the expression of β-lactam resistance (20, 24). Since at least two and perhaps multiple factors were subject to simultaneous change, it was possible that slime expression was linked to additional unrecognized and unknown virulence factors that were the actual determinants of pathogenicity. Such a system of pleiotropic phase variation of virulence factors has been described for *Bordetella pertussis* (discussed in reference 22); a similar system could exist for some strains of *S. epidermidis* (discussed in reference 22), since multiple virulence factors for *S. aureus* are known to be under coordinate control of a central regulatory gene such as *agr* (112) and *xpr* (130).

While the phenomenon of phase variation casts doubts on experiments demonstrating that slime is a virulence factor, recent observations regarding the related phenomenon of phenotypic modulation cast doubts on studies demonstrating that slime is not a virulence factor. Phenotypic modulation is another aspect of the *B. pertussis* model; in this case, the expression of certain phenotypic features is directly responsive to the microenvironment. (The distinction between phase variation and phenotypic modulation, as well as how these phenomena apply to *B. pertussis* and possibly *S. epidermidis*, is outlined in Fig. 6.) Deighton and Borland have recently discovered that the expression of slime is directly dependent upon the concentration of iron in the environment through a mechanism that appears to be identical to phenotypic modulation (35). These workers went on to propose that because of phenotypic modulation, the finding that a particular strain does not produce slime in vitro does not necessarily predict the production of slime in vivo. Phase variation and phenotypic modulation could explain the discordance between the microscopic observation that all infected medical devices are coated with a slimy layer of bacteria and the observation that many macroscopic infecting strains of CoagNS fail to produce slime in vitro.

PURIFICATION OF SLIME

Extracellular polysaccharides, such as the alginate of *Pseudomonas aeruginosa* and the mutans and fructans of *Streptococcus mutans*, mediate the attachment of these organisms to smooth surfaces in a bacterial layer morphologically identical to the slime of CoagNS. Like that of *P. aeruginosa* and *S. mutans*, several lines of evidence suggest that the essential matrix material of these structures is a polysaccharide. By transmission electron microscopy we have observed that slime-producing strains, specifically strains RP12 (29) (Fig. 5) and RP62A (21), were encased in an extracellular layer of material that stained with the polysaccharide-specific stain Alcian blue. The polysaccharide nature of this material was further evident from the selective destruction of slime by periodation (29, 93). Since then investigators have taken three paths to further isolate and identify the putative slime polysaccharide.

The most direct way to isolate slime is to simply extract polysaccharides from a slime-producing strain of CoagNS with the hope that the slime polysaccharide will be self-evident by its abundant presence in the extracts. This direct approach was the method chosen by Peters'

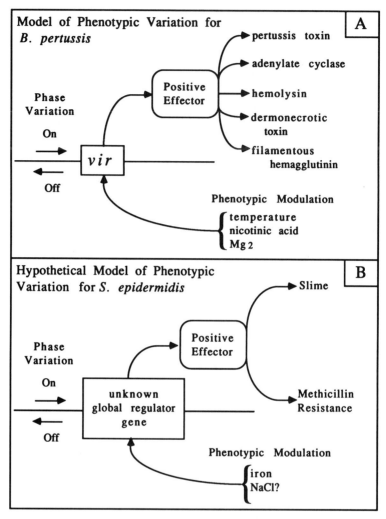

Figure 6. This figure diagrams the authors' hypothesis regarding the global regulation of the expression of slime for *S. epidermidis*. (Adapted from reference 24, with permission.) (A) The hypothesis is modeled on *B. pertussis*. For *B. pertussis*, a global regulator, the *vir* gene, controls the expression of a series of virulence factors and at least one adherence factor. *vir* is subject to two control mechanisms, a switching on and off through a spontaneous rearrangement of the chromosome (phase variation) at a rate of 10^{-6} and a direct induction in which *vir* is activated by specific environmental signals (phenotypic modulation). Accordingly, a phenotype may be expressed under permissive environmental conditions but not under restrictive conditions (phenotypic modulation) and also exist as a heterogeneous culture in which the majority of cells are in one phenotype but a minority have been switched to an alternate phenotype (phase variation) (discussed in reference

laboratory (Cologne), who were the first to try purifying slime (92, 116). By harvesting the KH11 organism from N-agar plates submerged in saline and disrupting the cells by sonication, these investigators obtained crude preparations of "extracellular slime substance" (ESS) (92). The crude material was further purified by passing the product over an anion-exchange column and extracting with increasing concentrations of salt. Peters identified the first two peaks of this extract, which were mannose and galactose rich, reacted with concanavalin A, and (by precoating polyethylene) inhibited early adherence, as the slime polysaccharide (92). Kotilainen and coworkers followed Peters' procedures and obtained a galactose/mannose/glucose-rich product from their strain, TU9711 (83). Immune serum developed in rabbits against the Kotilainen extract reacted with surface antigens on CoagNS; however, Western blots (immunoblots) did not detect any differences between slime-positive and slime-negative strains. With Peters' ESS preparations, Johnson et al. (75) have inhibited phagocytosis, Bykowska et al. have inhibited clotting (13), and Farber et al. have inhibited bacterial killing with vancomycin (47). Despite these accomplishments, the relationship of slime to ESS is uncertain. ESS preparations are only partially purified and contain both polysaccharides and proteins. Many ESS-producing organisms, including KH11, do not produce slime in laboratory cultures (20, 68, 116). Most importantly, both Drewry et al. (43) and Hussain et al. (70) have found that when ESS is prepared from agar-harvested bacteria—such as the preparations used by Peters and Kotilainen—the predominant component, a galactose-rich material, is really derived from the agar itself.

Drewry and coworkers have also tried the direct approach but failed to recover a convincing product from strain RP12 (43). Likewise, the direct approach was used by Hussain and coworkers (70), who avoided media contamination by harvesting RP62A and RP12 from synthetic media (69), disrupting the organisms by sonication, passing the material over a sizing column, collecting the void volume, and then passing the product over an anion-exchange column. The resulting extract from RP62A was glucose and glucosamine rich, while RP12 was glucose poor and glucosamine rich. Uronic acids were recovered from both prepara-

---

24). (B) The authors propose a similar system for RP62A in which both slime production and β-lactam resistance are subject to global regulation. Other unknown factors, including modulators of virulence and colonial morphology, may also be regulated with slime and β-lactam resistance. The authors' work (20) indicates that these factors are subject to phase variation at a rate of 1.1×10^{-5}; Deighton and Borland (35) have reported that these factors are also responsive to the presence of iron in the microenvironment, suggesting they might also be responsive to phenotypic modulation.

tions, and both preparations included high concentrations of protein, glycerol phosphate, and phosphorus, suggesting significant copurification of bacterial proteins and lipoteichoic acid (LTA) (70).

The second approach to the identification of the putative slime polysaccharide is to identify the material by functional analysis. As already described, this is the approach chosen by Pier and coworkers, who precoated silastic with bacterial extracts to prevent colonization, an approach that eventually led to the identification and purification of PS/A (136). Initially the Boston group believed they had discovered the slime polysaccharide, and there is still confusion on this point. Since the expression of this material does not correlate with the expression of slime (103), it would appear that the two phenomena are distinct. On the other hand, Muller and Pier have simultaneously interrupted the expression of slime and PS/A by insertion of a single transposon into the bacterial chromosome (101). This achievement is consistent with the two phenomena being identical, or it could mean that Muller and Pier simply interrupted a common regulatory gene or a key physiologic function required for both products.

The third approach, the one chosen by us, first required the creation of a slime-negative strain from a slime-positive strain; then all that was required was to compare the bacterial products of the two strains and identify the missing (and presumably slimy) materials. The most direct approach to this problem would have been single-point mutation of the chromosome, such as the mutations created by transposon-mediated mutagenesis. Until recently (101), however, such genetic systems for the CoagNS did not exist. Therefore, we sidestepped this limitation by searching for spontaneous mutants of RP62A that had lost the capacity to produce slime, discovering in the process that the production of slime was subject to reversible pleiotropic phase variation at a rate of 1×10^{-5}/ cell/generation (20). The rapid emergence and pleiotropic nature of the phase variants raised questions regarding the validity of any conclusions based entirely upon phase variants. Therefore, we produced a second set of strains, using the mutagen acriflavine to create chemical mutants of RP62A that no longer produced slime (9). Antigenic comparison of the lysozyme/lysostaphin crude extracts of the slime-producing parent against the derivative slime-nonproducing phase variant and chemical mutant allowed us to identify a particular antigen, the slime-associated antigen (SAA), which was only expressed by slime-producing strains of CoagNS (23). SAA is immunologically distinct from PS/A (23), has a high molecular weight (>100,000) (23), and resists heat and protease treatment (23) but is sensitive to periodation (unpublished observations of the authors). These findings demonstrate that SAA is a polysaccharide; therefore, we were not surprised that our initial chemical analysis found SAA to be 60% glucose (23). Since then we have learned that our initial findings were in error because of lysostaphin-mediated breakdown of the sizing column (unpublished observations of the authors). In subsequent preparations, using bacteria harvested from the synthetic media of Hussain and coworkers (69), we have found SAA to be glucose poor but rich in N-acetyl-glucosamine along with unidentified saccharides (unpublished observations of the authors), suggesting that this material may be similar to the slime extracts prepared by Hussain and coworkers (69).

PATHOGENIC FUNCTION OF SLIME PRODUCTION

Because of the conspicuous appearance of slime on electron micrographs and in laboratory culture, our presumption throughout the preceding discussion was that the pathogenic function of slime is to promote the colonization of medical devices. Kinetic studies of bacterial colonization suggest that this "cementing" role of slime is primarily important in the late stages of bacterial colonization, when the bacteria accumulate on the surface (23). On the basis of what we know about other systems, it appears likely that slime mediates this colonization by binding bacterial cells to cells, either through nonspecific mechanisms or possibly even through the binding of a bacterial lectin to a slime saccharide.

We have already noted that slime is one factor among many that promotes the colonization of smooth surfaces by CoagNS. The initial attachment of bacteria to the surface is dependent upon a variety of factors such as surface smoothness, hydrophobicity, PS/A, and the availability of bacterial adhesins to bind to targeted host proteins and platelets on the surface. Although these initial attachment factors clearly promote bacterial colonization, it is not necessarily true that the absence of these factors will prevent bacterial colonization; promoting bacterial colonization despite the absence of other colonization factors may be the true role of slime production in pathogenesis. For example, recalling that free-floating bacteria will always associate to some degree with any surface, one can visualize how if only a few organisms attach to the surface, these pioneering bacteria may be sufficient to colonize the surface of the device by multiplying in situ, creating a microcolony. Slime production could promote this colony formation by providing the structural integrity and positional stability of bacterial cells in the microcolony. Thus, slime-producing CoagNS could convert the inhospitable surface of a medical device into a receptive surface of a bacterial colony. This process is beautifully demonstrated by electron microscopy studies of in vitro colonization of n-butyl-2-cyanoacrylate by Olson, Ruseska, and Costerton (106) (Fig. 2). The appeal of this proposition is that it explains the capacity of slime-producing CoagNS to infect devices fabricated from a variety of materials, in a variety of settings.

The conspicuous appearance of slime has also suggested several alternative pathogenic mechanisms, which have been explored by different investigators. For example, slime could function as a capsule and impede phagocytosis by impairing opsonization, phagocytic engulfment (75, 141), or immune recognition. Slime could also promote antimicrobial resistance, directly by blocking the penetration of antibiotics into the bacterial cell or indirectly by maintaining the bacterial cell in an inactive resting state (46, 60, 128). Because these studies relied upon crude preparations of slime with suspect composition, only limited conclusions can be made regarding these possible functions; confirmation will require pure preparations of slime and strains with single point mutations of slime production.

RELEASE FROM THE SURFACE

It is axiomatic that in order to spread through an environment, all sessile life forms must have a stage in their life cycle when they are mobile. This principle applies to bacteria as well as to trees and barnacles. In all well-described bacterial adherence systems, as for example the pili-mediated adherence of *Escherichia coli* and *Neisseria gonorrhoeae* (reviewed in reference 28), a mechanism exists for the organisms to either display or not display the adherence factor. For both *E. coli* and *N. gonorrhoeae*, the expression of pili is turned on and off through a genetic mechanism of phase variation (reviewed in reference 28). Likewise, it now appears that for at least some CoagNS, the expression of slime production is turned on and off by both a genetic mechanism of phase variation and by environmental conditions, through a mechanism of phenotypic modulation.

We can now visualize the final stage of surface colonization by CoagNS. Following the establishment of a slime layer, nonadherent daughter cells escape from the slime layer either by switching off slime production or by exhaustion of the environmental conditions that support slime production. These nonadherent forms are then free to drift to new colonization sites to repeat the colonization process (see Fig. 1D).

CONCLUSION AND FUTURE DIRECTIONS

This leads us to the final question of this review. Because indwelling medical devices are of recent origin, how did the CoagNS evolve the necessary virulence factors to specifically infect these appliances? Several hypotheses can be constructed. It is conceivable that even though indwelling medical devices are of modern origin, there may have been sufficient time and patient exposure in hospitals for the evolution of a truly new pathogen. However, this seems unlikely, particularly considering that the CoagNS were noted to produce slime long before they became major nosocomial pathogens. It is more likely that the CoagNS were preadapted to exploit the microenvironment of indwelling medical devices. There are several possible sources for this preadaptation, but the possibilities are only speculative. Since the CoagNS normally reside on the skin, slime production and other adherence mechanisms could help the organism avoid desiccation and attach itself to the surface of the skin and hair. Likewise, smooth-surface adherence mechanisms could promote the transference of skin bacteria to tools and other objects and thereby promote bacterial dissemination by handling these materials. The most likely explanation for the existence of smooth-surface adherence mechanisms, however, lies outside of human experience. In addition to inhabiting the human skin, the CoagNS may also be marine organisms (62). This is important because the phenomenon of slime formation is a well-known attribute of marine organisms, which allows them to colonize the rocks and rubble of rivers, oceans, and lakes (reviewed in reference 28). Accordingly, the association of indwelling medical devices with slime-producing CoagNS may simply be a natural accident in which CoagNS mistake the microenvironment of the indwelling medical device for their natural habitat.

Although many questions persist regarding the true pathologic significance of slime production as well as other mechanisms that lead to the colonization of medical devices, significant progress has taken place in this field since the first edition of this book. With the recognition of phase variation, we can now explain some confusing aspects of the clinical microbiology of these organisms. Because of progress in this field, it is likely that in the near future, new material surfaces will be engineered that discourage colonization by staphylococci. Finally, with the purification of slime polysaccharides, experimental models utilizing these materials to monitor immune response and vaccinate animals have already been introduced for PS/A and are not far behind for SAA. It is likely that the near future will see these materials adapted to human medicine for badly needed new diagnostics and perhaps even protective vaccines.

Acknowledgments. We thank J. W. Costerton for his thoughtful review of this manuscript.

The laboratory investigations conducted by the authors were supported by the U.S. Department of Veterans Affairs and by the Italian National Research Council, Targeted Project "Prevention and Control of Disease Factor," Grant no. 9300769. W. A. S. is the recipient of an Associate Career Scientist award from the U.S. Department of Veterans Affairs.

REFERENCES

1. **Alexander, W., and D. Rimland.** 1987. Lack of correlation of slime production with pathogenicity in continuous ambulatory peritoneal dialysis peritonitis caused by coagulase-negative staphylococci. *Diagn. Microbiol. Infect. Dis.* **8:**215–220.
2. **Archer, G. L., N. Vishniavsky, and H. G. Stiver.** 1982. Plasmid pattern analysis of *Staphylococcus epidermidis* isolates from patients with prosthetic valve endocarditis. *Infect. Immun.* **35:**627–632.
3. **Baddour, L. M., L. P. Barker, G. D. Christensen, J. T. Parisi, and W. A. Simpson.** 1990. Phenotypic variation of *Staphylococcus epidermidis* in infection of transvenous endocardial pacemaker electrodes. *J. Clin. Microbiol.* **28:**676–679.
4. **Baddour, L. M., G. D. Christensen, M. G. Hester, and A. L. Bisno.** 1984. Production of experimental endocarditis by coagulase-negative staphylococci: variability in species virulence. *J. Infect. Dis.* **150:**721–727.
5. **Baddour, L. M., D. L. Smalley, A. P. Kraus, W. J. Lamoreaux, and G. D. Christensen.** 1986. Comparison of microbiologic characteristics of pathogenic and saprophytic coagulase-negative staphylococci from patients on continuous ambulatory peritoneal dialysis. *Diagn. Microbiol. Infect. Dis.* **5:**197–205.
6. **Baird-Parker, A. C.** 1965. The classification of staphylococci and micrococci from world wide sources. *J. Gen. Microbiol.* **38:**363–387.
7. **Baldassarri, L., W. A. Simpson, G. Donelli, and G. D. Christensen.** 1993. Variable fixation of staphylococcal slime by different histochemical fixatives. *Eur. J. Clin. Microbiol. Infect. Dis.* **12:**866–868.
8. **Bandyk, D. F., G. A. Berni, B. L. Thiele, and J. B. Towne.** 1984. Aortofemoral graft infection due to *Staphylococcus epidermidis*. *Arch. Surg.* **119:**102–108.
9. **Barker, L. P., W. A. Simpson, and G. D. Christensen.** 1992. Differential production of slime under aerobic and anaerobic conditions. *J. Clin. Microbiol.* **28:**2578–2579.
10. **Bayston, R., and S. R. Penny.** 1972. Excessive production of mucoid substance in *Staphylococcus* SIIA: a possible factor in colonisation of Holter shunts. *Dev. Med. Child Neurol.* **14**(Suppl. 27):25–28.
11. **Beaman, M., L. Solaro, D. Adu, and J. Michael.** 1987. Peritonitis caused by slime-producing coagulase-negative staphylococci in continuous ambulatory peritoneal dialysis. *Lancet* **i:**42.
12. **Beard-Pegler, M. A., C. L. Gabelish, E. Stubbs, C. Harbour, J. Robinson, M. Falk, R. Benn, and A. Vickery.** 1989. Prevalence of peritonitis-associated coagulase-negative staphylococci on the skin of continuous ambulatory peritoneal dialysis patients. *Epidemiol. Infect.* **102:**365–378.
13. **Bykowska, K., A. Ludwicka, Z. Wegrzynowicz, S. Lopaciuk, and M. Kopec.** 1985. Anticoagulant properties of extracellular slime substance produced by *Staphylococcus epidermidis*. *Thromb. Haemostasis* **54:**853–856.
14. **Cheesbrough, J. S., R. G. Finch, and R. P. Burden.** 1986. A prospective study of

the mechanisms of infection associated with hemodialysis catheters. *J. Infect. Dis.* **154**:579–589.

15. **Cheung, A. L., and V. Fischetti.** 1990. The role of fibrinogen in staphylococcal adherence to catheters *in vitro. J. Infect. Dis.* **161**:1177–1186.

16. **Chhatwal, G. S., K. T. Preissner, G. Muller-Berghaus, and H. Blobel.** 1987. Specific binding of the human S protein (vitronectin) to streptococci, *Staphylococcus aureus,* and *Escherichia coli. Infect. Immun.* **55**:1878–1883.

17. **Choo, M. H., D. R. Holmes, B. J. Gersh, J. D. Maloney, J. Meredith, J. R. Pluth, and J. Trusty.** 1981. Permanent pacemaker infections: characterization and management. *Am. J. Cardiol.* **48**:559–564.

18. **Christensen, G. D.** 1993. The sticky problem of *Staphylococcus epidermidis* sepsis. *Hosp. Pract.* **28**:27–36, 38.

19. **Christensen, G. D., L. M. Baddour, D. L. Hasty, J. H. Lowrance, and W. A. Simpson.** 1989. Microbial and foreign body factors in the pathogenesis of medical device infections, p. 27–59. *In* A. L. Bisno and F. A. Waldvogel (ed.), *Infections Associated with Indwelling Medical Devices,* American Society for Microbiology, Washington, D.C.

20. **Christensen, G. D., L. M. Baddour, B. M. Madison, J. T. Parisi, S. N. Abraham, D. L. Hasty, J. H. Lowrance, J. A. Josephs, and W. A. Simpson.** 1990. Colonial morphology of staphylococci on Memphis agar: phase variation of slime production, resistance to β-lactam antibiotics, and virulence. *J. Infect. Dis.* **161**:1153–1169.

21. **Christensen, G. D., L. M. Baddour, and W. A. Simpson.** 1987. Phenotypic variation of *Staphylococcus epidermidis* slime production in vitro and in vivo. *Infect. Immun.* **55**: 2870–2877.

22. **Christensen, G. D., L. M. Baddour, and W. A. Simpson.** 1990. Hypothetical model of phenotypic variation in staphylococci, p. 465–478. *In* T. Wadstrom, I. Eliasson, I. Holder, and A. Ljungh (ed.), *Pathogenesis of Wound and Biomaterial Associated Infections.* Springer-Verlag, London.

23. **Christensen, G. D., L. P. Barker, T. P. Mawhinney, L. M. Baddour, and W. A. Simpson.** 1990. Identification of an antigenic marker of slime production for *Staphylococcus epidermidis. Infect. Immun.* **58**:2906–2911.

24. **Christensen, G. D., L. P. Barker, W. A. Simpson.** Comparative virulence of chemical mutants and phase variants of a slime producing strain of *Staphylococcus epidermidis* in a mouse model of catheter infection. *In* T. Wadstrom (ed.), *Molecular Pathogenesis of Surgical Infections,* in press. Springer Verlag, London.

25. **Christensen, G. D., A. L. Bisno, J. T. Parisi, B. McLaughlin, M. G. Hester, and R. W. Luther.** 1982. Nosocomial septicemia due to multiply antibiotic-resistant *Staphylococcus epidermidis. Ann. Intern. Med.* **96**:1–10.

26. **Christensen, G. D., J. T. Parisi, A. L. Bisno, W. A. Simpson, and E. H. Beachey.** 1983. Characterization of clinically significant strains of coagulase-negative staphylococci. *J. Clin. Microbiol.* **18**:258–269.

27. **Christensen, G. D., and W. A. Simpson.** 1992. Gram-positive bacteria: pathogenesis of staphylococcal musculoskeletal infections, p. 57–78. *In* J. L. Esterhai, A. G. Gristina, and R. Poss (ed.), *Musculoskeletal Infection.* American Academy of Orthopaedic Surgeons, Park Ridge, Ill.

28. **Christensen, G. D., W. A. Simpson, and E. H. Beachey.** 1985. Microbial adherence in infections, p. 6–23. *In* G. L. Mandel, R. G. Douglas, and J. E. Bennett (ed.), *Principles and Practice of Infectious Diseases,* 2nd ed. John Wiley & Sons, Inc., New York.

29. **Christensen, G. D., W. A. Simpson, A. L. Bisno, and E. H. Beachey.** 1982. Adherence of slime-producing strains of *Staphylococcus epidermidis* to smooth surfaces. *Infect. Immun.* **37**:318–326.

30. **Christensen, G. D., W. A. Simpson, A. L. Bisno, and E. H. Beachey.** 1983. Experimental foreign body infections in mice challenged with slime producing *Staphylococcus epidermidis. Infect. Immun.* **40:**407–410.
31. **Christensen, G. D., W. A. Simpson, J. J. Younger, L. M. Baddour, F. F. Barrett, D. M. Melton, and E. H. Beachey.** 1985. Adherence of coagulase-negative staphylococci to plastic tissue culture plates: a quantitative model for the adherence of staphylococci to medical devices. *J. Clin. Microbiol.* **22:**996–1006.
32. **Chugh, T. D., G. J. Burns, H. J. Shuhaiber, and G. M. Bahr.** 1990. Adherence of *Staphylococcus epidermidis* to fibrin-platelet clots *in vitro* mediated by lipoteichoic acid. *Infect. Immun.* **58:**315–319.
33. **Davenport, D. S., R. M. Massanari, M. A. Pfaller, M. J. Bale, S. A. Streed, and W. J. Hierholzer, Jr.** 1986. Usefulness of a test for slime production as a marker for clinically significant infections with coagulase-negative staphylococci. *J. Infect. Dis.* **153:**332–339.
34. **Deighton, M. A., and B. Balkau.** 1990. Adherence measured by microtiter assay as a virulence marker for *Staphylococcus epidermidis* infections. *J. Clin. Microbiol.* **28:**2442–2447.
35. **Deighton, M. A., and R. Borland.** 1993. Regulation of slime production in *Staphylococcus epidermidis* by iron limitation. *Infect. Immun.* **61:**4473–4479.
36. **Deighton, M. A., V. A. Fleming, and C. J. Wood.** 1990. Slime production by coagulase-negative staphylococci causing single and recurrent episodes of peritonitis, p. 465–478. *In* T. Wadstrom, I. Eliasson, I. Holder, and A. Ljungh (ed.), *Pathogenesis of Wound and Biomaterial Associated Infections.* Springer-Verlag, London.
37. **Deighton, M. A., J. C. Franklin, W. J. Spicer, and B. Balkau.** 1988. Species identification, antibiotic sensitivity, and slime production of coagulase-negative staphylococci isolated from clinical specimens. *Epidemiol. Infect.* **101:**99–113.
38. **Deighton, M., S. Pearson, J. Capstick, D. Spelman, and R. Borland.** 1992. Phenotypic variation of *Staphylococcus epidermidis* isolated from a patient with native valve endocarditis. *J. Clin. Microbiol.* **30:**2385–2390.
39. **Denyer, S., M. C. Davies, J. A. Evans, R. G. Finch, D. G. E. Smith, M. H. Wilcox, and P. Williams.** 1990. Influence of carbon dioxide on the surface characteristics and adherence potential of coagulase-negative staphylococci. *J. Clin. Microbiol.* **28:**1813–1817.
40. **Diaz-Mitoma, F., G. K. M. Harding, D. J. Hoban, R. S. Roberts, and D. E. Low.** 1987. Clinical significance of a test for slime production in ventriculoperitoneal shunt infections caused by coagulase-negative staphylococci. *J. Infect. Dis.* **156:**555–560.
41. **Dobbins, J. J., D. Seligson, and M. J. Raff.** 1988. Bacterial colonization of orthopedic devices in the absence of clinical infection. *J. Infect. Dis.* **158:**203–205.
42. **Dougherty, S. H.** 1986. Implant infections, p. 276–289. *In* A. F. von Recum (ed.), *Handbook of Biomaterials Evaluation.* Macmillan Publishing Co., New York.
43. **Drewry, D. T., L. Galbraith, B. J. Wilkinson, and S. G. Wilkinson.** 1990. Staphylococcal slime: a cautionary tale. *J. Clin. Microbiol.* **28:**1292–1296.
44. **Dunne, W. M., D. B. Nelson, and M. J. Chusid.** 1987. Epidemiologic markers of pediatric infections caused by coagulase-negative staphylococci. *Pediatr. Infect. Dis. J.* **6:**1031–1035.
45. **Etienne, J., Y. Brun, N. E. Solh, V. Delorme, C. Mouren, M. Bes, and J. Fleurette.** 1988. Characterization of clinically significant isolates of *Staphylococcus epidermidis* from patients with endocarditis. *J. Clin. Microbiol.* **26:**613–617.
46. **Evans, R. C., and C. J. Holmes.** 1987. Effect of vancomycin hydrochloride on *Staphylococcus epidermidis* biofilm associated with silicone elastomer. *Antimicrob. Agents Chemother.* **31:**889–894.

47. **Farber, B. F., M. H. Kaplan, and A. G. Clogston.** 1990. *Staphylococcus epidermidis* extracted slime inhibits the antimicrobial action of glycopeptide antibiotics. *J. Infect. Dis.* **161**:37–40.

48. **Fidalgo, S., F. Vazquez, M. C. Mendoza, F. Perez, and F. J. Mendez.** 1990. Bacteremia due to *Staphylococcus epidermidis*: microbiologic, epidemiologic, clinical, and prognostic features. *Rev. Infect. Dis.* **12**:520–528.

49. **Fitzgerald, R. H., and D. R. Jones.** 1985. Hip implant infection. *Am. J. Med.* **78**(Suppl. 6B):225–228.

50. **Fleer, A., J. Verhoef, and A. P. Hernandez.** 1986. Coagulase-negative staphylococci as nosocomial pathogens in neonates: the role of host defense, artificial devices, and bacterial hydrophobicity. *Am. J. Med.* **80**(Suppl. 6B):161–165.

51. **Flock, J.-I., G. Froman, K. Jonsson, B. Guss, C. Signas, B. Nilsson, G. Raucci, M. Hook, T. Wadstrom, and M. Lindberg.** 1987. Cloning and expression of the gene for fibronectin-binding protein from *Staphylococcus aureus*. *EMBO J.* **6**:2351–2357.

52. **Franson, T. R., N. K. Sheth, H. D. Rose, and P. G. Sohnle.** 1984. Scanning electron microscopy of bacteria adherent to intravascular catheters. *J. Clin. Microbiol.* **20**: 500–505.

53. **Freeman, D. J., and F. R. Falkiner.** 1991. Coagulase-negative staphylococci and continuous ambulatory peritoneal dialysis. *Rev. Med. Microbiol.* **2**:98–104.

54. **Fuquay, J. I., D. T. Loo, and D. W. Barnes.** 1986. Binding of *Staphylococcus aureus* by human serum spreading factor in an in vitro assay. *Infect. Immun.* **52**:714–717.

55. **Gallimore, B., R. F. Gagnon, G. K. Richards.** 1988. Role of an intraperitoneal catheter implant in the pathogenesis of experimental *Staphylococcus epidermidis* peritoneal infection in renal failure mice. *Am. J. Nephrol.* **8**:334–343.

56. **George, R., L. Leibrock, and M. Epstein.** 1979. Long-term analysis of cerebrospinal fluid shunt infections. *J. Neurosurg.* **51**:804–811.

57. **Gnann, J. W., and C. G. Cobbs.** 1985. Infections of prosthetic valves and intravascular devices, p. 531–539. *In* G. L. Mandell, R. G. Douglas, and J. E. Bennett (ed.), *Principles and Practice of Infectious Diseases*, 2nd ed. John Wiley & Sons, Inc., New York.

58. **Gokal, R., J. M. Ramos, D. M. A. Francis, R. E. Ferner, T. H. J. Goodship, G. Proud, A. J. Bint, M. K. Ward, and D. N. S. Kerr.** 1982. Peritonitis in continuous ambulatory peritoneal dialysis. *Lancet* **ii**:1388–1391.

59. **Gristina, A. G., J. Dobbins, B. Giammara, J. C. Lewis, and W. C. De Vries.** 1988. Biomaterial-centered sepsis and the total artificial heart: microbial adhesion vs tissue integration. *JAMA* **259**:870–874.

60. **Gristina, A. G., R. A. Jennings, P. T. Naylor, Q. N. Myrvik, and L. X. Webb.** 1989. Comparative in vitro resistance of surface-colonizing coagulase-negative staphylococci. *Antimicrob. Agents Chemother.* **33**:813–816.

61. **Gunn, B. A.** 1989. Comparative virulence of human isolates of coagulase-negative staphylococci tested in an infant mouse weight retardation model. *J. Clin. Microbiol.* **27**:507–511.

62. **Gunn, B. A., and R. S. Colwell.** 1983. Numerical taxonomy of staphylococci isolated from the marine environment. *Int. J. Syst. Bacteriol.* **33**:751–759.

63. **Hall, R. T., S. L. Hall, W. G. Barnes, J. Izuegbu, M. Rogolsky, and I. Zorbas.** 1987. Characteristics of coagulase-negative staphylococci from infants with bacteremia. *Pediatr. Infect. Dis. J.* **6**:377–383.

64. **Herrmann, M., Q. J. Lai, R. M. Albrecht, D. F. Mosher, and R. A. Proctor.** 1993. Adhesion of *Staphylococcus aureus* to surface-bound platelets: role of fibrinogen/fibrin and platelet integrins. *J. Infect. Dis.* **167**:312–322.

65. **Herrmann, M., S. J. Suchard, L. A. Boxer, F. A. Waldvogel, and P. D. Lew.** 1991.

Thrombospondin binds to *Staphylococcus aureus* and promotes staphylococcal adherence to surfaces. *Infect. Immun.* **59:**279–288.

66. **Hogt, A. H., J. Dankert, J. A. de Vries, and J. Feijen.** 1983. Adhesion of coagulase-negative staphylococci to biomaterials. *J. Gen. Microbiol.* **129:**2959–2968.

67. **Holderbaum, D., G. S. Hall, and L. A. Ehrhart.** 1986. Collagen binding to *Staphylococcus aureus*. *Infect. Immun.* **54:**359–364.

68. **Hussain, M., C. Collins, J. G. M. Hastings, and P. J. White.** 1992. Radiochemical assay to measure the biofilm produced by coagulase-negative staphylococci on solid surfaces and its use to quantitate the effects of various antibacterial compounds on the formation of the biofilm. *J. Med. Microbiol.* **37:**62–69.

69. **Hussain, M., J. G. M. Hastings, and P. J. White.** 1991. A chemically defined medium for slime production by coagulase-negative staphylococci. *J. Med. Microbiol* **34:** 143–147.

70. **Hussain, M., J. G. M. Hastings, and P. J. White.** 1991. Isolation and composition of the extracellular slime made by coagulase-negative staphylococci in a chemically defined medium. *J. Infect. Dis.* **163:**534–541.

71. **Hussain, M., M. H. Wilcox, P. J. White, M. K. Faulkner, and R. C. Spencer.** 1992. Importance of medium and atmosphere type to both slime production and adherence by coagulase-negative staphylococci. *J. Hosp. Infect.* **20:**173–184.

72. **Inman, R. D., K. V. Gallegos, B. D. Brause, P. B. Redecha, and C. L. Christian.** 1984. Clinical and microbial features of prosthetic joint infection. *Am. J. Med.* **77:** 47–53.

73. **Ishak, M. A., D. H. M. Groschel, G. L. Mandel, and R. P. Wenzel.** 1985. Association of slime with pathogenicity of coagulase-negative staphylococci causing nosocomial septicemia. *J. Clin. Microbiol.* **22:**1025–1029.

74. **Ivey, F. M., C. A. Hicks, J. H. Calhoun, and J. T. Mader.** 1990. Treatment options for infected knee arthroplasties. *Rev. Infect. Dis.* **12:**468–478.

75. **Johnson, G. M., D. A. Lee, W. E. Regelmann, E. D. Gray, G. Peters, and P. G. Quie.** 1986. Interference with granulocyte function by *Staphylococcus epidermidis* slime. *Infect. Immun.* **54:**13–20.

76. **Jones, D., R. H. Deibel, and C. F. Niven.** 1963. Identity of *Staphylococcus epidermidis*. *J. Bacteriol.* **85:**62–67.

77. **Jones, P. G., R. L. Hopfer, L. Elting, J. A. Jackson, V. Fainstein, and G. P. Bodey.** 1986. Semiquantitative cultures of intravascular catheters from cancer patients. *Diagn. Microbiol. Infect. Dis.* **4:**299–306.

78. **Kaebnick, H. W., D. F. Bandyk, T. W. Bergamini, and J. B. Towne.** 1987. The microbiology of explanted vascular prosthesis. *Surgery* **102:**756–762.

79. **Karchmer, A. W., G. L. Archer, and W. E. Dismukes.** 1983. *Staphylococcus epidermidis* causing prosthetic valve endocarditis: microbiologic and clinical observations as guides to therapy. *Ann. Intern. Med.* **98:**447–455.

80. **Kloos, W. E., and M. S. Musselwhite.** 1975. Distribution and persistence of *Staphylococcus* and *Micrococcus* species and other aerobic bacteria on human skin. *Appl. Microbiol.* **30:**381–394.

81. **Kojima, Y., M. Tojo, D. A. Goldmann, T. D. Tosteson, and G. B. Pier.** 1990. Antibody to the capsular polysaccharide/adhesin protects rabbits against catheter-related bacteremia due to coagulase-negative staphylococci. *J. Infect. Dis.* **162:**435–441.

82. **Kotilainen, P.** 1990. Association of coagulase-negative staphylococcal slime production and adherence with the development and outcome of adult septicemias. *J. Clin. Microbiol.* **28:**2779–2785.

83. **Kotilainen, P., J. Maki, P. Oksman, M. K. Viljanen, J. Nikoskelainen, and P. Huovi-**

nen. 1990. Immunochemical analysis of the extracellular slime substance of *Staphylococcus epidermidis*. *Eur. J. Clin. Microbiol. Infect. Dis.* **9:**262–270.

84. **Kristinsson, K. G.** 1989. Adherence of staphylococci to intravascular catheters. *J. Med. Microbiol.* **28:**249–257.

85. **Kristinsson, K. G., R. C. Spencer, and C. B. Brown.** 1986. Clinical importance of production of slime by coagulase-negative staphylococci in chronic ambulatory peritoneal dialysis. *J. Clin. Pathol.* **39:**117.

86. **Kuusela, P., T. Vartio, M. Vuento, and E. B. Myhre.** 1985. Attachment of staphylococci and streptococci to fibronectin, fibronectin fragments, and fibrinogen bound to a solid phase. *Infect. Immun.* **50:**77–81.

87. **Kuypers, J. M., and R. Proctor.** 1989. Reduced adherence to traumatized rat heart valves by a low-fibronectin-binding mutant of *Staphylococcus aureus*. *Infect. Immun.* **57:**2306–2312.

88. **Lambe, D. W., K. P. Ferguson, J. L. Keplinger, C. G. Gemmell, and J. H. Kalbfleisch.** 1990. Pathogenicity of *Staphylococcus lugdunensis, Staphylococcus schleiferi,* and three other coagulase-negative staphylococci in a mouse model and possible virulence factors. *Can. J. Microbiol.* **36:**455–463.

89. **Locci, R., G. Peters, and G. Pulverer.** 1981. Microbial colonization of prosthetic devices. III. Adhesion of staphylococci to lumina of intravenous catheters perfused with bacterial suspensions. *Zentralbl. Bakteriol. Mikrobiol. Hyg. 1 Abt. Orig. B* **173:**300–307.

90. **Lopes, J. D., M. dos Reis, and R. R. Brentani.** 1985. Presence of laminin receptors in *Staphylococcus aureus*. *Science* **229:**275–277.

91. **Lowy, F. D., and S. M. Hammer.** 1983. *Staphylococcus epidermidis* infections. *Ann. Intern. Med.* **99:**834–839.

92. **Ludwicka, A., G. Uhlenbruck, G. Peters, P. N. Seng, E. D. Gray, J. Jelajaszewicz, and G. Pulverer.** 1984. Investigation on extracellular slime substance produced by *Staphylococcus epidermidis*. *Zentralbl. Bakteriol. Mikrobiol. Hyg. Ser. A* **258:**256–267.

93. **Mack, D., N. Siemssen, and R. Laufs.** 1992. Parallel induction by glucose of adherence and a polysaccharide antigen specific for plastic-adherent *Staphylococcus epidermidis:* evidence for functional relation to intercellular adhesion. *Infect. Immun.* **60:**2048–2057.

94. **Marples, R. R., J. F. Richardson, and M. J. de Saxe.** 1985. Four apparent outbreaks of prosthetic valve endocarditis caused by coagulase-negative staphylococci. *Zentralbl. Bakteriol. Suppl.* **14:**463–469.

95. **Marrie, T. J., and J. W. Costerton.** 1984. Morphology of bacterial attachment to cardiac pacemaker leads and power packs. *J. Clin. Microbiol.* **19:**911–914.

96. **Marrie, T. J., and J. W. Costerton.** 1984. Scanning and transmission electron microscopy of in situ bacterial colonization of intravenous and intraarterial catheters. *J. Clin. Microbiol.* **19:**687–693.

97. **Martin, M. A., M. A. Pfaller, R. M. Massanari, and R. P. Wenzel.** 1989. Use of cellular hydrophobicity, slime production, and species identification markers for the clinical significance of coagulase-negative staphylococcal isolates. *Am. J. Infect. Control* **17:**130–135.

98. **Martin, M. A., M. A. Pfaller, and R. P. Wenzel.** 1989. Coagulase-negative staphylococcal bacteremia. *Ann. Intern. Med.* **110:**9–16.

99. **Maxe, I., C. Ryden, T. Wadstrom, and K. Rubin.** 1986. Specific attachment of *Staphylococcus aureus* to immobilized fibronectin. *Infect. Immun.* **54:**695–704.

100. **McAllister, T. A., H. Mocan, A. V. Murphy, and T. J. Beattie.** 1987. Antibiotic susceptibility of staphylococci from CAPD peritonitis in children. *J. Antimicrob. Chemother.* **19:**95–100.

101. **Muller, E., J. Hubner, N. Gutierrez, S. Takeda, D. Goldmann, and G. B. Pier.** 1993. Isolation and characterization of transposon mutants of *Staphylococcus epidermidis* deficient in capsular polysaccharide/adhesin and slime. *Infect. Immun.* **61**:551–558, 1993.

102. **Muller, E., S. Takeda, D. A. Goldmann, and G. B. Pier.** 1991. Blood proteins do not promote adherence of coagulase-negative staphylococci to biomaterials. *Infect. Immun.* **59**:3323–3326.

103. **Muller, E., S. Takeda, H. Shiro, D. Goldmann, and G. B. Pier.** 1993. Occurrence of capsular polysaccharide/adhesin (PS/A) among clinical isolates of coagulase-negative staphylococci. *J. Infect. Dis.* **168**:1211–1218.

104. **Needham, C. A., and W. Stempsey.** 1984. Incidence, adherence, and antibiotic resistance of coagulase-negative *Staphylococcus* species causing human disease. *Diagn. Microbiol. Infect. Dis.* **2**:293–299.

105. **Odio, C., G. H. McCraken, and J. D. Nelson.** 1984. CSF shunt infections in pediatrics. *Am. J. Dis. Child.* **38**:1103–1108.

106. **Olson, M. E., I. Ruseska, and J. W. Costerton.** 1988. Colonization of n-butyl-2-cyano-acrylate tissue adhesive by *Staphylococcus epidermidis*. *J. Biomed. Mater. Res.* **22**:485–495.

107. **Pascual, A., A. Fleer, N. A. C. Westerdaal, and J. Verhoef.** 1986. Modulation of adherence of coagulase-negative staphylococci to teflon catheters *in vitro*. *Eur. J. Clin. Microbiol.* **5**:518–522.

108. **Passerini, L., K. Lam, J. W. Costerton, and E. G. King.** 1992. Biofilms on indwelling vascular catheters. *Crit. Care Med.* **20**:665–673.

109. **Patrick, C. C., M. R. Plaunt, S. V. Hetherington, and S. M. May.** 1992. Role of the *Staphylococcus epidermidis* slime layer in experimental tunnel tract infections. *Infect. Immun.* **60**:1363–1367.

110. **Paulsson, M., A. Ljungh, and T. Wadstrom.** 1992. Rapid identification of fibronectin, vitronectin, laminin, and collagen cell surface binding proteins on coagulase-negative staphylococci by particle agglutination assays. *J. Clin. Microbiol.* **30**:2006–2012.

111. **Paulsson, M., and T. Wadstrom.** 1990. Vitronectin and type-I collagen binding by *Staphylococcus aureus* and coagulase-negative staphylococci. *FEMS Microbiol. Immun.* **65**:55–62.

112. **Peng, H.-L., R. P. Novick, B. Kreiswirth, J. Kornblum, and P. Schlievert.** 1988. Cloning, characterization, and sequencing of an accessory gene regulator (*agr*) in *Staphylococcus aureus*. *J. Bacteriol.* **170**:4365–4372.

113. **Peters, G., R. Locci, and G. Pulverer.** 1981. Microbial colonization of prosthetic devices. II. Scanning electron microscopy of naturally infected intravenous catheters. *Zentralbl. Bakteriol. Mikrobiol. Hyg. 1 Abt. Orig. B* **173**:293–299.

114. **Peters, G., R. Locci, and G. Pulverer.** 1982. Adherence and growth of coagulase-negative staphylococci on the surfaces of intravenous catheters. *J. Infect. Dis.* **146**:479–482.

115. **Peters, G., F. Saborowski, R. Locci, and G. Pulverer.** 1984. Investigations on staphylococcal infection of transvenous endocardial pacemaker electrodes. *Am. Heart J.* **108**:359–365.

116. **Peters, G., F. Schumacher-Perdreau, B. Jansen, M. Bey, and G. Pulverer.** 1987. Biology of *Staphylococcus epidermidis* extracellular slime. *Zentralbl. Bakteriol. Suppl.* **16**:15–32.

117. **Ponce de Leon, S., S. H. Guenthner, and R. P. Wenzel.** 1986. Microbiologic studies of coagulase-negative staphylococci isolated from patients with nosocomial bacteremias. *J. Hosp. Infect.* **7**:121–129.

118. **Ponce de Leon, S., and R. P. Wenzel.** 1984. Hospital-acquired bloodstream infections with *Staphylococcus epidermidis*. *Am. J. Med.* **77**:639–644.

119. **Raad, I., W. Costerton, U. Sabharwal, M. Sacilowski, E. Anaissie, and G. P. Bodey.** 1993. Ultrastructural analysis of indwelling vascular catheters: a quantitative relationship between luminal colonization and duration of placement. *J. Infect. Dis.* **168:** 400–407.

120. **Righter, J.** 1987. Septicemia due to coagulase-negative *Staphylococcus* in a community hospital. *Can. Med. Assoc. J.* **137:**121–125.

121. **Ruiter, J. H., J. E. Degener, R. van Mechelen, and R. Bos.** 1985. Late purulent pacemaker pocket infection caused by *Staphylococcus epidermidis:* serious complications of *in situ* management. *PACE* **8:**903–907.

122. **Rupp, M. E., and G. L. Archer.** 1992. Hemagglutination and adherence to plastic by *Staphylococcus epidermidis. Infect. Immun.* **60:**4322–4327.

123. **Russell, P. B., J. Kline, M. C. Yoder, and R. A. Polin.** 1987. Staphylococcal adherence to polyvinyl chloride and heparin-bonded polyurethane catheters is species dependent and enhanced by fibronectin. *J. Clin. Microbiol.* **25:**1083–1087.

124. **Ryden, C., A. I. Yacoub, I. Maxe, D. Heinegard, A. Oldberg, A. Franzen, A. Ljungh, and K. Rubin.** 1989. Specific binding of bone sialoprotein to *Staphylococcus aureus* isolated from patients with osteomyelitis. *Eur. J. Biochem.* **184:**331–336.

125. **Schadow, K. W., W. A. Simpson, and G. D. Christensen.** 1988. Characteristics of adherence to plastic tissue culture plates of coagulase-negative staphylococci exposed to subinhibitory concentrations of antimicrobial agents. *J. Infect. Dis.* **157:**71–77.

126. **Schmidt, H., G. Naumann, and H. P. Putzke.** 1988. Detection of different fimbriae-like structures on the surface of *Staphylococcus saprophyticus. Zentralbl. Bakteriol. Hyg.* **268:**228–237.

127. **Sherertz, R. J. R. J. Falk, K. A. Huffman, C. A. Thomann, and W. D. Mattern.** 1983. Infections associated with subclavian Uldall catheters. *Arch. Intern. Med.* **143:** 52–56.

128. **Sheth, N. K., T. R. Franson, and P. G. Sohnle.** 1985. Influence of bacterial adherence to intravascular catheters on *in vitro* antibiotic susceptibility. *Lancet* **ii:**1266–1268.

129. **Skoutelis, A. T., R. L. Murphy, K. B. MacDonell, J. H. VonRoenn, C. D. Sterkel, and J. P. Phair.** 1990. Indwelling central venous catheter infections in patients with acquired immune deficiency syndrome. *J. Acquired Immune Defic. Syndr.* **3:**335–342.

130. **Smeltzer, M. S., M. E. Hart, and J. J. Iandolo.** 1993. Phenotypic characterization of *xpr,* a global regulator of extracellular virulence factors in *Staphylococcus aureus. Infect. Immun.* **61:**919–925.

131. **Stillman, R. I., R. P. Wenzel, and L. C. Donowitz.** 1987. Emergence of coagulase-negative staphylococci as major nosocomial bloodstream pathogens. *Infect. Control* **8:** 108–112.

132. **Switalski, L. M., P. Speziale, and M. Hook.** 1989. Isolation and characterization of a putative collagen receptor from *Staphylococcus aureus* strain Cowan I. *J. Biol. Chem.* **264:**21080–21086.

133. **Takeda, S., G. B. Pier, Y. Kojima, M. Tojo, E. Miller, T. Tosteson, and D. A. Goldmann.** 1991. Protection against endocarditis due to *Staphylococcus epidermidis* by immunization with capsular polysaccharide/adhesin. *Circulation* **84:**2539–2546.

134. **Tenney, J. H., M. R. Moody, K. A. Newman, S. C. Schimpf, J. C. Wade, J. W. Costerton, and W. P. Reed.** 1986. Adherent microorganisms on lumenal surfaces of long-term intravenous catheters: importance of *Staphylococcus epidermidis* in patients with cancer. *Arch. Intern. Med.* **146:**1949–1954.

135. **Timmerman, C. P., A. Fleer, J. M. Besnier, L. de Graaf, F. Cremers, and J. Verhoef.** 1991. Characterization of a proteinaceous adhesin of *Staphylococcus epidermidis* which mediates attachment to polystyrene. *Infect. Immun.* **59:**4187–4192.

136. **Tojo, M., N. Yamashita, D. A. Goldmann, and G. B. Pier.** 1988. Isolation and characterization of a capsular polysaccharide adhesin from *Staphylococcus epidermidis*. *J. Infect. Dis.* **157**:713–722.

137. **Vaudaux, P., D. Pittet, A. Haeberli, E. Huggler, U. E. Nydegger, D. P. Lew, and F. A. Waldvogel.** 1989. Host factors selectively increase staphylococcal adherence on inserted catheters: a role for fibronectin and fibrinogen or fibrin. *J. Infect. Dis.* **160**: 865–874.

138. **Vaudaux, P., D. Pittet, A. Haeberli, P. G. Lerch, J.-J. Morgenthaler, R. A. Proctor, F. A. Waldvogel, and D. P. Lew.** 1993. Fibronectin is more active than fibrin or fibrinogen in promoting *Staphylococcus aureus* adherence to inserted intravascular catheters. *J. Infect. Dis.* **167**:633–641.

139. **Vaudaux, P., R. Suzuki, F. A. Waldvogel, J. J. Morgenthaler, and U. E. Nydegger.** 1984. Foreign body infection: role of fibronectin as a ligand for the adherence of *Staphylococcus aureus*. *J. Infect. Dis.* **150**:546–552.

140. **Vaudaux, P. E., F. A. Waldvogel, J. J. Morgenthaler, and U. E. Nydegger.** 1984. Adsorption of fibronectin onto polymethylmethacrylate and promotion of *Staphylococcus aureus* adherence. *Infect. Immun.* **45**:768–774.

141. **Vaudaux, P. E., G. Zulian, E. Huggler, and F. A. Waldvogel.** 1985. Attachment of *Staphylococcus aureus* to polymethylmethacrylate increases its resistance to phagocytosis in foreign body infection. *Infect. Immun.* **50**:472–477.

142. **Wang, I.-w., J. M. Anderson, and R. E. Marchant.** 1993. *Staphylococcus epidermidis* adhesion to hydrophobic biomedical polymer is mediated by platelets. *J. Infect. Dis.* **167**:329–336.

143. **West, T. E., J. J. Walshe, C. P. Krol, and D. Amsterdam.** 1986. Staphylococcal peritonitis in patients on continuous peritoneal dialysis. *J. Clin. Microbiol.* **23**:809–812.

144. **Younger, J. J., G. D. Christensen, D. L. Bartley, J. C. H. Simmons, and F. F. Barrett.** 1987. Coagulase-negative staphylococci isolated from cerebrospinal fluid shunts: importance of slime production, species identification, and shunt removal to clinical outcome. *J. Infect. Dis.* **156**:548–554.

Infections Associated with Indwelling Medical Devices, 2nd ed.
Edited by Alan L. Bisno and Francis A. Waldvogel
© 1994 American Society for Microbiology, Washington, DC 20005

Chapter 4

Microbial Pathogenic Factors: Small Colony Variants

Richard A. Proctor

Small colony variants (SCVs) were reported in clinical specimens over 80 years ago (40). Since then, they have been reported many times and in many species, but their precise role in the pathogenesis of infectious diseases has not yet been fully defined. Recent data on *Staphylococcus aureus* SCVs suggest that they may cause persistent and recurrent infections as a result of their ability to survive within, but not lyse, the host cells.

Of interest, many of the metabolic characteristics of small colony variants are shared by organisms on biomaterial surfaces. When bacteria adhere to biomaterial surfaces, they undergo dramatic metabolic changes such as (i) slow growth (13, 23, 28, 76), (ii) decreased oxidative metabolism (52), and (iii) enhanced resistance to antibiotics (10, 13, 22, 23, 27, 34, 74, 76). As discussed below, SCVs also demonstrate decreased metabolism. This leads to slow growth (hence small colonies and increased resistance to cell wall-active antibiotics) and decreased antibiotic uptake (aminoglycoside import is dependent on an electrochemical gradient). Indeed, the parallels between SCVs and surface-bound organisms are strong, which allows one to speculate about whether some of the same mechanisms controlling the conversion to the SCV form are also occurring in adherent microorganisms. Because studies of surface-adherent organisms are more difficult to perform than studies of free-floating organisms, the lessons learned from stable *S. aureus* SCVs may well apply to organisms adherent to a biomaterial surface.

Richard A. Proctor • Department of Medical Microbiology and Immunology, University of Wisconsin, Madison, Wisconsin 53706.

SCVs have been reported from a wide range of organisms, including *S. aureus, Staphylococcus epidermidis, Pseudomonas aeruginosa, Salmonella typhimurium, Shigella* spp., *Brucella abortus, Escherichia coli, Lactobacillus acidophilus, Serratia marcescens,* and *Neisseria gonorrhoeae* (1–3, 6, 7, 11, 14, 17–21, 25, 26, 30–33, 35–37, 39, 42–44, 46, 48–50, 56–61, 63, 65–71, 75, 77–80, 83). The common phenotypic trait is slow growth, which leads to the development of microcolonies, usually defined as those more than 10-fold smaller than the normal colonies. Several other features are often found, including auxotrophies for hemin, thiamine, or menadione (*S. aureus, S. epidermidis, Salmonella typhimurium*) (1, 11, 18, 26, 37, 54, 57, 58, 60, 66, 67, 75, 80), decreased pigment formation (carotenoids in *S. aureus*, pyocyanin in *P. aeruginosa*) (6, 7, 19, 24, 38, 39, 54, 69, 79), decreased fermentation of sugars (*Shigella* spp., *S. aureus*) (20, 81), ability to revert to the parental phenotype (*Shigella* spp., *S. aureus, S. epidermidis*) (17, 19, 20, 50, 56, 70, 79, 82, 83), and decreased respiration (*Shigella* spp., *S. aureus*) (20, 81). The largest number of phenotypic characterizations and studies of SCV are available for staphylococcal species, and these organisms will be emphasized in the rest of this review. Of interest, several phenotypic characteristics vary simultaneously when *S. aureus* become SCVs; e.g., *S. aureus* SCVs are frequently nonhemolytic (14, 32, 50, 56, 79), fail to produce pigment (6, 19, 39, 54, 69, 79), produce only small amounts of coagulase (5, 32, 54, 56, 79), show decreased mannitol fermentation (6, 19, 37, 41, 50, 65), and display resistance to aminoglycoside antibiotics (1, 6, 11, 14, 18, 19, 43, 44, 48, 50, 54, 56, 68, 80).

SCVs are found in clinical specimens. *S. aureus* SCVs have been recovered, sometimes in pure culture, from abscesses (1, 30, 33, 43, 63, 65, 71), blood (1, 41, 56, 68, 78, 79), bones and joints (1, 11, 35), the pulmonary tract (17, 68, 78, 79), and soft tissues (17, 30, 35, 43, 44, 66, 71, 78). In animal studies, *S. aureus* SCVs cause disease and can be reisolated in pure culture (18, 48, 50, 54, 56, 79). Thus, *S. aureus* SCVs fulfill Koch's postulates. However, several studies performed with animal models suggest that *S. aureus* SCVs may be less virulent than normal strains (48, 50, 54, 56, 70, 79), as measured by lethal doses and fatality rates. This may in part be due to decreased serum resistance (79) and/or decreased rate of growth (1–3, 6, 7, 11, 14, 17–21, 25, 26, 30–33, 35–37, 39, 42–44, 46, 48–50, 56–61, 63, 65–71, 75, 77–80, 83). In spite of this apparent decreased virulence, *S. aureus* SCVs are able to persist as well as the parent strains in these animal models (2, 30, 48, 50, 79). This apparent contradiction between virulence and recovery from tissues may result from the ability of *S. aureus* SCVs to hide from host defenses, because of an intracellular locale (discussed below).

SCVs from a variety of genera and species have most frequently been isolated from patients and animals treated with antibiotics, especially aminoglycosides, but also sulfonamides and β-lactam antibiotics (1, 6, 11, 14, 17–19, 43, 44, 48, 50, 54, 68, 80). While many SCVs are unstable, i.e., revert to a rapidly growing phenotype, stable SCVs are most frequently isolated from patients and animals receiving antibiotics (1, 7, 11, 17, 18, 43, 44, 68) or from organisms cultured in the presence of antibiotics (5, 6, 17, 19, 39, 46, 50, 54, 56, 59, 77, 79, 80, 83). SCVs may be more resistant to antibiotics because of decreased uptake of drugs (aminoglycosides) (45, 47, 48) or because of the slow rate of growth (β-lactams). Nevertheless, SCVs have been isolated from patients who have not received antibiotics (11, 35, 56, 79) and in vitro by repeated subculture or from aged cultures (21, 31, 35, 69, 70).

The host environment may favor the selection of staphylococcal SVCs. Both *S. epidermidis* (2) and *S. aureus* (18, 48) SCVs have been harvested from rats and rabbits in the endocarditis model. While antibiotic selection may have played a role in these cases, we also have found that infecting cultured endothelial cells with wild type *S. aureus* leads to an enrichment for SCVs (J. M. Balwit and R. A. Proctor, unpublished data). This selection occurs within the intracellular milieu, as lysostaphin was continuously present in the culture medium, but in the absence of antibiotics as previously described (5, 73). In this tissue culture model, the number of organisms inoculated was 5×10^7, yet five relatively stable *S. aureus* SCVs were harvested, which is orders of magnitude higher than would be predicted compared with finding SCVs in broth or solid medium. The factor(s) in the host cells that causes this shift to SCVs is unknown.

The prevalence of SCVs in clinical specimens may be masked by the standard laboratory routines used to culture bacteria. Slow growth allows SCVs to be rapidly overgrown by normally growing organisms in liquid medium (division time of 180 versus 20 min), and SCVs may be missed on agar plates because the SCV colonies appear after 48 h, a time when the plates may have already been discarded. Also, SCVs tend to be unstable (17, 19, 50, 56, 70, 79, 82, 83). Even a small percentage of reversion at an early point in time would allow overgrowth by the more rapidly proliferating forms. Hence, only pure or stable cultures of SCVs would be likely to be found unless special efforts are made, e.g., primary plating of specimens onto solid medium, incubating cultures for at least 72 h, and reporting colonial variants to the physician. In our experience, SCVs are often found as mixtures of normal and SCV colony types. When the SCVs are further characterized and found to be the same as their more rapidly growing counterparts, laboratory personnel may discard the plates and not report these variants. Other factors that make

SCVs difficult to culture and identify are atypical colonial morphology (e.g., nonhemolytic, translucent colonies), unusual biochemical profiles (e.g., slowly coagulase positive, decreased sugar fermentation), and fastidious requirements for rapid growth (e.g., menadione, thiamine, CO_2 or hemin auxotrophy) (1, 5, 11, 30, 37, 39, 54, 59, 60, 63, 65–68, 71, 75, 80). Unless a tube coagulase test is performed and the test is incubated for 24 h, *S. aureus* SCVs may be reported to be coagulase negative. Nevertheless, two studies are available that suggest that *S. aureus* SCVs are found in 1 to 2% of clinical isolates (1, 79). The major drawback to these studies is that no primary plating was performed on these clinical isolates, resulting in the recovery of only relatively stable and/or pure cultures of SCVs. Thus, the frequency of SCV infections may have been underestimated in these two studies, and overall, they may be easily missed in the clinical laboratory because of atypical colony morphology, atypical biochemical profile, and slow, fastidious growth.

Of interest, we have recently described five consecutive *S. aureus* SCV clinical isolates and found that four of the strains had deficits in either menaquinone or hemin biosynthesis. The fifth isolate reverted to the rapidly growing form before it could be biochemically characterized. Of these five patients, two had infections that persisted for 27 and 53 years (55), and all five continued to have fever or other signs of active infection in spite of prolonged, intensive antibiotic therapy. In two cases, normal and SCV phenotypes were isolated and shown to be clonal by field-inversion gel electrophoresis. Thus, clinical *S. aureus* SCV isolates with defects in electron transport cause persistent infections that resist antibiotic therapy. In previous reports, *S. aureus* or *S. epidermidis* have been found to cause persistent, resistant, and recurrent infections in animal models (18, 48, 56, 79) and in humans (2, 17, 30, 35, 41, 50, 79).

Recently, *S. aureus* SCVs have been found to persist within cultured cells (5). The basis for this persistence is thought to be due to the reduced production of alpha-toxin (formerly called alpha-hemolysin). The importance of alpha-toxin production for endothelial cell lysis has been previously established by using site-directed mutants in the alpha-toxin gene (73). The alpha-toxin-negative mutants, but not the parent strain, were able to persist within cultured endothelial cells. While the mechanism for decreased production of alpha-toxin by *S. aureus* SCVs is unknown, most laboratory and clinical *S. aureus* SCVs produce nonhemolytic colonies (5, 14, 32, 45, 48, 50, 54, 56), whereas almost all normally growing *S. aureus* clinical isolates are strongly hemolytic.

One possible insight into the mechanism for reduced alpha-toxin production in *S. aureus* SCVs is a strong correlation between a disrupted electron transport chain and alpha-toxin production (5). A review of the literature shows that *S. aureus* SCVs, as well as other SCVs from other species (e.g., *E. coli*, *S. epidermidis*, *Salmonella* sp., and *P. aeruginosa*), show reduced electron transport activity assessed by decreased respiration, decreased methylene blue dye reduction, decreased oxidative metabolism of sugars, reduced ATP production, or decreased tetrazolium dye reduction (11, 15, 16, 19, 20, 26, 39, 58, 59, 67, 80). Reversal of SCV phenotype of *S. aureus* SCVs by adding compounds that can be utilized to repair the defect in electron transport simultaneously enhances alpha-toxin production (5, 55). Compounds that have been tested are menadione, a water-soluble vitamin K derivative, and hemin. Hemin is used in cytochrome biosynthesis, and menadione is isoprenylated to form menaquinone (8, 37, 72) (Fig. 1). Both menaquinone and cytochromes are components of the electron transport system in *S. aureus*. Of note, extensively characterized *S. aureus* hemin biosynthetic mutants demonstrate an SCV phenotype, including decreased coagulase activity, aminoglycoside resistance, decreased pigmentation, slow growth, and reduced hemolytic activity (45). Finally, anaerobic growth of five strongly hemolytic *S. aureus* clinical isolates on rabbit blood agar produced nonhemolytic colonies (72a). Anaerobic growth down-regulates menaquinone biosynthesis in *S. aureus* (8) and electron transport. Taken together, these

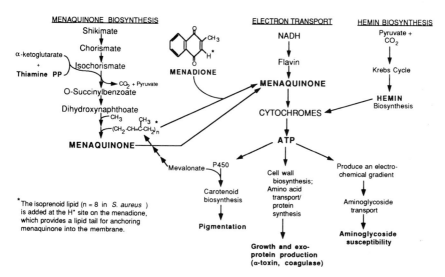

Figure 1. A hypothetical model for alterations in hemin and menaquinone biosynthesis causing the small colony variant phenotype of *S. aureus*.

observations show that alpha-toxin production is dependent upon electron transport.

One possible link between decreased alpha-toxin production and electron transport could arise from the reduced availability of amino acids that are needed for protein synthesis, because all amino acids in *S. aureus* are imported via ATP-dependent mechanisms (64). Reduced availability of ATP would decrease the rate of protein synthesis, which is consistent with *S. aureus* SCVs showing little hemolytic activity as well as being weakly coagulase positive, i.e., only small amounts are produced. An alternative mechanism could be reduced transport of alpha-toxin (45), but this suggestion is controversial as other workers find that alpha-toxin is not actively exported from *S. aureus* (9). Also, *S. aureus* SCVs are slowly coagulase positive, showing that at least one exoprotein is released. Thus, by regulating the electron transport system activity, *S. aureus* may demonstrate two populations of organisms: an aggressive (alpha-toxin producing) subpopulation that causes acute destruction of host tissues and a quiescent subpopulation (i.e., SCVs) that can persist within the protective environment of host cells yet cause recurrent disease when the electron transport chain is reconstituted.

Down-regulation of the electron transport system can also account for many of the other phenotypic characteristics of *S. aureus* SCVs in addition to reduced alpha-toxin production (Fig. 1). Pigment formation (6, 19, 54, 63, 69, 79) and aminoglycoside transport (15, 16) require ATP and an intact electron transport system. The yellow carotenoid pigments that give *S. aureus* colonies their characteristic color require ATP for their biosynthesis (38). Similarly, aminoglycoside uptake by *S. aureus* is an energy-dependent process that requires ATP and an electrochemical gradient that is produced via the electron transport system (45, 47, 48). Also, decreased availability of ATP would lead to slow growth, and hence small colonies, because of the large number of ATP molecules used in cell wall biosynthesis, e.g., lipoteichoic acid biosynthesis alone may account for 5% of the total ATP used by staphylococci (29). Finally, a block in electron transport would inhibit the mannitol fermentative pathway of *S. aureus*, making the SCV organisms mannitol negative (6, 19, 37, 41, 50, 65).

The *S. aureus* SCVs from our five patients, from clinical isolates reported in other studies, and from animal models are defective in electron transport (1, 11, 18, 29, 54, 55, 66). This raises the question of why electron transport variants are found when many other defects in metabolism could produce slow growth and reduce alpha-toxin production. Several factors may play a role. First, the pathway that is interrupted must be nonessential for bacterial survival. *S. aureus* and other bacterial species routinely survive without electron transport when grown anaerobically, as long as glucose is available. Of interest, menaquinone biosynthesis is the component that is down-regulated under anaerobic conditions in *S. aureus* (8). In contrast, defects in amino acid metabolism are often lethal without an exogenous supply of the missing amino acid. As long as a sufficient supply of glucose is available, nonoxidative ATP production is sufficient for organism survival; thus, electron transport is an optional pathway. Second, the defect must not be repaired by a substance readily available from the host. For example, vitamins (thiamine and menadione) and hemin are in limited supply within host cells (12, 53, 62). This allows the organism to maintain an SCV phenotype. While an *S. aureus* tryptophan auxotroph grew slowly on artificial medium (thus producing small colonies), it grew rapidly within cultured endothelial cells and readily lysed the monolayer (4). Third, the ability to revert to the parental phenotype would permit reversion to a more aggressive (and therefore clinically apparent) form. As the biosynthesis of menaquinone and hemin are not constitutively expressed, this allows for variation in the electron transport chain activity. Thus, the combination of a nonessential pathway that can be regulated by the microorganism and that cannot be supplemented by substances within the intracellular milieu of the host cells may account for the predominance of electron-transport-deficient strains in clinical SCV isolates.

In summary, SCVs are found in clinical specimens. While their overall prevalence has not been firmly established, problems in discovering and identifying these organisms may underestimate their prevalence. A hypothetical model that accounts for most of the known characteristics of *S. aureus* SCVs is shown in Fig. 1. From the previous literature and our recent observations, clinical *S. aureus* SCVs isolates are auxotrophic for compounds that are biosynthesized into components of the electron transport system in almost all cases when biochemical characterization is performed. Menadione and hemin are the two most frequent substances that reverse the *S. aureus* SCV phenotype. In addition, thiamine is a cofactor used in menadione biosynthesis (8) and CO_2 may be involved in the synthesis of the porphyrin ring found in hemin (some *S. aureus* SCVs can be stimulated to grow by supplementing with either CO_2 or hemin [55]). Reduced activity of the electron transport system can account for most of the features typically seen in *S. aureus* SCVs, e.g., a reduction in available ATP would slow growth (cell wall biosynthesis uses large quantities of ATP), reduce pigment formation (ATP is required for carotenoid biosynthesis), and decrease aminoglycoside transport. Therefore, by down-regulating the biosynthesis of a nonessential pathway, *S. aureus* SCVs can produce multiple phenotypic changes that may lead to increased survival within the host cells, and reversal of the SCV phenotype may form the basis for recrudescent infections. Whether this is found with other bacterial genera is yet to be determined.

REFERENCES

1. **Acar, J. F., F. N. Goldstein, and P. Lagrange.** 1978. Human infections caused by thiamine- or menadione-requiring *Staphylococcus aureus*. *J. Clin. Microbiol.* **8:**142–147.
2. **Baddour, L. M., G. D. Christensen, J. H. Lowrance, and W. A. Simpson.** 1989. Pathogenesis of experimental endocarditis. *Rev. Infect. Dis.* **11:**452–463.
3. **Baddour, L. M., W. A. Simpson, J. J. Weems, Jr., M. M. Hill, and G. D. Christensen.** 1988. Phenotypic selection of small-colony variant forms of *Staphylococcus epidermidis* in the rat model of endocarditis. *J. Infect. Dis.* **157:**757–763.
4. **Balwit, J. M.** 1992. Intracellular persistence of a *Staphylococcus aureus* small-colony variant. M.S. thesis. University of Wisconsin—Madison.
5. **Balwit, J. M., P. van Langevelde, J. M. Vann, and R. A. Proctor.** Gentamicin-resistant, menadione and hemin auxotrophic *Staphylococcus aureus* persist within cultured endothelial cells. *J. Infect. Dis.*, in press.
6. **Barbour, R. G. H.** 1950. Small colony variants ("G" forms) produced by *Staphylococcus pyogenes* during the development of resistance to streptomycin. *Aust. J. Exp. Biol. Med. Sci.* **28:**411–420.
7. **Bayer, A. S., D. C. Norman, and K. S. Kim.** 1987. Characterization of *Pseudomonas aeruginosa* isolated during unsuccessful therapy of experimental endocarditis. *Antimicrob. Agents Chemother.* **31:**70–75.
8. **Bentley, R., and R. Meganathan.** 1982. Biosynthesis of vitamin K (menaquinone) in bacteria. *Microbiol. Rev.* **46:**241–280.
9. **Bhakdi, S. (Institute of Medical Microbiology, University of Giessen, Giessen, Germany).** Personal communication.
10. **Bisno, A. L.** 1989. Infections of central nervous system shunts, p. 93–109. *In* A. L. Bisno and F. A. Waldvogel (ed.), *Infections Associated with Indwelling Medical Devices.* American Society for Microbiology, Washington, D.C.
11. **Borderon, E., and T. Horodniceanu.** 1976. Mutants déficients à colonies naines de *Staphylococcus:* étude de trois souches isolées chez des malades porteurs d'ostéo synthèses. *Ann. Inst. Pasteur Microbiol.* **127A:**503–514.
12. **Borgna-Pignatti, C., P. Marradi, L. Pinelli, N. Monetti, and C. Patrini.** 1989. Thiamine-responsive anemia in DIDMOAD syndrome. *J. Pediatr.* **114:**405–410.
13. **Brown, M. R., P. J. Collier, and P. Gilbert.** 1990. Influence of growth rate on susceptibility to antimicrobial agents: modification of the cell envelope and batch and continuous culture studies. *Antimicrob. Agents Chemother.* **34:**1623–1628.
14. **Browning, C. H., and H. S. Adamson.** 1950. Stable dwarf-colony forms produced by *Staphylococcus pyogenes*. *J. Pathol. Bacteriol.* **62:**499–500.
15. **Bryan, L. E., and S. Kwan.** 1981. Aminoglycoside-resistant mutants of *Pseudomonas aeruginosa* deficient in cytochrome *d*, nitrate reductase, and aerobic transport. *Antimicrob. Agents Chemother.* **19:**958–964.
16. **Bryan, L. E., and H. M. van den Elzen.** 1977. Effects of membrane-energy mutations and cations on streptomycin and gentamicin accumulation by bacteria: a model for entry of streptomycin and gentamicin in susceptible and resistant bacteria. *Antimicrob. Agents Chemother.* **12:**163–177.

17. **Bulger, R. J.** 1967. A methicillin-resistant strain of *Staphylococcus aureus*. Clinical and laboratory experience. *Ann. Intern. Med.* **67**:81–89.

18. **Chambers, H. F., and M. M. Miller.** 1987. Emergence of resistance to cephalothin and gentamicin during combination therapy for methicillin-resistant *Staphylococcus aureus* endocarditis in rabbits. *J. Infect. Dis.* **155**:581–585.

19. **Chin, Y. M., and S. A. Harmon.** 1971. Genetic studies of kanamycin resistance in *Staphylococcus aureus*. *Jpn. J. Microbiol.* **15**:417–423.

20. **Chinn, B. D.** 1936. Characteristics of small colony variants with special reference to *Shigella paradysenteriae sonne*. *J. Infect. Dis.* **59**:137–151.

21. **Chinn, B. D.** 1936. Characteristics of small colony variants of *Shigella paradysenteriae sonne* and *Staphylococcus aureus*. *Proc. Soc. Exp. Biol. Med.* **34**:237–238.

22. **Chuard, C., M. Herrmann, P. Vaudaux, F. A. Waldvogel, and D. P. Lew.** 1991. Successful therapy of experimental chronic foreign-body infection due to methicillin-resistant *Staphylococcus aureus* by antimicrobial combinations. *Antimicrob. Agents Chemother.* **35**:2611–2616.

23. **Chuard, C., P. Vaudaux, F. A. Waldvogel, and D. P. Lew.** 1993. Susceptibility of *Staphylococcus aureus* growing on fibronectin-coated surfaces to bactericidal antibiotics. *Antimicrob. Agents Chemother.* **37**:625–632.

24. **Colien, F. E.** 1935. A study of microbic variation in a yellow pigment-producing coccus. *J. Bacteriol.* **30**:301–321.

25. **Colwell, C. A.** 1946. Small colony variants of *Escherichia coli*. *J. Bacteriol.* **52**:417–422.

26. **Devriese, L. A.** 1973. Hemin-dependent mutants isolated from methicillin-resistant *Staphylococcus aureus* strains. *Antonie van Leeuwenhoek J. Microbiol. Serol.* **39**:33–40.

27. **Dworkin, R., G. Modin, S. Kunz, O. Rich, O. Zak, and M. Sande.** 1990. Comparative efficacies of ciprofloxacin, pefloxacin, and vancomycin in combination with rifampin in a rat model of methicillin-resistant *Staphylococcus aureus* chronic osteomyelitis. *Antimicrob. Agents Chemother.* **34**:1014–1016.

28. **Evans, D. J., D. G. Allison, M. R. W. Brown, and P. Gilbert.** 1991. Susceptibility of *Pseudomonas aeruginosa* and *Escherichia coli* biofilms toward ciprofloxacin: effect of specific growth rate. *J. Antimicrob. Chemother.* **27**:177–184.

29. **Fischer, W. (Institute for Biochemistry, University of Erlangen, Erlangen, Germany).** Personal communication.

30. **Goudie, J. G., and R. B. Goudie.** 1955. Recurrent infection by a stable dwarf-colony variant of *Staphylococcus aureus*. *J. Clin. Pathol.* **8**:284–287.

31. **Hadley, P., and H. Carapetian.** 1933. A study of the infective qualities possessed by G phase pleomorphism and filterability. *J. Bacteriol.* **25**:94–96.

32. **Hale, J. H.** 1947. Studies on staphylococcal mutation: characterization of the "G" (gonidial) variant and factors concerned in its production. *Br. J. Exp. Pathol.* **28**:202–210.

33. **Hale, J. H.** 1951. Studies on *Staphylococcus* mutation: a naturally occurring "G" gonidial variant and its carbon dioxide requirements. *Br. J. Exp. Pathol.* **32**:307–313.

34. **Henry, N. K., M. S. Rouse, A. L. Whitesell, M. E. McConnell, and W. R. Wilson.** 1987. Treatment of methicillin-resistant *Staphylococcus aureus* experimental osteomyelitis with ciprofloxacin or vancomycin alone or in combination with rifampin. *Am. J. Med.* **82**(Suppl. 4A):73–75.

35. **Hoffstadt, R. E., and G. P. Youmans.** 1932. *Staphylococcus aureus*: dissociation and its relation to infection and to immunity. *J. Infect. Dis.* **51**:216–242.

36. **Huddleson, I. F., and B. Baltzer.** 1952. The characteristics and dissociation pattern of type G (micro-colony type) of *Brucella arbortus*, p. 64–83. *Studies in Brucellosis, III. A Series of Five Papers*. Michigan State College, East Lansing, Mich.

37. **Jensen, J.** 1957. Biosynthesis of hematin compounds in a hemin requiring strain of *Micrococcus pyogenes* var. *aureus*. *J. Bacteriol.* **73**:324–333.

38. **Joyrce, G. H., and D. C. White.** 1971. Effects of benso(a)pyrene and piperonyl butoxide on formation of respiratory system, phospholipids, and carotenoids of *Staphylococcus aureus. J. Bacteriol.* **106:**403–411.

39. **Kaplan, M. L., and W. E. Dye.** 1976. Growth requirements of some small-colony-forming variants of *Staphylococcus aureus. J. Clin. Microbiol.* **4:**343–348.

40. **Kolle, W., and H. Hetsch.** 1911. *Die Experimentelle Bacteriologie und die Infectionskrankheiten mit Besonderer Berücksichtigung der Immunitätslehre,* 3rd ed., vol. 1. Urban und Schwarzenberg, Berlin.

41. **Koneman, E. W., S. D. Allen, V. R. Dowell, Jr., and H. M. Sommers.** 1979. *Color Atlas and Textbook of Diagnostic Microbiology,* 2nd ed., p. 264–265. J. B. Lippincott, Philadelphia.

42. **Kopeleff, N.** 1934. Dissociation and filtration of *Lactobacillus acidophilus. J. Infect. Dis.* **55:**368–389.

43. **Lacy, R. W.** 1969. Dwarf-colony variants of *Staphylococcus aureus* resistant to aminoglycoside antibiotics and to a fatty acid. *J. Med. Microbiol.* **2:**187–197.

44. **Lacy, R. W., and A. A. B. Mitchell.** 1969. Gentamicin-resistant *Staphylococcus aureus. Lancet* ii:1425–1426.

45. **Lewis, L. A., K. Li, M. Bharosay, M. Cannella, V. Jorgenson, R. Thomas, D. Pena, M. Velez, B. Pereira, and A. Sassine.** 1990. Characterization of gentamicin-resistant respiratory-deficient (Res⁻) variant strains of *Staphylococcus aureus. Microbiol. Immunol.* **34:**587–605.

46. **Li, K., J. J. Farmer III, and A. Coppola.** 1974. A novel type of resistant bacteria induced by gentamicin. *Trans. N.Y. Acad. Sci.* **36:**396–415.

47. **Miller, M. H., S. C. Edberg, L. J. Mandel, F. C. Behar, and N. H. Steigbigel.** 1980. Gentamicin uptake in wild type and aminoglycoside-resistant small colony mutants of *Staphylococcus aureus. Antimicrob. Agents Chemother.* **18:**722–729.

48. **Miller, M. H., M. A. Wexler, and N. H. Steigbigel.** 1978. Single and combination antibiotic therapy of *Staphylococcus aureus* experimental endocarditis: emergence of gentamicin mutants. *Antimicrob. Agents Chemother.* **14:**336–343.

49. **Morton, H. E., and J. Shoemaker.** 1945. The identification of *Neisseria gonorrhoeae* by means of bacterial variation and the detection of small colony forms in clinical material. *J. Bacteriol.* **50:**585–590.

50. **Musher, D. M., R. E. Baughn, G. B. Templeton, and J. N. Minuth.** 1977. Emergence of variant forms of *Staphylococcus aureus* after exposure to gentamicin and infectivity of the variants in experimental animals. *J. Infect. Dis.* **136:**360–369.

51. **Nydahl, B. C., and W. L. Hall.** 1965. The treatment of staphylococcal infection with nafcillin with a discussion of staphylococcal nephritis. *Ann. Intern. Med.* **63:**27–43.

52. **O'Rourke, S. V., J. F. Monthony, and D. T. Stitt.** 1991. A study of nutritional requirements of methicillin sensitive and resistant *Staphylococcus aureus* strain types. *Program Abstr. 31st Intersci. Conf. Antimicrob. Agents Chemother.,* abstr. 168.

53. **Padmanaban, G., V. Venkateswar, and P. N. Rangarajan.** 1989. Haem as a multifunctional regulator. *Trends Biochem. Sci.* **14:**492–496.

54. **Pelletier, L. L., Jr., M. Richardson, and M. Feist.** 1979. Virulent gentamicin-induced small colony variants of *Staphylococcus aureus. J. Lab. Clin. Med.* **94:**324–334.

55. **Proctor, R. A., P. van Langevelde, J. Maslow, M. Kristjansson, and R. Arbeit.** 1993. *Staphylococcus aureus* small colony variants can cause persistent and resistant infections. *Program Abstr. 33rd Intersci. Conf. Antimicrob. Agents Chemother.,* abstr. 1162.

56. **Quie, P. G.** 1969. Microcolonies (G variants) of *Staphylococcus aureus. Yale J. Biol. Med.* **41:**394–403.

57. **Sasarman, A., and T. Horodniceanu.** 1967. Locus determining normal colony formation on the chromosome of *Escherichia coli* K12. *J. Bacteriol.* **94:**1268–1269.

58. **Sasarman, A., K. E. Sanderson, M. Surdeanu, and S. Sonea.** 1970. Hemin-deficient mutants of *Salmonella typhimurium*. *J. Bacteriol.* **102:**531–536.

59. **Sasarman, A., M. Surdeanu, V. Portelance, R. Dobardzic, and S. Sorrea.** 1971. Classification of vitamin K-deficient mutants of *Staphylococcus aureus*. *J. Gen. Microbiol.* **65:** 125–130.

60. **Sasarman, A., M. Surdeanu, J. Sabados, V. Greceanu, and T. Horodniceanu.** 1968. Menaphthone requiring mutants of *Staphylococcus aureus*. *Rev. Can. Biol.* **23:**333–340.

61. **Schnitzer, R. J., L. J. Canagni, and M. Back.** 1943. Resistance of small colony variants (G forms) of a *Staphylococcus* toward the bacteriostatic activity of penicillin. *Proc. Soc. Exp. Biol. Med.* **53:**75–78.

62. **Shearer, M. J., P. T. McCarthy, O. E. Crampton, and M. B. Mattock.** 1987. The assessment of human vitamin K status from tissue measurements, p. 437–452. *In* J. W. Suttie (ed.), *Current Advances in Vitamin K Research*. Elsevier, New York.

63. **Sherris, J. C.** 1952. Two small colony variants of *Staphylococcus aureus* isolated in pure culture from closed infected lesions and their carbon dioxide requirements. *J. Clin. Pathol.* **5:**354–355.

64. **Short, S. A., D. C. White, and H. R. Kaback.** 1972. Active transport in isolated bacterial membrane vesicles. V. The transport of amino acids by membrane vesicles prepared from *Staphylococcus aureus*. *J. Biol. Chem.* **247:**298–304.

65. **Slifkin, M., L. P. Merkow, S. A. Kreuzberger, C. Engwall, and M. Pardo.** 1971. Characterization of CO_2 dependent microcolony variants of *Staphylococcus aureus*. *Am. J. Clin. Pathol.* **56:**584–592.

66. **Sompolinsky, D., M. Cohen, and G. Ziv.** 1974. Epidemiological studies on thiamineless dwarf-colony variants of *Staphylococcus aureus* as etiologic agents of bovine mastitis. *Infect. Immun.* **9:**217–228.

67. **Sompolinsky, D., Z. E. Geller, and S. Segal.** 1967. Metabolic disorders in thiamineless dwarf strains of *Staphylococcus aureus*. *J. Gen. Microbiol.* **48:**205–213.

68. **Spagna, V. A., R. J. Fass, R. B. Prior, and T. G. Slama.** 1978. Report of a case of bacterial sepsis caused by a naturally occurring variant form of *Staphylococcus aureus*. *J. Infect. Dis.* **138:**277–278.

69. **Swingle, E. L.** 1934. Studies on small colony variants of *Staphylococcus aureus*. *Proc. Soc. Exp. Biol. Med.* **31:**891–893.

70. **Swingle, E. L.** 1935. Studies on a small colony variant of *Staphylococcus aureus*. *J. Bacteriol.* **29:**467–490.

71. **Thomas, M. E. M., and J. H. Cowlard.** 1955. Studies on a CO_2-dependent *Staphylococcus*. *J. Clin. Pathol.* **8:**288–291.

72. **Tien, W., and D. C. White.** 1968. Linear sequential arrangement of genes of the biosynthetic pathway of protoheme in *Staphylococcus aureus*. *Proc. Natl. Acad. Sci. USA* **61:** 1392–1398.

72a. **Van Langevelde, P., and R. A. Procter.** Unpublished results.

73. **Vann, J. M., R. A. Proctor.** 1988. Cytotoxic effects of ingested *Staphylococcus aureus* on bovine endothelial cells: role of *S. aureus* α-hemolysin. *Microb. Pathog.* **4:**443–453.

74. **Vergères, P., and J. Blaser.** 1992. Amikacin, ceftazidime, and flucloxacillin against suspended and adherent *Pseudomonas aeruginosa* and *Staphylococcus epidermidis* in an in vitro model of infection. *J. Infect. Dis.* **165:**281–289.

75. **Weinberg, E. D.** 1950. Vitamin requirements of dwarf colony variants of bacteria. *J. Infect. Dis.* **87:**299–306.

76. **Widmer, A. F., A. Wiestner, R. Frei, and W. Zimmerli.** 1991. Killing of nongrowing and adherent *Escherichia coli* determines drug efficacy in device-related infections. *Antimicrob. Agents Chemother.* **35:**741–746.

77. **Wilson, S. G., and C. C. Sanders.** 1976. Selection and characterization of strains of *Staphylococcus aureus* displaying unusual resistance to aminoglycosides. *Antimicrob. Agents Chemother.* **10:**519–525.

78. **Wise, R. I.** 1956. Small colonies (G variants) of staphylococci: isolation from cultures and infections. *Ann. N.Y. Acad. Sci.* **65:**169–174.

79. **Wise, R. I., and W. W. Spink.** 1954. The influence of antibiotics on the origin of small colony (G variants) of *Micrococcus pyogenes* var. *aureus. J. Clin. Invest.* **33:**1611–1622.

80. **Yegian, D., G. Gallo, and M. W. Toll.** 1959. Kanamycin resistant staphylococcus mutants requiring hemin for growth. *J. Bacteriol.* **78:**10–12.

81. **Youmans, G. P.** 1937. Production of small colony variants of *Staphylococcus aureus. Proc. Soc. Exp. Biol. Med.* **36:**94–98.

82. **Youmans, G. P., and E. Delves.** 1942. The effect of inorganic salts on the production of small colony variants by *Staphylococcus aureus. J. Bacteriol.* **44:**127–136.

83. **Youmans, G. P., E. H. Williston, and M. Simon.** 1945. Production of small colony variants of *Staphylococcus aureus* by the action of penicillin. *Proc. Soc. Exp. Biol. Med.* **58:**56–57.

Infections Associated with Indwelling Medical Devices, 2nd ed.
Edited by Alan L. Bisno and Francis A. Waldvogel
© 1994 American Society for Microbiology, Washington, DC 20005

Chapter 5

Infections of Central Nervous System Shunts

Alan L. Bisno and Linda Sternau

For over four decades, neurosurgeons have inserted prosthetic devices within the central nervous system (CNS) for a variety of clinical indications. The most common usage by far has been to divert cerebrospinal fluid (CSF) in patients with hydrocephalus. Although ventricular fluid has been diverted to a number of other bodily sites (e.g., gallbladder, pleura, and ureter), at present virtually all CSF shunts are either ventriculojugular (atrial; VA) or ventriculoperitoneal (VP). On occasions when the need for decompression is judged to be acute and self-limited, an external ventricular drainage system may be utilized.

A second major indication for the insertion of a CNS prosthetic device is to continuously monitor intracranial pressure (ICP) in patients who have experienced a variety of acute cerebral insults or who have intracerebral mass lesions. These devices, which include subarachnoid screws, intraventricular catheters, and cup catheters, are usually inserted for a relatively limited time period. Intraventricular (ventriculostomy) catheters may also be therapeutic in temporarily lowering the ICP by removing small amounts of CSF.

Indwelling CNS reservoirs are employed for the administration of therapeutic agents that penetrate the blood-brain barrier poorly and which, when given systemically in requisite dosages, cause unacceptable organ damage. Such intraventricular therapy is employed on occasion for the treatment of a limited number of CNS neoplasms and infections.

Infection is the foremost complication of CSF shunt implantation.

Alan L. Bisno and Linda Sternau • Veterans Affairs Medical Center and University of Miami School of Medicine, Miami, Florida 33125.

Such infections are of particular concern because of the threat that they pose to cerebral function. CSF shunt infections may lead to meningitis, ventriculitis, ventricular compartmentalization, and cortical mantle thinning as well as subdural empyema and seizures. Shunt infections have been shown to be the single complication that correlates with mental retardation and deterioration of mental capacity (36). The treatment of shunt infections requires extension of the hospital stay by 2 or 3 weeks and additional surgery. CNS infections can also be especially lethal to the immunocompromised host.

Shunt infections, as well as the resultant morbidity and mortality, have substantially decreased over the past three decades. Infection rates have been reported as high as 31% (25, 32, 34, 40). However, most series in the last decade report rates of 1 to 10% (12, 14, 39, 43, 49, 55). Many factors have been associated with increased risk of infection, including the age of patient, etiology of hydrocephalus, the type of shunt implanted, and the surgeon's experience. Other factors that have been suggested include the timing of operation, duration of surgery, number of people in the operating room, and the skin and shunt material preparation.

Most of the reported series of CSF shunt infections are of infant and pediatric populations, as the majority of devices are placed or revised for congenital hydrocephalus. Within this group, it is clear that infants under 6 months of age experience rates of infection that are two to three times greater than those observed in older children. The infection rate may be even higher in the myelomeningocele patient requiring a shunt in the first week of life. Ammirati and Raimondi (3) found a 48% infection rate in those patients shunted in the first week compared with 24% in the second to eighth weeks after birth. Likewise, premature infants with intraventricular hemorrhage (IVH) have by far the highest shunt infection rate (3).

A higher incidence of shunt infection has also been found in the geriatric population. In a 25-year experience, George et al. (18) reported that persons 60 years of age and older had a higher incidence of shunt infections (16.7%) than did other adults (6.8%) or infants (13.6%). They also found that about 80% of infections occurred within 1 month of surgery.

It is unclear whether the infection rate varies among the types of shunt (VA, VP, ventriculoureteral, or ventriculopleural). What is clear is that the manifestations of infections of these various shunt types are very different and that some are more significant than others. The complication of "shunt nephritis" following septicemia with a VA shunt, for example, has led most neurosurgeons today to use the peritoneum as their first choice for distal placement.

The highest risk of infection occurs in shunt reinsertion after a previous infection. This may represent a relapse of the original infection because of either inadequate treatment or a residual vegetative source that reinoculates the system. Alternatively, a new pathogen may be introduced via the external CSF drainage system. Moreover, a variety of local anatomic or systemic immunologic abnormalities may predispose an individual patient to reinfection.

Infections also complicate the external ventricular drainage systems utilized for ICP monitoring. Aucoin et al. (5) studied 255 patients undergoing ICP monitoring for a variety of disorders, including intracerebral hemorrhage, open and closed trauma, and tumors. Infections observed included ventriculomeningitis, osteomyelitis, and wound suppuration. There was an overall infection rate of 11%, compared with a rate of 6% in patients undergoing craniotomy alone. The infection rate was 7.5% in patients with a subarachnoid screw, 14.9% in patients with a subdural cup catheter, and 21.9% in patients with an intraventricular (ventriculostomy) catheter. The great majority of infections observed with the last device were ventriculomeningitis. Mayhall et al. (33) undertook a prospective epidemiologic study of ventriculostomy-related ventriculitis or meningitis in 172 consecutive neurosurgical patients between April 1979 and June 1981. The rate of infection was 11%. Risk factors for infection included neurosurgical operations, ICP of 20 mm Hg or more, and ventricular catheterization for more than 5 days. Both intracerebral hemorrhage and irrigation of the intracranial catheter predisposed to the development of infection associated with pressure monitors (6, 33).

ETIOLOGY AND PATHOGENESIS

The bacteria responsible for most shunt infections are commensal organisms with low virulence. The organisms most frequently causing infections of indwelling CNS prostheses are the coagulase-negative staphylococci. The majority of these are likely to be *Staphylococcus epidermidis*, although it is not clear in many reports whether modern methods of taxonomy (22), which differentiate more than two dozen species of coagulase-negative staphylococci, were employed. The second most frequent pathogen is *Staphylococcus aureus*. A variety of other gram-positive organisms, including viridans streptococci, *Streptococcus pyogenes*, enterococci, corynebacteria, and propionibacteria, may be involved. Less frequently, *Haemophilus influenzae* and gram-negative enteric bacteria (*Esche-*

richia coli, Klebsiella spp., and a variety of others [48]) may be the culprits. Infection with gram-negative bacilli has been observed somewhat more frequently in patients with ventriculoureteral or lumboureteral shunts. Gram-negative species are also more common in VP shunts when there is compromise of the intestinal integrity. This is occasionally seen following percutaneous trochar placement of peritoneal ends.

The factors responsible for infections of CNS prosthetic devices are poorly defined. Several observations, however, buttress the impression that most such infections are due to the implantation of the organism at the time of surgery or to the contamination of the device by ward personnel during manipulation. These observations include the facts that most infections occur within the first few weeks after surgery, that irrigation of the system is a risk factor for infection of intracranial monitors, and that the most frequent pathogens are common skin flora.

The predominant role of coagulase-negative staphylococci in CNS prosthetic infections undoubtedly relates to their ecologic niche as a major constituent of normal cutaneous flora. There may, however, be certain biologic properties of these organisms that equip them particularly well for infection at this site. Much has been written in this volume of the extracellular slime substance of *S. epidermidis* (see chapters 2 and 3). The potential clinical relevance of this substance was first commented upon by Bayston and Penny (8), who noted excessive production of a "mucoid substance" in coagulase-negative staphylococci isolated from CNS Holter shunts. Two reports suggest that bacterial adherence properties or elaboration of slime may be important factors in the persistence of intracranial foreign body infections due to coagulase-negative staphylococci. Younger et al. (59) studied 85 strains of coagulase-negative staphylococci isolated from CNS shunts, of which 51 were believed to represent pathogens and 34 were believed to represent contaminants. The strains were assayed spectrophotometrically for their ability to adhere to tissue culture plates and were then classified as adherent or nonadherent by defined criteria. Adherent strains comprised a significantly higher proportion of isolates from true infections than from contamination. Moreover, infections due to nonadherent organisms were significantly more likely to be cured by antibiotics alone (without removal of the colonized shunt) than were infections due to adherent organisms. Diaz-Mitoma et al. (13) found that obstruction of VP shunts and failure to cure the infections by antibiotics alone were both more frequent when infectious episodes were due to slime-producing coagulase-negative staphylococci.

These studies are in accord with the general clinical experience that staphylocccal infections cannot usually be treated in situ with antibiotics alone but require replacement of the shunt. This is likely due, at least in part, to the role of glycocalyceal material in protecting bacteria from host defenses and antimicrobial agents. Perhaps assays of glycocalyx production might provide insight into those infections that could be managed more conservatively. At present, however, there exist neither the standardized techniques for quantitatively measuring slime production at a clinically useful level nor the prospective data to support such an approach.

CLINICAL MANIFESTATIONS

The manifestations of CNS shunt infections are highly variable. The most common presentation is a nonspecific one consisting of fever, nausea, vomiting, malaise, or signs of increased ICP (47). The last suggests obstruction or malfunction of the shunt. In the majority of cases these symptoms appear within a few weeks to months of insertion. Erythema along the shunt tract or obvious wound infection may also be evident, generally in patients who develop their infections in the immediate postoperative period. Although photophobia may be present, classic signs of meningeal irritation are present in no more than one-third of VP and VA shunt infections (47). This is because in patients with obstructive hydrocephalus, CSF cannot pass into the subarachnoid space, and even in patients with communicating hydrocephalus, the placement of a shunt may lead eventually to functional closure of the aqueduct of Sylvius (24).

In patients with VP shunts, an inflammatory exudate may lead to loculation of CSF, resulting in the formation of a peritoneal cyst (40). These cysts are often palpable in infants and are visualized by ultrasonography (Fig. 1) or computed tomography. The cysts may be sterile, but when their presence is coupled with fever or other symptoms indicative of infection, the VP shunt should be considered a possible focus. In some instances infections of VP shunts present with signs and symptoms indicative of acute peritonitis. The signs may be generalized, or if the infection is restricted to a loculated cyst, they may be localized.

At times, patients infected with organisms representative of normal skin flora, such as coagulase-negative staphylococci and *Propionibacterium* spp. (anaerobic or aerotolerant diphtheroids), may pursue an extremely indolent clinical course. Such patients may exhibit only intermittent low-grade fever and malaise with little or no change in spinal fluid cell count, glucose, or protein. Under such circumstances the physician must be careful to differentiate CNS shunt infections from intercurrent viral or bacterial infections of the upper respiratory, urinary, or gastroin-

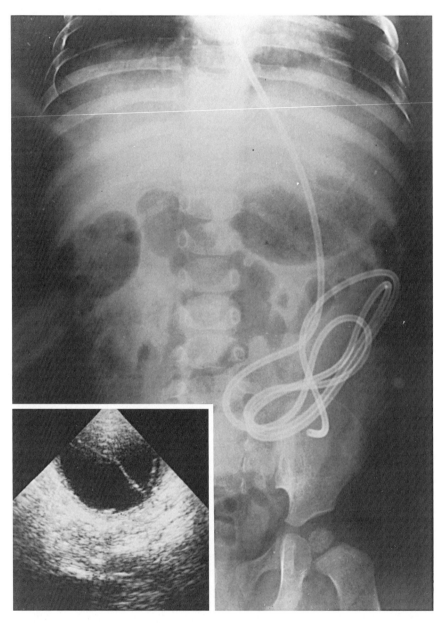

Figure 1. Peritoneal cyst in an 11-month-old hydrocephalic infant with a malfunction of a ventriculoperitoneal shunt. The X ray shows the distal tip of the shunt catheter coiled in the left lower quadrant of the abdomen. The sonogram (inset) demonstrates that the catheter is contained within an echo-free, cystic mass. (Courtesy of Thomas F. Boulden, LeBonheur Children's Medical Center, Memphis, Tenn.)

testinal tract. Occasional patients with ventriculovascular shunts, but not those with shunts to the peritoneum or other sites, develop a form of acute glomerulonephritis known as "shunt nephritis." In nearly all of these cases the infecting organism has been *S. epidermidis*, although occasional instances have been due to corynebacteria and listerias. The condition is characterized clinically by fever, edema, malaise, hepatosplenomegaly, hypocomplementemia, anemia, azotemia, hematuria, and proteinuria (10). Pathological findings consist of mesangial hypercellularity and granular deposits of immunoglobulins and complement along the glomerular membrane. These findings, considered characteristic of immune complex glomerulonephritis, are presumably due to the continuous bacteremia associated with VA shunt infections.

Infections of ICP-monitoring devices often occur in patients with altered sensorium. As is the case in CNS shunt infections, signs of meningeal irritation are not usually present; therefore, fever is the most frequent indication of the presence of infection. Clinical diagnosis is further complicated, however, by the fact that these patients are often critically ill and have many other potential sources of nosocomial and community-acquired infection.

The diagnosis of infections associated with indwelling CNS prostheses is dependent primarily upon culture of CSF from the system itself. In the case of CNS shunts, fluid should be obtained for Gram stain and culture directly from the shunt reservoir. In indolent infections in which the initial Gram stain is nondiagnostic, fluid should be cultured anaerobically as well as aerobically. Some indolent organisms, especially diphtheroids, may be fastidious and require more than 3 days for growth. Blood cultures are nearly always positive in patients with VA shunts who have not had recent antibiotics, but such cultures are positive in a minority of patients with VP shunts. Urine cultures are revealing in patients with ventriculoureteral or lumboureteral shunts but not otherwise. Leukocytosis in the peripheral blood and pleocytosis, hypoglycorrhachia, and markedly increased protein concentration in the CSF are helpful confirmatory findings. As indicated previously, these abnormalities are often mild or absent entirely.

MANAGEMENT OF INFECTIONS

Details of the management of infections associated with CNS shunts are complex, depending as they do on the nature of the shunt (usually VP or VA), the infecting organism and its antimicrobial susceptibility, the severity of the clinical manifestations, the age of the patient (open or closed fontanelles), and the urgency of maintaining continuous access to the ventricular system. Furthermore, there are few controlled studies, and experienced clinicians hold widely differing opinions. With these caveats, the following general guidelines seem to be reasonable.

Upon clinical suspicion of the occurrence of a CNS shunt infection, attempts should be made to arrive at a specific microbiologic diagnosis by culture and Gram stain of CSF obtained from the shunt reservoir and from any local area of purulence and by culture of blood. A shunt tap, or sample from an external ventriculostomy, should be performed with the utmost attention paid to sterile technique. This should generally be performed by a neurosurgeon or physician who is familiar with the technique and underlying hardware. In the febrile patient with remote shunt surgery, other potential sources of infection should be ruled out as completely as possible prior to performing a shunt tap. This avoids the risk of contaminating the shunt system in a bacteremic patient.

When performing a percutaneous needle tap, the area around the shunt reservoir is shaved, and the surrounding hair should be taped out of the way. The scalp area is prepared using povidone-iodine solution followed by alcohol and then draped. A 21-gauge butterfly needle or Huber needle is placed into the reservoir (or valve if no reservoir is present). An opening and closing pressure should be recorded with a manometer. CSF sample aliquots should be allowed to drip into sterile vials. Aspiration of CSF should be discouraged to avoid debris being pulled into the ventriculostomy catheter. If only 1 ml of CSF can be obtained, it should be reserved for Gram stain, culture, and sensitivity testing. If additional fluid is obtained, it can be used for a cell count with differential and determination of CSF glucose and protein.

Cultures should be held for 7 days. Antibiotic therapy should also be instituted, and this is usually administered intravenously and often intraventricularly via the shunt. When definitive clinical or laboratory evidence of infection is obtained, one of the major and immediate decisions to be made is whether to remove the infected shunt. Removal obviously extirpates a critical nidus of infection but also eliminates a convenient route for intraventricular administration of antimicrobial agents and leaves the hydrocephalic patient subject to the dangers of increased ICP. In practice, there are the following three options: (i) remove the shunt, utilize an external ventricular drainage device or ventricular taps for decompression (and, if desired, for antibiotic administration), and institute systemic antibiotics; (ii) remove the infected shunt, replace it immediately with a new indwelling device, and institute systemic (and, if desired, intraventricular) antibiotics; and (iii) leave the shunt in place and treat with systemic (with or without intraventricular) antibiotics. James et al. (25) treated 10 patients by each of these strategies. The patients were children ranging in age from 2 months to 7.5 years with hydrocephalus of various etiologies, and all had shunts which drained into the peritoneal cavity. All patients received antibiotics both intravenously and intraventricularly. Clinical and bacteriologic cures were achieved in all 20 patients in group i, 9 of 10 in group ii, but only 3 of 10 in group iii. The mean durations of hospitalization were 24.7 ± 17, 32.7 ± 8, and 47 ± 37 days for groups A, B, and C, respectively.

A large number of studies have now been reported in which one or more of these strategies have been utilized (Table 1). Obviously, pooling of studies conducted at different times and places by different investigators using various patient populations and clinical protocols is fraught

Table 1. Shunt infection cure rates with various therapeutic modalities[a]

Reference	No. cured/no. treated		
	Antibiotics alone without shunt removal	Antibiotics and immediate replacement with a new shunt	Antibiotics and shunt removal, insertion of EVD,[b] or repeated ventricular aspirates
Schoenbaum et al. (47)	5/28		25/26
Odio et al. (39)	10/13		46/46
Salmon (45)		5/10	
Sells et al. (48)	1/8	1/6	9/9
James et al. (26)	3/10	9/10	10/10
Venes (52)		6/9	3/3
Perrin and McLaurin (41)		6/6	
James et al. (25)	4/11	11/13	16/17
Wald and McLaurin (53)	15/20		
Mates et al. (32)	6/7		
Shurtleff et al. (50)	2/26	6/22	19/19
Morrice and Young (37)	4/14	19/23	14/18
Nicholas et al. (38)		21/27	
Frame and McLaurin (17)	8/11		
Forward et al. (15)	8/15		13/13
Schimke et al. (46)	4/11		
Luthardt (30)	1/17		
Callaghan et al. (11)	0/4		
Walters et al. (55)	20/48	30/35	24/32
Younger et al. (59)	4/11		34/34
Total (success rate)	95/254 (37)[c]	114/161 (71)	213/227 (94)

[a] Modified from Yogev (57) with permission.
[b] EVD, Extraventricular device.
[c] Numbers within parentheses indicate percentages.

with hazard. Nevertheless, it is impressive that 94% of the 227 infections treated with shunt removal and insertion of an external drainage device or repeated ventricular taps were cured, compared with 71% of 161 infections treated with immediate shunt replacement. Poor results (37% cure rate) were achieved in the 254 infections in which shunts were left in place. Given these data, the first strategy is recommended for most patients with CNS shunt infections. The second alternative, removal of the shunt with immediate replacement, may be more appropriate for certain patients, such as infants or uncooperative patients who might dislodge or contaminate an external system, or patients who require simultaneous drainage of more than one CSF-containing cavity (24).

Are there any patients in whom the catheter might be left in place? In patients with extremely low-grade infections—judged by mild clinical symptomatology and modest derangement of CSF values, some authorities may begin a trial of systemic and intraventricular antibiotics, recognizing that it will be successful in only a minority of cases. In this circumstance it is mandatory to follow closely the clinical course and CSF Gram stain, culture, and cell counts of the patient. Unless the cultures become sterile promptly and remain so and all other indicators suggest continued improvement, the shunt should be removed. It has been suggested (32), on the basis of quite limited data, that infections occurring early in the postoperative period might be more amenable to treatment with antimicrobial agents alone. Data reviewed above (13, 59) suggest that shunt infections caused by coagulase-negative staphylococci that fail to exude measurable amounts of slime or to adhere well to tissue culture plates might be more readily cured without removal of the prosthetic device. This concept, however, remains a subject for future research.

Another alternative, which has become more popular in treatment of infections of VP shunts, is externalizing the distal end of the peritoneal shunt (35). This technique offers several advantages including (i) a single surgical procedure, (ii) ready access for CSF sampling, (iii) diversion of infected CSF out of the CNS, and (iv) maintained CSF flow with a valve still proximal, to prevent CSF overdrainage.

Using local anesthesia, a small incision is made over the distal shunt catheter on the chest wall and attached to a closed external drainage bag. While externalized, CSF cultures are obtained until the CSF is again sterile. Thereafter, surveillance CSF cultures are obtained twice a week to be certain the CSF is negative before a new shunt is inserted. Usually 7 to 10 days is sufficient, with appropriate intravenous antibiotic coverage and external CSF drainage. The new shunt is generally placed at a distant site. If the patient had significant peritonitis, it may be best to place the new shunt into the atrium. The old system is then removed, and antibiotics are continued for 24 h and then stopped.

The choice of antimicrobial therapy must be individualized, depending upon the clinical appearance of the patient, CSF findings, and local patterns of antimicrobial susceptibility. If the patient does not appear to be acutely ill, the initial Gram stain of CSF fails to reveal microorganisms, and abnormalities in the spinal fluid concentrations of neutrophils, protein, and glucose are modest, therapy may be initiated with antistaphylococcal antibiotics. Penicillinase-resistant penicillins, such as oxacillin, or cephalosporins that penetrate the blood-brain barrier in the presence of inflammation (e.g., cefuroxime, ceftriaxone) may be employed. The latter would also be effective against many strains of gram-negative enteric bacilli (e.g., *E. coli* and *Klebsiella* spp.). Neither penicillinase-resistant penicillins nor cephalosporins will be effective, however, against methicillin-resistant strains of coagulase-negative staphylococci and *S. aureus*, which are becoming increasingly prevalent nosocomial pathogens. In institutions wherein such bacteria are known to be common causes of shunt infections, it is prudent to initiate therapy with vancomycin while awaiting bacteriologic data. Sulfamethoxazole-trimethoprim (SXT) and rifampin are also effective in vitro against many strains of methicillin-resistant staphylococci. The former may be given orally or intravenously and the latter may be given orally, and both penetrate well into the CSF. These agents may at times be useful as ancillary therapy. Rifampin in particular has been used successfully in combination with other agents, at least in anecdotal case reports (19, 44). This is analogous to the use of rifampin in prosthetic valve endocarditis due to coagulase-negative staphylococci. The drug must not be used as a single agent because of the rapid development of resistance. Many strains of methicillin-resistant staphylococci are also susceptible in vitro to ciprofloxacin and other quinolones.

A wide variety of choices is available for the systemic treatment of gram-negative infections. A number of the newer expanded-spectrum cephalosporins (e.g., cefuroxime, cefotaxime, ceftriaxone, ceftazidine) achieve therapeutic concentrations in CSF after intravenous administration in patients with inflamed meninges. There has been experience with intraventricular administration of a number of "gram-negative" antibiotics, including cephalothin, cefazolin, gentamicin, and amikacin. Experience with intraventricular administration of the newer cephalosporins is, however, limited.

Once the infected shunt has been removed, might not systemic antibiotics alone be adequate for cure of the infection? There is a paucity of data addressing this point in the literature. Some authorities are content to use systemic antibiotics alone, providing the patient is pursuing a benign clinical course. Others, however, prefer to treat CNS shunt infections with both systemic and intraventricular antibiotics because of patient-to-patient variability in antibiotic concentrations achieved in CSF after intravenous therapy alone. This is particularly true for individuals who might have inflammation or scarring of the choroid plexus and ependyma as a result of their underlying cerebral diseases. Moreover, aminoglycosides and a number of the cephalosporins do not adequately penetrate the blood-brain barrier, even in the presence of inflammation.

The use of intraventricular antibiotics is not without hazard. There is considerable variability in intraventricular concentrations achieved after standard dosages (27). Attainment of excessively high intraventricular antimicrobial levels has been associated with neurotoxicity, both in experimental animals (21) and in humans (16). CNS toxicity associated with antibiotic preservative has been reported. Therefore, preservative-free gentamicin or vancomycin is generally recommended (30). There is considerable variation in the doses of intraventricular antibiotics employed by different groups. Intraventricular dosages of some of the more commonly used beta-lactam and aminoglycoside antibiotics have been recommended by James (24) and by Kaufman and McLone (28). For vancomycin, McLaurin and Frame (35) recommend total daily doses of 10 mg for newborns and 20 mg for children. Data on the pharmacokinetics of intraventricular vancomycin are extremely scanty (20, 42). Reesor et al. (42) recommend starting with an empiric dose of 8 to 10 mg. Hirsch et al. (20), however, noted a peak CSF vancomycin level of 80.6 μg/ml 2 h after an initial instillation of 7.5 mg into an Ommaya reservoir. Arroyo and Quindlen (4) gave 10 mg of intraventricular vancomycin for 10 days to an adult patient and documented a marked accumulation of the drug in the CSF (606 μg/ml). It is thus highly advisable to monitor CSF levels of antibiotics administered intraventricularly.

In patients treated with shunt removal and insertion of an external drainage device and in whom clinical and microbiologic response is optimal, intravenous and, if elected, intraventricular therapy should continue for a minimum of 7 days. Intraventricular antibiotics should be administered every 24 h. If spinal fluid and blood cultures collected 48 h after discontinuance of antibiotics are sterile, the CNS shunt may be replaced. There is also the occasional patient in whom the shunt is removed and is no longer required. This may be due to a decreased CSF production following infection or a recovery of CSF absorption after the initial instillation of the shunt. These rare patients need to be monitored with serial CT scans to be certain that the hydrocephalus does not recur. In patients treated with the removal of the infected shunt and reinsertion of a new shunt in the same operation, 3 weeks of intravenous and 2 weeks of twice-daily intrashunt antibiotics are recommended (24).

The principles enunciated above for the management of CNS shunt infections apply as well to infections associated with ICP-monitoring devices. That is, the infecting device should be removed and appropriate antibiotic therapy should be instituted. Systemic therapy alone is adequate for the treatment of infections associated with devices placed in a subdural location unless a subdural empyema forms. In the case of ventriculostomy infections, the reinsertion of an external device in a separate site for intraventricular antibiotic administration may be necessary (24). Occasionally, the patient may have positive CSF cultures but a minimal CSF pleocytosis, which may reflect colonization of the catheter. Removal of the catheter and several days of antibiotics may be successful alone.

ANTIMICROBIAL PROPHYLAXIS

The use of antimicrobial agents in the perioperative period in the hope of preventing infection has become standard for patients receiving prosthetic heart valves or hips. Numerous studies have been published that purport to evaluate the utility of antimicrobial agents in preventing infections associated with CNS shunts (1, 2, 6, 7, 12, 18, 23, 29, 31, 34, 45, 54, 56, 57, 61). Unfortunately, the studies have often been uncontrolled and retrospective. Moreover, it has been difficult for any one group to assemble enough patients to obtain definitive results, given the fact that the current rate of shunt infections in most centers is below 10%. Such data as do exist are conflicting. Only a few selected studies will be mentioned here. Yogev et al., in a report published only in abstract form (58), randomized 190 pediatric patients undergoing placement of VP shunts to receive either nafcillin (50 mg/kg every 6 h for five doses), the same regimen plus rifampin (10 mg/kg every 12 h for three doses), or a saline placebo. Prophylaxis was started 13 h preoperatively, and patients were followed for at least 6 months. Shunt infections developed in 6 of 84 (7.1%) patients in the placebo group versus 2 of 106 (1.9%) in the two treatment groups ($P = 0.07$). Although the results did not achieve the generally accepted level of statistical significance, they were intriguing and suggested that a larger study might be necessary to settle the issue.

Two other studies examined the efficacy of SXT prophylaxis and reached opposite conclusions. Wang et al. (56) randomized 120 children undergoing VP shunt surgery at the Hospital for Sick Children, Toronto,

Ontario, Canada, to receive either a placebo or SXT (5 mg of trimethoprim per kg in combination with 25 mg of sulfamethoxazole per kg intravenously during the hour preceding surgery and 8 and 16 h postoperatively). Although the mean period of follow-up was 11 months, some patients without complications were followed for as little as 1 month. Shunt infections occurred in 4 of 55 (7.3%) recipients of SXT and in 5 of 65 (7.6%) controls. Thus, the authors concluded that perioperative prophylaxis with SXT was ineffectual. Blomstedt (9) likewise conducted a randomized, double-blind trial of SXT in patients undergoing shunting operations or ventriculostomy at the University Central Hospital, Helsinki, Finland. A total of 122 patients undergoing VA shunts were randomly assigned to receive either a placebo or SXT intravenously. The active drug was given as an infusion of 160 mg of trimethoprim and 400 mg of sulfamethoxazole at the time of arrival in the operating room and every 12 h thereafter for three doses. Patients who had undergone an external ventriculostomy received either a placebo or a dose of SXT every 12 h until the drainage tube was removed and then three additional doses. Among patients receiving VA shunts, 14 of 60 patients developed infections, while only 4 of 62 antibiotic recipients were infected ($P <$ 0.01). Among the 52 patients undergoing ventriculostomy only, there were no significant differences in infection rates between the SXT and placebo groups, but these devices were usually in place for only a day, and only one infection was observed in each treatment group.

As regards the data on efficacy of SXT prophylaxis for CNS shunt infections, it should be pointed out that there were certain major differences between the Toronto and Helsinki studies. The Toronto study included only VP shunts, and most patients were in the first decade of life. Indeed, one-third of the patients were less than 1 year of age. In contrast, the Helsinki study involved only VA shunts, and patients less than 12 years of age were excluded from participation. Follow-up in the Helsinki study was for a minimum of 6 months, while some patients in Toronto had a rather brief follow-up. In both studies the definition of infection appeared to depend upon positive bacteriologic cultures, although the clinical symptomatology prompting those cultures was either vaguely described (56) or completely omitted (9). An aspect of the Finnish study worth noting was the high infection rate (23%) in the placebo group.

In a more recently published study, Walters et al. (54) compared rifampin-trimethoprim prophylaxis to placebo in a prospective, randomized trial involving 243 patients undergoing 300 CSF shunting procedures. Although there was a lower infection rate in the antibiotic recipients (12% versus 19%), the results were not conclusive because of the higher than expected incidence of infection in both groups.

Two brief reports detail retrospective analyses of experiences with vancomycin prophylaxis. One group (60) analyzed experiences before and after the institution of a single 5-mg intraventricular injection of vancomycin at the time of surgery for insertion of VP shunts. The second group (51) compared infection rates at their institution in children receiving vancomycin prophylaxis for neurosurgical shunt procedures and in those who did not receive such medication. The prophylactic regimen consisted of an intrathecal dose of 10 mg given during the operation and intravenous doses given 4 and 6 h after the operation. However, there were only 14 patients in the no-prophylaxis group. Neither of these retrospective analyses found that intravenous vancomycin prophylaxis was beneficial. However, they were neither prospective, randomized, nor controlled, and one of the studies had too few untreated patients to allow any conclusions to be drawn. Bayston et al. (7) did attempt a prospective study of vancomycin prophylaxis. Half of the 158 patients were randomized to receive 10 mg of vancomycin into the ventricular system during hydrocephalus shunt surgery. The number of infections observed in both treatment and control groups, however, was too small to allow assessment of efficacy.

An intriguing approach has been taken by Choux et al. (12), who suggest that a "team approach" surgical protocol, with only one dose of antibiotics, reduced their shunt infection rate from 7.75% to 1.04%. This protocol emphasizes the surgical preparation and technique: in the preoperative period they recommend a careful evaluation of the general medical condition and skin integrity, with no shaving except in older children. In the operating room (OR), shunts should be done early in the day before any other neurosurgical cases, neonates should be treated before older children, and no more than four shunts should be placed per day. The operation should take 20 to 40 min and only four people should be allowed in the OR: the surgeon, assistant, anesthesiologist, and circulating nurse—no scrub nurse. The surgeon should be an experienced shunt surgeon. The shunt material should be opened only at the last moment, and the valve should not be tested. They recommend only two skin incisions and a quality skin closure. Although prophylactic antibiotics (oxacillin) were given 30 min prior to skin incision and the shunt materials were rinsed in gentamicin prior to implantation, the contribution of such prophylaxis to the low infection rate is unknown.

This protocol underscores an important surgical principle that less operating room time, less OR staff and traffic, and less manipulation of the foreign body implanted into the body provide the best means of prevention of shunt infection. The authors recommend using an iodine-impregnated adhesive plastic drape (3 MI obon drape) and handling all shunt materials with instruments (rather than with hands) to decrease the chance of skin flora contamination. This no-touch technique has long been advocated by Venes (52), who was a pioneer in the prevention of shunt infections.

The reports cited illustrate the current perplexity in the medical literature over the efficacy of prophylaxis. At present, one can only conclude that there is no scientifically valid, independently confirmed body of evidence to indicate that any particular prophylactic regimen is effective in preventing infections associated with CNS shunts.

SUMMARY AND CONCLUSIONS

There has been a marked lowering of the incidence of infections associated with the insertion of indwelling CNS prosthetic devices over the past 30 years, presumably as a result of improvements in technique and materials. Nevertheless, infection remains a significant hazard for patients requiring these devices. Most infections are due to gram-positive cocci, particularly *S. epidermidis,* and occur within the first few weeks to months after implantation. The clinical presentation can be quite variable, depending upon the nature of the prosthetic device, the age and condition of the patient, and the infecting microorganism. Both accurate diagnosis and appropriate treatment depend upon the isolation and identification of the infecting organism, which is usually most readily isolated from the device itself. In most instances cure of the infection requires removal of the infecting device (or, in VP shunts, externalization of the distal end) plus appropriate antimicrobial therapy. However, well-designed, controlled trials of various forms of management are lacking. Likewise, only a few of the numerous reports of antimicrobial prophylaxis for infections of CNS shunts meet generally agreed-upon criteria for an acceptable clinical trial. At present, the efficacy of such prophylaxis remains to be determined.

REFERENCES

1. **Ajir, F., A. B. Levin, and T. A. Duff.** 1981. Effect of prophylactic methicillin on cerebrospinal fluid shunt infections in children. *Neurosurgery* **9:**6–8.
2. **Alvarez-Garijo, J. A., and M. V. Mengual.** 1982. Infection rate with and without prophylactic antibiotic therapy after shunt insertion for hydrocephalus. *Monogr. Neural Sci.* **8:**66–68.
3. **Ammirati, M., and A. J. Raimondi.** 1987. Cerebrospinal fluid shunt infections in children. *Child's Nerv. Syst.* **3:**106–109.

4. Arroyo, J. C., and E. A. Quindlen. 1983. Accumulation of vancomycin after intraventricular infusions. *South. Med. J.* **76:**1554–1555.

5. Aucoin, P. J., H. R. Kotilainen, N. M. Gantz, R. Davidson, P. Kellogg, and B. Stone. 1986. Intracranial pressure monitors: epidemiologic study of risk factors and infections. *Am. J. Med.* **80:**369–376.

6. Bayston, R. 1975. Antibiotic prophylaxis in shunt surgery. *Dev. Med. Child Neurol.* **17**(Suppl. 35):99–103.

7. Bayston, R., C. Bannister, V. Boston, R. Burman, B. Burns, F. Cooke, R. Cooke, R. Cudmore, R. Fitzgerald, C. Goldberg, et al. 1990. A prospective randomized controlled trial of antimicrobial prophylaxis in hydrocephalus shunt surgery. *Z. Kinderchir.* **45**(Suppl. 1):5–7.

8. Bayston, R., and S. R. Penny. 1972. Excessive production of mucoid substance in *Staphylococcus* SIIA: a possible factor in colonization of Holter shunts. *Dev. Med. Child Neurol.* **14**(Suppl. 27):25–28.

9. Blomstedt, G. C. 1985. Results of trimethoprim-sulfamethoxazole prophylaxis in ventriculostomy and shunting procedures: a double-blind randomized trial. *J. Neurosurg.* **62:**694–697.

10. Bolton, W. K., M. A. Sande, D. E. Normansell, B. C. Sturgill, and F. B. Westervelt, Jr. 1975. Ventriculojugular shunt nephritis with *Corynebacterium bovis*. Successful therapy with antibiotics. *Am. J. Med.* **59:**417–423.

11. Callaghan, R. P., S. J. Cohen, and G. T. Stewart. 1961. Septicemia due to colonization of Spitz-Holter valves by staphylococci: five cases treated with methicillin. *Br. Med. J.* **5229:**860–863.

12. Choux, M., L. Genitori, D. Lang, and G. Lena. 1992. Shunt implantation: reducing the incidence of shunt infection. *J. Neurosurg.* **77:**875–880.

13. Diaz-Mitoma, F., G. K. Hardin, D. J. Hoban, R. S. Roberts, and D. E. Low. 1987. Clinical significance of a test for slime production in ventriculoperitoneal shunt infections caused by coagulase-negative staphylococci. *J. Infect. Dis.* **156:**555–560.

14. Erashin, Y., D. G. McLone, B. B. Storrs, and R. Yogev. 1989. Review of 3,017 procedures for the management of hydrocephalus in children. *Concepts Pediatr. Neurosurg.* **9:**21–28.

15. Forward, K. R., H. D. Fewer, and H. G. Stiver. 1983. Cerebrospinal fluid shunt infections: a review of 35 infections in 32 patients. *J. Neurosurg.* **59:**389–394.

16. Fossieck, B., Jr., and R. H. Parker. 1974. Neurotoxicity during intravenous infusion of penicillin: a review. *J. Clin. Pharmacol.* **14:**504–512.

17. Frame, P. T., and R. L. McLaurin. 1984. Treatment of CSF shunt infections with intrashunt plus oral antibiotic therapy. *J. Neurosurg.* **60:**354–360.

18. George, R., L. Leibrock, and M. Epstein. 1979. Long-term analysis of cerebrospinal fluid shunt infections: a 25 year experience. *J. Neurosurg.* **51:**804–811.

19. Gombert, M. E., S. H. Landesman, M. L. Corrado, S. C. Stein, E. T. Melvin, and M. Cummings. 1981. Vancomycin and rifampin therapy for *Staphylococcus epidermidis* meningitis associated with CSF shunts. *J. Neurosurg.* **55:**633–636.

20. Hirsch, B. E., M. Amodio, A. I. Einzig, R. Halevy, and R. Soeiro. 1991. Instillation of vancomycin into a cerebrospinal fluid reservoir to clear infection: pharmacokinetic considerations. *J. Infect. Dis.* **163:**197–200.

21. Hodges, G. R., I. Watanabe, P. Singer, S. Rengachary, D. Reeves, D. R. Jusetesen, S. E. Worley, and E. P. Gephardt, Jr. 1981. Central nervous system toxicity of intraventricularly administered gentamicin in adult rabbits. *J. Infect. Dis.* **143:**148–155.

22. Holt, J. G., N. R. Krieg, P. H. A. Snead, J. T. Staley, and S. T. Williams (ed.). 1994. *In Bergey's Manual of Determinative Bacteriology,* 9th ed., p. 527–558. Williams & Wilkins, Baltimore.

23. **Ignelzi, R. J., and W. M. Kirsch.** 1975. Follow-up analysis of ventriculoperitoneal and ventriculoatrial shunts for hydrocephalus. *J. Neurosurg.* **42:**679–682.
24. **James, H. E.** 1984. Infections associated with cerebrospinal fluid prosthetic devices, p. 23–41. *In* B. Sugarman and E. J. Young (ed.), *Infections Associated with Prosthetic Devices.* CRC Press, Inc., Boca Raton, Fla.
25. **James, H. E., J. W. Walsh, H. D. Wilson, and J. D. Connor.** 1982. Management of cerebrospinal fluid shunt infections: a clinical experience. *Monogr. Neural Sci.* **8:**75–77.
26. **James, H. E., J. W. Walsh, H. D. Wilson, J. D. Connor, J. R. Bean, and P. A. Tibbs.** 1980. Prospective randomized study of therapy in cerebrospinal fluid shunt infection. *Neurosurgery* **7:**459–463.
27. **James, H. E., H. D. Wilson, J. D. Connor, and J. W. Walsh.** 1982. Intraventricular cerebrospinal fluid antibiotic concentrations in patients with intraventricular infections. *Neurosurgery* **10:**50–54.
28. **Kaufman, B. A., and D. G. McLone.** 1991. Infections of cerebrospinal fluid shunts, p. 561–585. *In* W. M. Scheld, R. J. Whitley, and D. T. Durack (ed.), *Infections of the Central Nervous System.* Raven Press, New York.
29. **Lambert, M., A. E. MacKinnon, and A. Vaishnav.** 1984. Comparison of two methods of prophylaxis against CSF shunt infection. *Z. Kinderchir.* **39:**109–110.
30. **Luthardt, T.** 1970. Bacterial infections in ventriculo-aricular shunt systems. *Dev. Med. Child Neurol.* **12**(Suppl. 22):105–109.
31. **Malis, L. I.** 1979. Prevention of neurosurgical infection by intraoperative antibiotics. *Neurosurgery* **5:**339–343.
32. **Mates, S., J. Glaser, and K. Shapiro.** 1982. Treatment of cerebrospinal fluid shunt infections with medical therapy alone. *Neurosurgery* **11:**781–783.
33. **Mayhall, C. G., N. H. Archer, V. A. Lamb, A. C. Spadora, J. W. Baggett, J. D. Ward, and R. K. Narayan.** 1984. Ventriculostomy-related infections. A prospective epidemiologic study. *N. Engl. J. Med.* **310:**553–559.
34. **McCullough, D. C., J. G. Kane, J. H. Presper, and M. Wells.** 1980. Antibiotic prophylaxis in ventricular shunt surgery. I. Reduction of operative infection rates with methicillin. *Child's Brain* **7:**182–189.
35. **McLaurin, R. L., and P. T. Frame.** 1987. Treatment of infection of cerebrospinal fluid shunts. *Rev. Infect. Dis.* **9:**595–603.
36. **McLone, D. G., D. Czyzewski, A. J. Raimondi, and R. C. Sommers.** 1982. Central nervous system infections as a limiting factor in the intelligence of children with myelomeningocoele. *Pediatrics* **70:**338.
37. **Morrice, J. J., and D. G. Young.** 1974. Bacterial colonization of Holter valves: a ten-year survey. *Dev. Med. Child Neurol.* **16**(Suppl. 32):85–90.
38. **Nicholas, J. L., I. M. Kamal, and H. B. Eckstein.** 1970. Immediate shunt replacement in the treatment of bacterial colonization of Holter valves. *Dev. Med. Child Neurol.* **12**(Suppl. 22):110–113.
39. **Odio, C., G. H. McCracken, Jr., and J. D. Nelson.** 1984. CSF shunt infections in pediatrics. A seven year experience. *Am. J. Dis. Child.* **138:**1103–1108.
40. **Parry, S. W., J. F. Schuhmacker, and R. C. Llewellyn.** 1975. Abdominal pseudocysts and ascites formation after ventriculoperitoneal shunt procedures. Report of four cases. *J. Neurosurg.* **43:**476–480.
41. **Perrin, J. C., and R. L. McLaurin.** 1967. Infected ventriculoatrial shunts: a method of treatment. *J. Neurosurg.* **27:**21–26.
42. **Reesor, C., A. W. Chow, A. Kureishi, and P. J. Jewesson.** 1988. Kinetics of intraventricular vancomycin in infections of cerebrospinal fluid shunts. *J. Infect. Dis.* **158:**1142–1143.

43. **Renier, D., J. Lacombe, A. Pierre-Kahn, C. Sainte-Rose, and J. F. Hirsch.** 1984. Factors causing acute shunt infection—computer analysis of 1,174 operations. *J. Neurosurg.* **61:**1072–1078.

44. **Ring, J. C., K. L. Cates, K. K. Belani, T. L. Gaston, R. J. Sveum, and S. C. Marker.** 1979. Rifampin for CSF shunt infections caused by coagulase-negative staphylococci. *J. Pediatr.* **95:**317–319.

45. **Salmon, J. H.** 1972. Adult hydrocephalus: evaluation of shunt therapy in 80 patients. *J. Neurosurg.* **37:**423–428.

46. **Schimke, R. T., P. H. Black, V. H. Mark, and M. N. Swartz.** 1961. Indolent *Staphylococcus albus* or *aureus* bacteremia after ventriculoantristomy: role of foreign body in its initiation and perpetuation. *N. Engl. J. Med.* **264:**264–270.

47. **Schoenbaum, S. C., P. Gardner, and J. Shillito.** 1975. Infections of cerebrospinal fluid shunts: epidemiology, clinical manifestations, and therapy. *J. Infect. Dis.* **131:**543–552.

48. **Sells, C. J., D. B. Shurtleff, and J. D. Loeser.** 1977. Gram-negative cerebrospinal fluid shunt-associated infections. *Pediatrics* **59:**614–618.

49. **Shapiro, S., J. Boaz, M. Kleiman, J. Kalsbeck, and J. Mealey.** 1988. Origin of organisms infecting ventricular shunts. *Neurosurgery* **22:**868–872.

50. **Shurtleff, D. B., E. L. Foltz, R. D. Weeks, and J. Loeser.** 1974. Therapy of *Staphylococcus epidermidis:* infections associated with cerebrospinal fluid shunts. *Pediatrics* **53:**55–62.

51. **Slight, P. H., K. Gundling, S. A. Plotkin, L. Schut, D. Bruce, and L. Sutton.** 1985. A trial of vancomycin for prophylaxis of infections after neurosurgical shunts. *N. Engl. J. Med.* **312:**921.

52. **Venes, J. L.** 1976. Control of shunt infection: report of 150 consecutive cases. *J. Neurosurg.* **45:**311–314.

53. **Wald, S. L., and R. L. McLaurin.** 1980. Cerebrospinal fluid antibiotic levels during treatment of shunt infections. *J. Neurosurg.* **52:**41–46.

54. **Walters, B. C., L. Goumnerova, H. J. Hoffman, E. B. Hendrick, R. P. Humphreys, and C. Levinton.** 1992. A randomized controlled trial of perioperative rifampin/trimethoprim in cerebrospinal fluid shunt surgery. *Child's Nerv. Syst.* **8:**253–257.

55. **Walters, B. C., H. J. Hoffman, E. B. Hendrick, and R. P. Humphreys.** 1984. Cerebrospinal fluid shunt infection. Influences on initial management and subsequent outcome. *J. Neurosurg.* **60:**1014–1021.

56. **Wang, E. E., C. G. Prober, B. E. Hendrick, H. J. Hoffman, and R. P. Humphreys.** 1984. Prophylactic sulfamethoxazole and trimethoprim in ventriculoperitoneal shunt surgery: a double-blind, randomized, placebo-controlled trial. *JAMA* **251:**1174–1177.

57. **Yogev, R.** 1985. Cerebrospinal fluid shunt infections: a personal view. *Pediatr. Infect. Dis. J.* **4:**113–118.

58. **Yogev, R., F. Shinco, and D. McLone.** 1983. Prophylaxis for ventriculo-peritoneal shunt surgery with nafcillin alone or in combination with rifampin. *Program Abstr. 23rd Intersci. Conf. Antimicrob. Agents Chemother.*, abstr. 664.

59. **Younger, J. J., G. D. Christensen, D. L. Bartley, J. C. Simmons, and F. Barrett.** 1987. Coagulase-negative staphylococci isolated from cerebrospinal fluid shunts: importance of slime production, species identification, and shunt removal to clinical outcome. *J. Infect. Dis.* **156:**548–554.

60. **Younger, J. J., J. C. Simmons, and F. F. Barrett.** 1987. Failure of single-dose intraventricular vancomycin for cerebrospinal fluid shunt surgery prophylaxis. *Pediatr. Infect. Dis. J.* **6:**212–213.

61. **Yu, H. C., and R. H. Patterson, Jr.** 1973. Prophylactic antimicrobial agents after ventriculoatriostomy for hydrocephalus. *J. Pediatr. Surg.* **5:**881–885.

Infections Associated with Indwelling Medical Devices, 2nd ed.
Edited by Alan L. Bisno and Francis A. Waldvogel
© 1994 American Society for Microbiology, Washington, DC 20005

Chapter 6

Ocular Infections

Ann Sullivan Baker and Oliver D. Schein

Ocular infections attributed to foreign bodies may be categorized by the anatomic location of the infection. Foreign body-associated infections of the lid and orbit are chiefly secondary to trauma. Corneal infections due to contact lens use account for the preponderance of foreign body infections of the anterior segment of the eye. Endophthalmitis associated with cataract surgery or with foreign bodies introduced by trauma is an important cause of infections of the posterior segment of the eye. This chapter will address each of these areas but will concentrate on microbial keratitis secondary to contact lens use and endophthalmitis after surgical or traumatic perforation of the eye.

CORNEAL AND SCLERAL INFECTIONS

The key inciting event in microbial keratitis is a defect in the corneal epithelium. This occurs commonly in contact lens-associated infections as discussed below. It may also occur as a sequela to a foreign body introduced by minor trauma. Although the majority of these infections are bacterial, suspicion for fungal keratitis must be maintained, especially when the foreign body originates in an agricultural setting. Corneal

Ann Sullivan Baker • Infectious Disease Service, Massachusetts Eye & Ear Infirmary, and Massachusetts General Hospital, Boston, Massachusetts 02114, and Harvard Medical School, Boston, Massachusetts 02115. **Oliver D. Schein** • Cornea Service and Dana Center for Preventive Ophthalmology, The Wilmer Eye Institute, The Johns Hopkins University, Baltimore, Maryland 21287-9019.

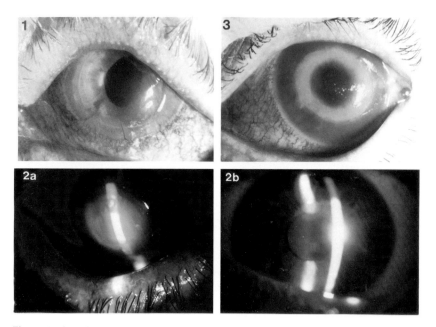

Figure 1. *Serratia marcescens* suture abscess 18 months after penetrating keratoplasty.

Figure 2. (a) Acute-presentation, *P. aeruginosa* corneal ulcer associated with extended-wear soft contact lens. (b) Same case 3 months after treatment; note corneal scarring in visual axis. Final visual acuity, 20/50.

Figure 3. *Acanthamoeba* keratitis in daily-wear soft lens user; ring epithelial defect and stromal infiltrate.

infections may also originate from suture abscesses (Fig. 1) in the postoperative setting, typically after cataract extraction or corneal transplantation (penetrating keratoplasty). Both topical antibiotic therapy and removal of the suture are usually necessary for resolution of the infection. Scleral infections associated with foreign bodies result either from contiguous spread from the cornea or in association with external prostheses used in retinal detachment surgery. Combined corneoscleritis is frequently pseudomonal and carries a very poor visual prognosis (1). Silicone sponge implants are prosthetic devices that are placed under the conjunctiva and over the sclera encircling the equator of the globe (scleral buckle) in cases of retinal detachment. The postoperative infection rate for this procedure is on the order of 0.58 to 4% (26, 30, 34). Staphylococci, both coagulase positive and coagulase negative, predominate in these infections. Removal of the implant, irrigation, and administration of topical antibiotics are the mainstay of treatment. Systemic antibiotics are of limited use because of the relative avascularity of the sclera.

CONTACT LENS-ASSOCIATED INFECTIONS

Background

Contact lenses have three principal uses. By far the most frequent use is the correction of common refractive errors, where they replace the use of spectacles and offer sharper acuity and a greater field of vision. Lenses used for this purpose of correcting common myopia and hyperopia are often described as "cosmetic" contact lenses. "Aphakic" contact lenses refers to lenses used after cataract surgery. These are becoming less frequent in light of the great popularity and success of intraocular lenses. A third, and more specialized, function is the "bandage," or "therapeutic," contact lens. This is a large, soft contact lens that is fitted to promote epithelialization of the corneal surface in the setting of a variety of ocular surface diseases. It serves a protective, rather than a refractive, function in this capacity.

The overwhelming majority of contact lenses in use today are cosmetic. In 1986, it was estimated that there were approximately 18.2 million Americans wearing contact lenses. Of these, about 5 million wore hard or gas-permeable contact lenses, 9.1 million wore daily-wear soft contact lenses, and 4.1 million wore extended-wear soft contact lenses (33). The contact lens industry currently estimates that there are approximately 24 million Americans wearing contact lenses. Much of the growth in contact lens use between 1986 and 1993 has been attributed by industry to the use of disposable soft contact lenses. These are currently felt to account for approximately 20% of new contact lens fits. Complications occurring with contact lens use range from minor irritations to the subject of this section, the potential for the permanent loss of vision from microbial keratitis.

The pathogenesis of infections associated with contact lenses differs somewhat from that of other prosthesis-related infections discussed in this book, in that trauma to and abrasion of the corneal surface contribute greatly to the disease process. Although it is recognized that microbial keratitis can occur with the use of any kind of contact lens, it is widely acknowledged that the risk is greater with overnight lens use. Over the past 3 years a number of controlled studies have been performed addressing risk factors for ulcerative keratitis among contact lens wearers (9, 18, 48, 71). These studies have been remarkably consistent in their indictment of overnight wear of contact lenses. The first study to be reported on the relative risk of ulcerative keratitis among users of daily-wear and extended-wear soft contact lenses was a multicenter case-control study in the United States (71). This study found an overall relative risk of keratitis of approximately 4 to 1 for extended-wear lens users compared with daily-wear soft lens users. However, lens type does not accurately predict actual lens wear, since many extended-wear lens users use them only during the day and many of those with daily-wear lenses occasionally wear them overnight. When lens wearers were distinguished according to their overnight use of lenses, the users of extended-wear lenses who wore them overnight had a risk 10 to 15 times as great as the users of daily-wear lenses who did not, and users of daily-wear lenses who sometimes wore them overnight had 9 times the risk of the users of such lenses who did not. For users of overnight lenses, the risk of ulcerative keratitis was incrementally related to the extent of overnight wear. At present there are approximately 18.2 million Americans who wear contact lenses; of these, about 5 million wear hard or gas-permeable lenses, 9.1 million use daily-wear soft contact lenses, and 4.1 million use extended-wear soft contact lenses (33).

A companion study (66) provided estimates of the incidence of ulcerative keratitis for use of daily-wear soft lenses and extended-wear soft lenses (overnight). A rate of approximately one case of ulcerative keratitis per 2,500 daily-wear soft lens users per year was estimated. For overnight lens wear, a rate of approximately one case per 300 users per year was estimated. Similar relative risks of extended-wear versus daily-wear lens use have since been documented in a controlled study from England (48). More recent controlled studies, which have included populations wearing the newer disposable contact lenses have documented that disposable soft lens users (who in general also wear their lenses overnight) share with conventional extended-wear lens users the same increased risks relative to those of daily-wear lens users (9, 48). These studies, one performed in the United States (9) and the other performed in England (48), indicated a 13- to 17-fold relative risk for disposable lens use, compared with daily-wear soft or rigid gas-permeable lens use. It appears that most of this risk can be explained by overnight wear rather than by any specific effect of the lens material itself. Many of these controlled studies have examined the adequacy of lens care hygiene as a potential risk factor for ulcerative keratitis among contact lens wearers. Interestingly, despite the emphasis placed on hygiene by practitioners and the industry, the finding of any protective effect has been at best marginal in controlled studies. In summary, then, the overwhelming, predisposing risk factor for ulcerative keratitis among contact lens wearers is over-night wear.

Clinical Features

In ophthalmologic parlance the terms microbial keratitis and micro-bial corneal ulceration are used interchangeably. Pain, photophobia, de-creased visual acuity, and discharge are the chief patient complaints. On examination, the hallmark of this condition is the presence of a corneal epithelial defect with an underlying infiltrate in the corneal stroma (Fig. 2a). There are specific conditions in which the infiltrate may be localized at the outset to the epithelium, but these are exceptional. The spectrum of disease at presentation ranges from infiltrates of less than 1 mm in diameter and depth to diffuse corneal infiltration and perforation. Large infiltrates are frequently accompanied by a mucopurulent discharge and a hypopyon, a layering of sterile inflammatory debris in the anterior chamber of the eye. Although there are frequently some clues from the clinical examination, the association of particular organisms with specific clinical presentations is notoriously unreliable and has limited use in the choice of treatment options.

The precise location of the infiltrate should be documented by slit lamp examination before the initiation of steps for diagnosis and treat-ment. The diameter and configuration of the infection, its relationship to the visual axis, its depth in the cornea, and the presence of associated eye conditions should be noted, and if possible, photography should be performed. Corneal scrapings for microscopy and culture are the sine qua non for diagnosis. Scrapings are typically performed with a sterile spatula or scalpel blade at the slit lamp after topical anesthesia.

Superficial epithelial and inflammatory tissue is debrided, and ef-forts are made to shave specimens from both the bed and the leading edge of the ulcer crater. Under usual circumstances cultures are plated onto blood and chocolate agar, thioglycolate broth, and Sabouraud me-dium. A glass slide is prepared for Gram stain, and several extra slides are kept in reserve in case special stains prove to be necessary. If fungal infection is suspected, a Giemsa or methenamine silver stain may be performed, as well as a Calcofluor white preparation. Calcofluor white is a dye that binds to a variety of polysaccharides in the cell walls of fungi and the cysts of amoebae, allowing them to fluoresce under UV light for rapid identification. In setting where these more unusual infec-tions are suspected, Calcofluor white provides the possibility for rapid diagnosis with a greater sensitivity and specificity than conventional stains (46).

The choice of initial antibiotic therapy reflects the organism most

Table 1. Culture-positive corneal infections related to and unassociated with contact lens wear from 1982 to 1985 at the Massachusetts Eye & Ear Infirmary

Organism	Number (%) of infections		
	CL[a] associated ($n = 53^b$)	No CL ($n = 140^b$)	Total ($n = 193^b$)
Gram-positive cocci			
Staphylococcus aureus	14 (26)	35 (25)	49 (25)
Coagulase-negative staphylococci	3 (6)	9 (6)	12 (6)
Streptococcus pneumoniae	4 (8)	17 (12)	21 (11)
Beta-hemolytic streptococci	2 (4)	7 (5)	9 (5)
Viridans group streptococci	4 (8)	6 (4)	10 (5)
Enterococci	1 (2)	0	1 (1)
Other	1 (2)	0	1 (1)
Gram-positive bacilli (corynebacteria)	1 (2)	13 (9)	14 (7)
Gram-negative bacilli			
Pseudomonas aeruginosa	13 (25)	16 (11)	29 (15)
Pseudomonas maltophilia	1 (2)	0	1 (1)
Other Pseudomonas spp.	1 (2)	0	1 (1)
Serratia marcescens	2 (4)	7 (5)	9 (5)
Klebsiella oxytoca	1 (2)	6 (4)	7 (4)
Klebsiella pneumoniae	0	1 (1)	1 (1)
Proteus mirabilis	0	3 (2)	4 (2)
Morganella morganii	1 (2)	2 (1)	3 (2)
Enterobacter aerogenes	1 (2)	0	1 (1)
Acinetobacter calcoaceticus	1 (2)	0	1 (1)
Moraxella spp.	0	11 (8)	11 (5)
Other	0	5 (4)	5 (4)
Fungi			
Candida sp.	1 (2)	7 (5)	8 (4)
Aspergillus spp.	0	1 (1)	1 (1)
Amoebae			
Acanthamoeba spp.	2 (4)	0	1 (1)
Other	0	1 (1)	1 (1)

[a] CL, Contact lens.
[b] In several cases more than one organism was cultured.

commonly associated with contact lens use. Table 1 illustrates experience with corneal infection at the Massachusetts Eye & Ear Infirmary and compares the microbiology of contact lens- and non-contact lens-associated microbial keratitis.

Gram-positive cocci and *Pseudomonas* species predominate, and amoebal and fungal infections are relatively rare. These findings have been quite consistent in the literature (2, 20, 38, 55, 61). Given a high likelihood of these organisms, there is a strong rationale for initial broad-spectrum therapy pending final culture results (6). Historically, the standard initial treatment for presumed bacterial keratitis has been combined topical treatment with fortified aminoglycoside (gentamicin or tobramycin at 14 mg/ml) and fortified cefazolin (50 to 150 mg/ml). For sight-threatening disease, these drops are given on an inpatient basis every 15 to 60 min, depending on the severity of infection. The choice of antibiotic and the frequency of administration can then be modified at 24 to 48 h in accordance with the clinical response.

These initial fortified antibiotics provide excellent broad-spectrum coverage and corneal penetration. Over the past several years, there has been an increasing tendency to use topical quinolone antibiotics as initial treatment for microbial keratitis. These agents have broad-spectrum coverage and good corneal penetration, and they can be used in concentrations available from standard pharmacies, as opposed to the fortified preparations that must be specially compounded by experienced pharmacists. There is, however, some concern among corneal specialists about the use of topical quinolones in light of their reduced efficacy against streptococci. To date, there have been no controlled studies comparing any of the topical quinolones with traditional fortified treatment.

Subconjunctival antibiotic injections do not deliver a greater antibiotic concentration to the corneal stroma than do fortified drops, and they are quite painful. Generally, these injections are reserved for instances of scleral infection or noncompliance with topical medications or occasionally for children who will not allow drops to be given. Antibiotic treatment is continued for 7 to 14 days, with a dosage schedule determined by clinical response and physician judgment. Broad-spectrum antibiotics are maintained in culture-negative cases where stabilization of the process has been achieved. The antibiotic choice is clearly modified depending on culture results. In cases of severe keratitis associated with contact lens use, the presumption of *Pseudomonas* species is often made, and topical ticarcillin or piperacillin (6 mg/ml) may be added empirically to the initial treatment. If the clinical condition of the patient deteriorates on treatment, repeat scrapings are performed. If these cultures are also negative, consideration should be given to corneal punch biopsy to provide deep tissue necessary for pathologic and microbiologic assay of more unusual or fastidious organisms.

In addition to antibiotics, cycloplegics are routinely given to eliminate ciliary spasm and hence improve comfort. The use of topical steroid as adjunctive treatment of microbial keratitis is controversial. In general, topical steroids are not used in the initial treatment of bacterial keratitis. Anecdotal reports of recurrence or recrudescence of pseudomonal keratitis with topical steroid use have led some corneal specialists to discourage steroid use entirely in the presence of this or other similarly virulent organisms. However, loss of corneal substance because of ongoing inflammation with associated collagenase and proteolytic enzyme release frequently occurs even after the ulcer has been sterilized. Therefore, the judicious use of low-dose topical steroids in this setting may be helpful in reducing scarring.

In cases of limited corneal perforation, cyanoacrylate tissue adhesive is used to seal the wound to prevent the complications that attend the loss of the anterior chamber or the extrusion of intraocular contents. Substantial central perforations require penetrating keratoplasty; peripheral perforations can be managed with patch grafts of donor corneal or scleral tissue. Long-term visual loss in microbial keratitis is related to the size of the resultant scar after successful treatment and its location with respect to the visual axis. Central scars significantly affecting acuity require keratoplasty for correction. Eyes that have suffered perforations are at risk over the short term for endophthalmitis and over the long term for glaucoma and cataract. Infections that spread to the sclera have a very poor prognosis. In their analysis of 60 cases requiring inpatient treatment, Donnenfeld et al. (20) reported that 60% regained visual acuity of 20/40 or better, 15% required penetrating keratoplasty because of significant corneal scarring, and almost 4% eventually required enucleation, underscoring the potential severity of the condition. However, it must be noted that the majority of patients will present with small infiltrates outside the visual axis and will enjoy a complete recovery with outpatient antibiotic treatment. Figure 2 illustrates the presentation, course, and medical treatment of a severe, nonperforating corneal infection with *Pseudomonas aeruginosa* associated with a soft cosmetic contact lens.

Fungal keratitis has also been reported in association with contact lens use (7, 82). Although these infections are often severe and resistant to medical treatment, they are thankfully rare. However, our experience has been that fungus is likely to be associated with therapeutic (bandage) lens use, where the ocular surface is already compromised and where topical, chronic antibiotic and steroid use is frequently predisposing. Natamycin (5% suspension), amphotericin B drops (0.1 to 1.0% concentration), topical or subconjunctival miconazole (10 mg/ml), and oral fluconazole and itraconazole are the chief antibiotics used, with the choice dependent on culture results.

Acanthamoeba keratitis associated with contact lens use has received much attention in both the medical and the lay press over the past several years. Although a rare infection, it can be difficult to diagnose and treat.

Acanthamoeba sp. is a free-living amoeba existing in both trophozoite and cyst forms that presumably gains access to the eye from contaminated solution or water. A fully developed case has a characteristic ring stromal infiltrate (Fig. 3) that on scraping will yield the organism on Calcofluor white staining or via culture on *Escherichia coli*-enriched agar. Early cases of *Acanthamoeba* keratitis are much more difficult to recognize because a dendritiform epithelial picture may predominate, which can mimic many other corneal conditions (44). A standard for medical treatment has not been firmly established. However, it is evident that intensive topical treatment with 0.1% propamidine, neomycin, and 1% miconazole in various combinations has been successful in achieving a medical cure in a number of cases (14, 22, 35, 42, 56, 85). In mild epithelial cases, debridement can be diagnostic and curative; however, in more severe cases, medical therapy often fails, and penetrating keratoplasty is necessary. Recurrent amoebic keratitis has also been reported after corneal transplantation (5).

Predisposing Factors

As previously discussed, overnight wear of contact lenses is the principal predisposing factor for lens-related microbial keratitis. Microbial keratitis associated with contact lens use requires both the presence of pathogenic organisms in sufficient quantity to overcome local defenses and a break in the corneal epithelium to allow penetration into the corneal stroma. Although *Neisseria gonorrhoeae*, *Corynebacterium diphtheriae*, and *Neisseria meningitidis* are capable of penetrating intact corneal epithelium, the organisms commonly associated with microbial keratitis require an epithelial defect to gain access to the stroma. Local protective ocular factors include both the flushing action of tears and their immunological constituents, immunoglobulins (chiefly secretory immunoglobulin A), lysozyme, and lactoferrin. The conjunctiva also contains the full cellular equipment necessary for humoral and cell-mediated responses.

Normal conjunctival flora are chiefly coagulase-negative staphylococci and micrococci. Gram-negative organisms are rare, and pseudomonal colonization appears to be on the order of 1% or less (37, 45, 50, 69, 72). Cosmetic contact lens use itself is not believed to alter the conjunctival microbial flora (37, 50, 69, 72); however, contact lens storage cases and solutions are frequently contaminated with a wide range of microorganisms and are presumed to be the source of the infections (13, 15, 21, 41, 55, 63, 82).

Identical physiologic properties, antibiograms, serotypes, and plasmid profiles have been described for *P. aeruginosa* isolated from corneal ulcers and in-use saline solutions (49). In a recent, systematic study of contact lens product contamination, Donzis et al. (21) found that 52 of 100 asymptomatic contact lens wearers had contaminated lens care systems; 13% of in-use commercial solutions and 46% of lens cases were contaminated. All bottles of in-use homemade saline (12 patients) were contaminated and included two isolations of *Acanthamoeba* spp. Gram-negative rods were detected in 26 patients, including 12 patients with *Pseudomonas* species. Similar patterns of contamination were found for hard, soft, daily-wear, and extended-wear lenses.

Bacteria are capable of adhering directly to soft contact lenses, and it appears that this adherence is maximized by lenses coated with mucin and protein (77). *P. aeruginosa* has been shown to adhere to both worn and unworn soft contact lenses, although it is unclear whether *Pseudomonas* species have a preferential ability to bind in comparison with other bacteria (10, 24). In a recent study, Fleiszig et al. found that *P. aeruginosa* adherence to epithelial cells is enhanced in those who use extended-wear soft contact lenses (25).

Lens wear produces microabrasions to the corneal epithelial surface that allow ambient pathogenic organisms to penetrate. Lenses that are too tightly fitted, overworn, or inadequately cleaned or that in some fashion compromise the epithelium likely contribute to infection; however, the relative contributions of these factors are unknown. In acanthomoeba keratitis, swimming with contact lenses in place and the use of homemade saline have been indentified as behavioral risk factors (76), while in the more common bacterial corneal ulcers, particular cleaning regimens, length of lens wear, and other related activities have not been specifically identified.

Prevention

The overwhelming risk factor for microbial keratitis among lens wearers is overnight wear. It has recently been estimated (70a) that approximately 50% of ulcerative ketatitis among users of daily-wear lenses can be attributed directly to overnight wear, as can 75% of cases among users of extended-wear lenses, either conventional or disposable. Therefore, given current contact lens technology, the most effective way to reduce the incidence of these infections is to discourage overnight wear of lenses. It is also appropriate to educate consumers more thoroughly about potential risks and lens hygiene.

A recent Food and Drug Administration survey of contact lens users (33) found, for example, that an alarming number of subjects could not recall the length of lens wear suggested by their prescriber, confused the purpose of their care products, and were unaware of possible adverse consequences. Better education of patients, closer attention to routine lens care habits, and vigilance against a consumer attitude that contact lenses are harmless cosmetic devices will likely decrease the frequency of microbial keratitis. Once an infection has become established, the final outcome is heavily dependent on the degree of infiltration at the time of initial treatment. Any contact lens-wearing subject who experiences the acute onset of ocular pain, decreased vision, and a red eye should remove the lens and seek ophthalmologic attention promptly.

ENDOPHTHALMITIS ASSOCIATED WITH CATARACT SURGERY

The number of intraocular lenses (IOLs) implanted in the United States has been increasing exponentially. It is estimated that more than 3.5 million implants were performed between 1978 and 1986, with 929,000 implants in 1985 alone (16, 74). Presently, approximately 1.3 million lenses are implanted yearly.

IOL implantation was introduced by Ridley, an English ophthalmologist, in 1949. He noted that polymethacrylate fragments in the eyes of World War II flight crews did not cause much tissue reaction. Close to 90% of all implantations today involve posterior chamber IOLs (Fig. 4).

The incidence of endophthalmitis after cataract removal and implantation of IOLs has been reported to be about 0.1 to 0.3% (75), but only a few large series and a small number of case reports have been published

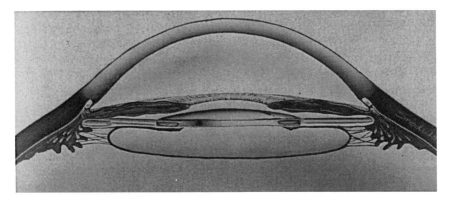

Figure 4. Schematic illustration of a sagittally sectioned anterior segment containing ciliary-fixated posterior chamber lens. The loops course in front of the peripheral flaps of the anterior capsule and insert into the angle or groove formed by the junction of the iris root and the ciliary body. (Krystyna S. Rodulski, artist; courtesy of David J. Apple, Charleston, S.C. Reprinted with permission [4].)

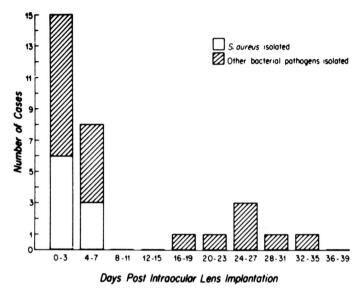

Figure 5. Isolation of bacterial pathogens related to onset of initial symptoms of endophthalmitis following intraocular lens implantation. (Reprinted with permission [81].)

(23, 67, 80, 81, 86). The history, indications, and complications of IOL implantation have been reviewed by Liesegang (43).

A review of 30 cases by Weber et al. at the Massachusetts Eye & Ear Infirmary showed that 77% of cases of endophthalmitis after lens implantation occurred within 7 days of initial cataract surgery and that all cases in this series occurred within 32 days (81) (Fig. 5). Driebe et al. described 83 cases of endophthalmitis with IOLs involving a decade of experience at the Bascom Palmer Eye Institute during the period that cataract surgery underwent a major change from intracapsular to extracapsular procedures (23). A problem with the cataract section was believed to contribute to the development of endophthalmitis in 22% of the patients. Two risk factors were identified. The first involved the wound and included problems such as poor closure, suture problems, and wound leaks. Problems with the vitreous constituted the second risk factor, either vitreous loss or persistent vitreous to the cataract wound. Ideally the vitreous cavity is not violated with the extracapsular technique.

Endophthalmitis after lens implantation may also occur in an epidemic fashion; organisms have included *P. aeruginosa, Candida* species, and *Paecilomyces lilacinus,* the last resulting from use of a contaminated batch of neutralizing solution (28, 51, 54, 64, 79, 80). Endophthalmitis occurring in an epidemic fashion has not yet been associated with the contamination of IOLs.

To date, there have not been reports of seeding of IOLs in patients with systemic (endogenous) infection. IOLs may not act in the same manner as foreign bodies, within or in contact with the vascular compartment, which may serve as a nidus for pathogens from transient or prolonged bacteremia. The aqueous-blood barrier is reestablished within 12 weeks after ocular surgery and may be responsible for limiting secondary bacterial seeding of the globe (36).

Apple et al. evaluated IOL infections at the Center for IOL Research in Utah (4). *Staphylococcus aureus* was detected on both the optic and haptic (loop) with the scanning electron microscope, as well as at the junction of the loop and the optic (Fig. 6).

Several cases of infection after extracapsular cataract extraction have been reported in which subsequent pathologic analyses identified the organisms and found the infection to be localized or confined to the lens capsular sac (3, 52) (Fig. 7). The most common offending organisms were gram-positive pleomorphic bacilli; in several cases, the bacteria were identified by Meisler et al. as *Propionibacterium acnes* (52). This entity has been described by Piest et al. as a "localized endophthalmitis" (65). Metabolic products from the organisms are released from the capsular bag, the anterior segment, and the vitreous. A synergistic reaction may occur between these organisms and retained lens cortical remnants that may cause or exacerbate a hypersensitivity reaction. The pathogenesis of localized endophthalmitis has nothing to do with the type of IOL fixation (lens capsular sac or ciliary sulcus); rather, the simple presence of a capsular sac after extracapsular cataract extraction is the prerequisite for the clinical condition.

P. acnes endophthalmitis seems to be even more delayed in onset and prolonged in course than that caused by coagulase-negative staphylococci, the more widely recognized organisms in indolent postoperative endophthalmitis (59, 70). In a laboratory model of *P. acnes* endophthalmitis, Nobe et al. found that inflammation was more prolonged in the pseudophakic eye (57). The lens may act as a nidus to attract *P. acnes*. *P. acnes* may then act together with residual lens cortical material to produce postoperative inflammation, manifested as uveitis or endophthalmitis.

More recently, Cusumano and associates at the University Eye Hospital in Bonn have described a membrane-like coating of giant cells on the optic (17). They have found slime-producing and non-slime-producing organisms. Menikoff evaluated a case-control study at the N.Y. Eye &

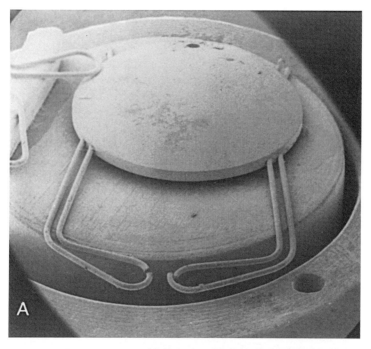

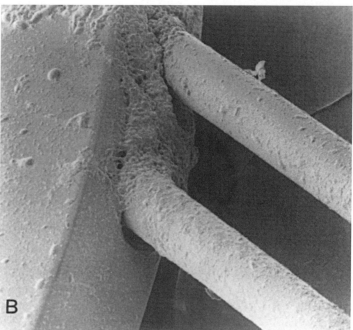

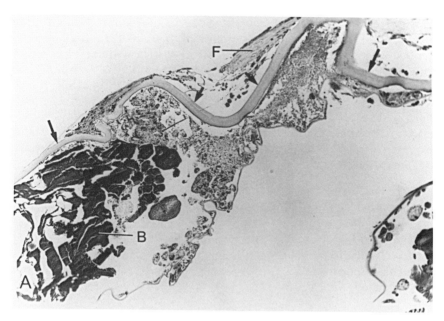

Figure 7. Photomicrograph of the capsular sac removed from the eye of a 71-year-old patient implanted with a posterior chamber lens who was well for 6 months until posterior capsular opacification developed. An Nd:YAG laser capsulotomy was performed. After this procedure the eye developed a severe, diffuse inflammation diagnosed as probable endophthalmitis. The IOL and the lens capsular sac were removed. Note the portion of the lens capsule (arrows) and the fibrous metaplasia (F) of residual lens cortex. The lightly stained material is residual necrotic lens substance. The deeply stained basophilic material (B) at the left is gram positive and represents necrotic organisms. (Gram stain; original magnification, ×30. Courtesy of Francis W. Price, Jr., Indianapolis, Ind. Reprinted with permission [4].)

Figure 6. (A) A scanning electron micrograph of an Optical Radiation Corp. Model II Stableflex lens implanted in a patient who subsequently developed a *Staphylococcus aureus* endophthalmitis. (Original magnification, ×10). (B) Higher-power scanning electron micrograph of one of the loop-optic junctions of the lens seen in panel A, showing extensive deposition of cells and other biological substances on the surface of the loop and optic. This finding is commensurate with the surrounding inflammatory reaction. The infection in this case was long standing, and the IOL was removed when the condition recurred. (Original magnification, ×100. Courtesy of David J. Apple. Reprinted with permission [4].)

Ear Infirmary; his group corroborated the risk of communication with the vitreous cavity and subsequent endophthalmitis (53). They also described an increased risk of infection with an IOL made of polypropylene. Raskin, at the same institution, used quantitative techniques to evaluate the adherence of *Staphylococcus epidermidis* to two IOL types: lenses with polypropylene haptics and all polymethyl methacrylate (68). Finally, Jansen et al. from Cologne reported a case of late-onset *S. epidermidis* endophthalmitis with massive colonization on the lens loop and from the vitreous (39). Clonal identity of all four isolates was confirmed by plasma DNA analysis.

Presentation

The most common presenting symptoms of pseudophakic endophthalmitis are ocular pain, decreased vision, headache, and photophobia. The most common signs of infection include lid swelling, conjunctival injection and discharge, corneal edema, cells and flair in the anterior chamber, hypopyon, and poor or absent retinal red reflex. Most patients are afebrile (Table 2).

Table 2. Presenting symptoms, signs, and laboratory findings for 30 patients with endophthalmitis[a]

Findings at presentation	No. of patients
Symptoms	
Pain in the eye	22
Decreased visual acuity	17
Discharge	7
Headache	5
Red eye	4
Photophobia	2
Signs	
Lid edema	10
Conjunctival injection	20
Corneal edema/haze/striae	20
Anterior chamber cells and flare	23
Hypopyon	21
Absent of poor reflex	22
Elevated ocular tension	5
Temperature > 37.8°C	0
Laboratory data[b]	
Bands >10%	1

[a] From reference 81.
[b] The leukocyte count in the patients ranged from 5,600 to 18,300/mm, with a mean (+ SD) of 11,300 (+ 3,010)/mm.

Table 3. Organisms associated with pseudophakic endophthalmitis[a,b]

Organism	No. of isolates
S. aureus	8
Coagulase-negative staphylococci	16
Streptococcus spp.	
Enterococcus spp.	1
Alpha-hemolytic	1
Proteus mirabilis	1
Mixed	
P. acnes	1
Coagulase-negative staphylococci	3
S. aureus	1
Streptococci, group D	1
Total	33

[a] 30 patients.
[b] Reprinted with permission from reference 81.

Bacteriology

Coagulase-negative staphylococci and *S. aureus* are the most common organisms associated with pseudophakic endophthalmitis (23, 81). *S. epidermidis* (coagulase-negative staphylococcus) was the most common organism, accounting for 58% of the isolates in the series of Weber et al. and 38% in the series of Dreibe and associates. *S. aureus* accounted for 31% in the Weber series; other pathogens include *Proteus mirabilis*, enterococci, and alpha-hemolytic streptococci. Multiple strains were isolated from four patients. Infections with gram-positive pathogens and anaerobic bacteria such as *P. acnes* have also been reported (60) (Table 3).

Diagnosis

Vitreous cultures are essential in evaluating endophthalmitis; anterior chamber cultures may be negative in the presence of positive vitreous cultures (81, 86). Cultures are obtained by passing a fine needle through the pars plana into the vitreous cavity and aspirating the contents. Alternatively, a vitrectomy may be performed. Intravitreal antibiotics are delivered empirically at the same procedure.

Therapy

Although it has been suggested that in cases of pseudophakic endophthalmitis the IOL should be removed, there is no evidence to support this notion. The surgical removal of an IOL in an inflamed eye is a difficult and hazardous procedure; this procedure risks hemorrhage and retinal tears (79). A review of the literature suggests that most patients can be cured without lens removal and that, in fact, removal of the lens does not lead to an improved visual outcome. It has been shown that experimentally induced *S. aureus* pseudophakic endophthalmitis in rabbits can be cured through the use of intraocular antibiotics alone (36). Pseudophakic endophthalmitis or its treatment was associated with an increased incidence of late retinal detachment in the series of Weber et al.; three patients suffered this complication, which has been reported to occur in 0.3 to 0.9% of patients after IOL implantation (84). In about 9% of the cases of *P. acnes* infection, the capsule and the lens may ultimately need to be removed.

The treatment of choice for pseudophakic endophthalmitis is intravitreal antibiotics such as vancomycin (1 mg) and amikacin (400 µg). The use of intravitreal steroid is routine in many practices; this may decrease membrane formation and subsequent traction on the retina. Topical antibiotics such as cefazolin (33 mg/ml) or vancomycin (15 mg/ml) plus tobramycin (14 mg/ml) are often instilled into the conjunctival sac two or three times a day. High-dose systemic antibiotics such as vancomycin (1 to 2 g/day) are given to most patients. Although this is still controversial, some are treating with intravitreal antibiotics only. The length of intravenous antibiotic therapy depends on the clinical status of the patient and the organism. For coagulase-negative staphylococcal infections, 3 to 5 days of systemic antibiotics are usually adequate; 12 to 14 days are recommended for fulminant infections due to *S. aureus*, streptococci, gram-negative bacteria, or fungi. Repeat intraocular antibiotic in 2 or 3 days may also be necessary in these more fulminant cases. Some retina surgeons also give steroids systemically for 5 to 7 days. The new quinolones may play a role in systemic therapy of susceptible organisms. The antibiotic of choice in *Aspergillus* or *Candida* endophthalmitis is amphotericin B, which is administered both into the vitreous (5 to 10 µg) and intravenously (29). Oral fluconazole (800 mg or more) may be efficacious as a long-term follow-up antibiotic for *Candida* endophthalmitis (62).

Vitrectomy, or evacuation of the contents of the vitreous, remains a controversial issue. Vitrectomy has the advantage of obtaining a better sample for culture, allowing visualization of the fungus, removing bacteria and leukocytes, allowing for better distribution of intravitreal antibiotics, and eliminating the vitreous matrix for inflammatory membrane formation. The risks of vitrectomy include retinal detachment and bleeding. In cases of fulminant *S. aureus*, streptococcal, gram-negative, or fungal endophthalmitis, the value of vitrectomy with removal of the abscess appears to outweigh the risk of the procedure.

Prevention

Cleaning of the lids and lashes is appropriate prior to cataract removal and IOL placement. Preoperatively, topical antibiotics may reduce the incidence of endophthalmitis; a 5% betadine solution applied to the ocular surface, and a 10% iodine wash of the lids at the time of surgery are useful procedures (73). For the repeat eye surgery, or for the diabetic or immunocompromised patient, preoperative systemic antibiotics (1 to 2 h) prior to surgery, such as cefotetan, cefazolin, or vancomycin, may be useful.

POSTTRAUMATIC ENDOPHTHALMITIS

Posttraumatic endophthalmitis occurs after penetrating injury to the globe. It is difficult to determine the incidence of endophthalmitis after penetrating trauma; a retrospective analysis of 257 cases revealed an incidence of 7.4% (8). Intraocular foreign bodies add an increased risk of posttraumatic endophthalmitis. A metal object contaminated with dust or other foreign material may be contaminated with bacteria such as *Bacillus* or *Acinetobacter* species or may allow the entry of lid conjunctival flora such as coagulase-negative staphylococci and streptococci; wood or other vegetable matter may harbor fungi (47, 78).

A survey of 198 patients with intraocular foreign bodies was reviewed from Pakistan (40). The most common cause was a flying particle while a hand hammer was being used, followed by fragments of bomb and mine blasts. Intraorbital foreign bodies occurred in 76 eyes, and intraocular foreign bodies occurred in 132 eyes; irreparable damage caused 13 eyes (6.2%) to be enucleated. Ten eyes developed severe endophthalmitis or panophthalmitis requiring evisceration. No single organism, with the exception of *Bacillus cereus*, predominates in posttraumatic endophthalmitis; *Bacillus* species are more common in posttraumatic endophthalmitis, with a 10-fold increase in frequency (19, 32, 58). Therapy for traumatic endophthalmitis is similar to that for endophthalmitis after lens implantation. However, antibiotics to cover *B. cereus* should be given intravitreally as well as intravenously. Thus, vancomycin (1 mg) and amikacin (400 µg) are instilled in the vitreous. Similarly, vancomycin (1 to 2 g/day) or clindamycin (600 to 900 mg) is given intravenously at 8-h intervals, in addition to gentamicin. Tetanus status should also be ascertained.

Finally, computer-assisted tomographic scanning or magnetic resonance imaging may be useful in evaluating the presence of foreign bodies.

LID AND ORBIT INFECTIONS

Foreign body-associated lid and orbit infections are mainly secondary to trauma. Inflammatory signs may persist after initial drainage and antibiotic therapy. Typically, the foreign body is incompletely removed and a granuloma slowly forms, presenting with erythema or a chronically draining fistula months to years later.

One case was described in detail of a young boy who fell into a rosebush at the age of 1 year (12). He developed seizures and unilateral exophthalmos several years later. Skull films revealed a ringlike calcification in the anterior cranial fossa above the roof of the right orbit. A chronic frontal brain abscess was found, which contained *S. aureus* and *Enterobacter* organisms as well as vegetable matter.

Typically, the organisms involved in orbital trauma include skin flora such as staphylococci, anaerobic streptococci, and *P. acnes*. Evaluation should also include computer-assisted tomographic scanning or magnetic resonance imaging to confirm that all foreign material has been drained (31). Antibiotic therapy should be directed toward the organisms on Gram stain and final cultures and sensitivities. Two weeks of intravenous or oral therapy or both would be the usual length of treatment.

REFERENCES

1. **Alfonso, E., K. R. Kenyon, L. D. Ormerod, R. Stevens, M. Wagoner, and D. M. Albert.** 1987. Pseudomonas corneoscleritis. *Am. J. Ophthalmol.* **103:**90–97.
2. **Alfonso, E., S. Mandelbaum, M. J. Fox, and R. K. Foster.** 1986. Ulcerative keratitis associated with contact lens wear. *Am. J. Ophthalmol.* **101:**429–433.
3. **Apple, D. J., N. Mamalis, R. L. Steinmetz, R. C. Loftfield, A. S. Crandall, R. J. Olson.** 1984. Phacoanaphylactic endophthalmitis associated with extracapsular cataract extraction and posterior chamber intraocular lens. *Arch. Ophthalmol.* **102:** 1528–1532.
4. **Apple, D. J., N. Mamalis, R. J. Olson, M. C. Kinkaid.** 1989. Inflammation, p. 237–254. *In Intraocular Lenses. Evaluation, Designs, Complications and Pathology.* Williams & Wilkins, Baltimore.
5. **Baum, J., and D. Albert.** 1985. Case records of the Massachusetts General Hospital. A 29 year old native of India with bilateral ulcerative keratitis. *N. Engl. J. Med.* **312:** 634–641.
6. **Baum, J. L.** 1979. Initial therapy of suspected microbial corneal ulcers. I. Broad antibiotic therapy based on prevalence of organisms. *Surv. Ophthalmol.* **24:**97–105.
7. **Berger, R. I., and B. S. Streeten.** 1981. Fungal growth in aphakic soft contact lenses. *Am. J. Ophthalmol.* **91:**630–633.

8. Brinton, G. S., R. A. Hyndiuk, T. M. Topping, T. M. Aaberg, F. H. Reeger, and G. W. Abrams. 1984. Post traumatic endophthalmitis. *Arch. Ophthalmol.* **102**:547–550.

9. Buehler, P. O., O. D. Schein, J. F. Stamler, D. D. Verdier, and J. Katz. 1992. The increased risk of ulcerative keratitis among disposable soft contact lens users. *Arch. Ophthalmol.* **110**:1555–1558.

10. Butrus, S. I., S. A. Klotz, and R. P. Misra. 1987. Pseudomonas attachment to new hydrogel lenses. *Arch. Ophthalmol.* **105**:106–109.

11. Carlson, A. N., M. R. Tetz, and D. J. Apple. 1989. Infectious complications of modern cataract surgery and intraocular lens implantation. Infections of prosthetic devices. *Infect. Dis. Clin. North Am.* **3**:339–354.

12. Castleman, B. R., E. Scully, and B. U. McNeely. 1973. Case records of MGH. *N. Engl. J. Med.* **288**:674–679.

13. Chalupa, E. H., A. Swarbrick, B. A. Holden, and J. Sjostrand. 1987. Severe corneal infections associated with contact lens wear. *Ophthalmology* **94**:17–22.

14. Cohen, E. J., H. W. Buchanan, P. A. Laugbhrea, C. P. Adams, P. G. Galentine, G. S. Visvesvara, R. Folberg, J. J. Arentsen, and R. P. Laibson. 1985. Diagnosis and management of Acanthamoeba keratitis. *Am. J. Ophthalmol.* **92**:1471–1479.

15. Cohen, E. J., P. R. Laibson, J. J. Arentsen, and C. S. Clemons. 1987. Corneal ulcer associated with cosmetic extended wear soft contact lenses. *Ophthalmology* **94**:109–113.

16. Crawford, B. A., and D. V. Kaufman. 1984. Environmental standards for introcular lens implantation. *Aust. J. Ophthalmol.* **12**:49–55.

17. Cusamano, A., B. Massino, and M. Spitznas. 1991. Is chronic intraocular inflammation after lens implantation of bacterial origin. *Ophthalmology* **98**:1703–1710.

18. Dart, J. K. G., F. Stapleton, and D. Minassian. 1991. Contact lenses and other risk factors in microbial keratitis. *Lancet* **338**:650–653.

19. Davey, R. T., Jr., and W. B. Tauber. 1987. Post-traumatic endophthalmitis: the emerging role of Bacillus cereus infection. *Rev. Infect. Dis.* **9**:110–123.

20. Donnenfeld, E. D., E. J. Cohen, J. J. Arentsen, G. I. Genvert, and P. R. Laibson. 1986. Changing trends in contact lens associated corneal ulcers: an overview of 116 cases. *CLAO J.* **12**:145–149.

21. Donzis, P. B., B. J. Mondino, B. A. Weissman, and D. A. Bruckner. 1987. Microbial contamination of contact lens care systems. *Am. J. Ophthalmol.* **104**:325–333.

22. Driebe, W. T., G. A. Stern, E. J. Epstein, et al. 1988. Acanthamoeba keratitis: potential role for topical clotrimazole in combination chemotherapy. *Arch. Ophthalmol.* **106**:1196–1201.

23. Driebe, W. T., Jr., S. Mandelbaum, R. K. Foster, L. K. Schwartz, and W. W. Culbertson. 1986. Pseudophakic endophthalmitis, diagnosis and management. *Ophthalmology* **93**:442–448.

24. Duran J. A., M. F. Refojo, I. K. Gibson, and K. R. Kenyon. 1987. Pseudomonas attachment to new hydrogel lenses. *Arch. Ophthalmol.* **105**:106–109.

25. Fleiszig, S. M. J., N. Efron, and G. B. Pier. 1992. Extended contact lens wear enhances Pseudomonas aeruginosa adherence to human corneal epithelium. *Invest. Ophthalmol. Visual Sci.* **33**:2908–2916.

26. Folk, J. C., J. Cutkomp, and F. Koontz. 1987. Bacterial scleral abscesses after retinal buckling operations. *Ophthalmology* **94**:1148–1154.

27. Galentine, P. G., E. J. Cohen, R. P. Laibson, C. P. Adams, R. Michaud, and J. J. Arentsen. 1984. Corneal ulcers associated with contact lens wear. *Arch. Ophthalmol.* **102**:891–894.

28. Gerding, D. N., B. J. Poley, W. H. Hall, D. P. LeWin, and M. D. Clark. 1979. Treatment of Pseudomonas endophthalmitis associated with prosthetic intraocular lens implantation. *Am. J. Ophthalmol.* **88**:902–908.

29. **Gilbert, C. M., and M. A. Novak.** 1984. Successful treatment of postoperative Candida endophthalmitis in an eye with an intraocular lens implant. *Am. J. Ophthalmol.* **97:** 593–595.

30. **Hahn, Y. S., A. Lincoff, H. Lincoff, and I. Kreissig.** 1979. Infection after sponge implantation for scleral buckling. *Am. J. Ophthalmol.* **87:**180–185.

31. **Harris, G. J., and A. Syvertsen.** 1981. Multiple projection computed tomography in orbital disorders. *Ann. Ophthalmol.* **13:**183–188.

32. **Hemady, R., M. Zaltas, B. Paton, C. S. Foster, and A. S. Baker.** 1990. Bacillus-induced endophthalmitis: new series of 10 cases and review of the literature. *Br. J. Ophthalmol.* **74:**26–29.

33. **Herman, C. L.** 1987. An FDA survey of U.S. contact lens wearers. *Contact Lens Spectrum* **July:**89–92.

34. **Hilton, G. F., and R. H. Wallyn.** 1978. The removal of scleral buckles. *Arch. Ophthalmol.* **96:**2061–2063.

35. **Hirst, L. W., W. R. Green, W. Merz, C. Kauman, G. S. Visvesvara, A. Jensen, and M. Howard.** 1984. Management of acanthamoeba keratitis: a case report and a review of the literature. *Ophthalmology* **91:**1105–1111.

36. **Hopen, G., B. J. Mondino, D. Kizy, and J. Lipkowitz.** 1982. Intraocular lenses and experimental bacterial endophthalmitis. *Am. J. Ophthalmol.* **94:**402–407.

37. **Hovding, G.** 1981. The conjunctival and contact lens bacterial flora during lens wear. *Acta Ophthalmol.* **59:**387–401.

38. **Hyndiuk, R. A., D. N. Skorich, and E. M. Burd.** 1986. Bacterial keratitis, p. 303–330. *In* K. F. Tabbara and R. A. Hyndiuk (ed.), *Infections of the Eye.* Little, Brown & Co., Boston.

39. **Jansen, B., C. Hartmann, F. Schumacker-Perdreau, and G. Peters.** 1991. Late onset endophthalmitis associated with intraocular lens: a case of molecularly proved S. epidermidis etiology. *Br. J. Ophthalmol.* **75:**440–441.

40. **Khan, M. D., N. Kundi, Z. Mohammed, and A. F. Nazeer.** 1987. A 6½ year study of intraocular and intraorbital foreign bodies in the Northeast Frontier Province—Pakistan. *Br. J. Ophthalmol.* **71:**716–719.

41. **Krachner, J. H., and J. J. Purcell, Jr.** 1978. Bacterial corneal ulcers in cosmetic soft contact lens wearers. *Arch. Ophthalmol.* **96:**57–61.

42. **Larkin, D. D. F., and J. K. G. Dart.** 1988. Treatment of Acanthamoeba keratitis: potential role for topical clotrimazole in combination chemotherapy. *Arch. Ophthalmol.* **106:** 1196–1201.

43. **Liesegang, T. J.** 1984. Cataracts and cataract operations. *Mayo Clin. Proc.* **59:**556–567, 622–632.

44. **Lindquist, T. D., N. A. Sher, and D. J. Doughman.** 1988. Clinical signs and medical therapy of early acanthamoeba keratitis. *Arch. Ophthalmol.* **106:**73–77.

45. **Locatcher-Khorazo, D., and E. Gutierrez.** 1972. The bacterial flora of the healthy eye, p. 14. *In* D. Locatcher-Khorazo and B. C. Seegal (ed.), *Microbiology of the Eye.* The C. V. Mosby Co., St. Louis.

46. **Marines, H. M., M. S. Osato, and R. L. Font.** 1987. The value of calcofluor white in the diagnosis of mycotic and acanthamoeba infections of the eye and ocular adnexa. *Ophthalmology* **94:**23–25.

47. **Mark, D. B., and M. W. Gaynon.** 1983. Trauma induced endophthalmitis caused by Acinetobacter anitratus. *Br. J. Opthalmol.* **67:**124–126.

48. **Matthews, T. D., D. G. Frazer, D. C. Minassian, C. F. Radford, and J. F. G. Dart.** 1992. Risks of keratitis and patterns of use with disposable contact lens users. *Arch. Ophthalmol.* **110:**1555–1558.

49. **Mayo, M. S., S. L. Cook, R. L. Schlitzer, M. A. Ward, L. A. Wilson, and D. G. Ahearn.** 1986. Antibiograms, serotypes, and plasmid profiles of *Pseudomonas aeruginosa* associated with corneal ulcers and contact lens wear. *J. Clin. Microbiol.* **24:**372–376.
50. **McBride, M. E.** 1979. Evaluation of microbial flora of the eye during wear of soft contact lenses. *Appl. Environ. Microbiol.* **37:**233–236.
51. **McCray, E., N. Rampell, S. L. Solomon, W. W. Bond, W. J. Marone, and D. O. O'Day.** 1986. Outbreak of *Candida parapsilosis* endophthalmitis after cataract extraction and intraocular lens implantation. *J. Clin. Microbiol.* **24:**625–628.
52. **Meisler, D. M., A. G. Palestine, D. W. Vastine, D. R. Demartini, B. F. Murphy, W. J. Reinhart, Z. N. Zakov, J. T. McMahon, and T. P. Cliffel.** 1986. Chronic Propionibacterium endophthalmitis after extracapsular cataract extraction and intraocular lens implantation. *Am. J. Ophthalmol.* **102:**733–739.
53. **Menikoff, J. A., M. G. Speaker, M. Marmor, and E. Raskin.** 1991. A case-control study of risk factors for postoperative endophthalmitis. **98:**1761–1768.
54. **Miller, G. R., G. Rebell, R. C. Magoon, S. M. Kulvin, and R. K. Forster.** 1978. Intravitreal antimycotic therapy and the cure of mycotic endophthalmitis caused by a Paecilomyces lilacinus contaminated pseudophakos. *Ophthalmic Surg.* **9(6):**54–63.
55. **Mondino, B. J., B. A. Weissman, M. D. Farb, and T. H. Pettit.** 1986. Corneal ulcers associated with daily-wear and extended wear contact lenses. *Am. J. Ophthalmol.* **102:** 58–65.
56. **Moore, M. B., J. P. McCulley, M. M. Luckenback, H. Gelender, C. Newton, M. S. McDonald, and G. S. Visvesvara.** 1985. Acanthamoeba keratitis associated with soft contact lenses. *Am. J. Ophthalmol.* **100:**389–395.
57. **Nobe, J. R., S. M. Finegold, L. L. Rife, M. A. C. Edelstein, and R. E. Smith.** 1987. Chronic anaerobic bacteria endophthalmitis in pseudophakic rabbit eyes. *Invest. Ophthalmol. Visual Sci.* **28:**259–263.
58. **O'Day, D. M., R. S. Smith, and C. R. Gregg.** 1981. The problem of Bacillus species infection with special emphasis on the virulence of Bacillus. *Ophthalmology* **88:**833–838.
59. **Ormerod, L. D., D. D. Ho, L. E. Becker, R. J. Cruise, H. I. Grohar, B. G. Paton, A. R. Frederick, T. M. Topping, J. J. Weiter, S. M. Buzney, R. A. Ling, and A. S. Baker.** 1993. Endophthalmitis caused by the coagulase-negative staphylococci. Disease spectrum and outcome. *Ophthalmology* **100:**715–723.
60. **Ormerod, L. D., G. B. Paton, J. Haaf, T. M. Topping, and A. S. Baker.** 1987. Chronic anaerobic bacteria endophthalmitis. *Ophthalmology* **94:**799–808.
61. **Ormerod, L. D., and R. E. Smith.** 1986. Contact lens-associated microbial keratitis. *Arch. Ophthalmol.* **104:**79–83.
62. **Park, S. S., D. J. D'Amico, B. Paton, and A. S. Baker.** 1993. Treatment of exogenous candida endophthalmitis in rabbits with oral fluconazole or combination fluconazole and flucytosine. ARVO Annual Meeting Abstract Issue. May #1258.
63. **Patrinely, J. R., K. R. Wilhelmus, J. M. Rubin, and J. E. Key.** 1985. Bacterial keratitis associated with extended wear soft contact lenses. *CLAO J.* **11:**234–236.
64. **Pettit, T. H., R. J. Olson, R. Y. Foos, and W. J. Martin.** 1980. Fungal endophthalmitis following intraocular lens inplantation. A surgical epidemic. *Arch. Ophthalmol.* **98:** 1025–1039.
65. **Piest, K. L., M. V. Kincaid, M. R. Tetz, D. J. Apple, W. A. Roberts, and F. W. Price, Jr.** 1987. Localized endophthalmitis: a newly described cause of the so-called toxic lens syndrome. *J. Refractive Surg. Cataract* **13:**498–510.
66. **Poggio, E. C., P. W. Glynn, O. D. Schein, V. A. Scardino, J. M. Seddon, and K. R. Kenyon.** 1989. The incidence of ulcerative keratitis among users of daily-wear and extended-wear soft contact lenses. *N. Engl. J. Med.* **321:**779–783.

67. Puliafito, C. A., A. S. Baker, J. Haaf, and C. S. Foster. 1982. Infectious endophthalmitis: review of 36 cases. *Ophthalmology* **89**:921–929.
68. Raskin, E. W., M. G. Speaker, S. A. McCormick, D. Wong, J. A. Menikoff, and R. Palton-Henrion. 1993. Influence of haptic material on the adherence of staphylococci to intraocular lenses. *Arch. Ophthalmol.* **111**:250–253.
69. Rauschi, R. T., and J. J. Rogers. 1978. The effect of hydrophilic contact lens wear on the bacterial flora of the human conjunctiva. *Int. Contact Lens Clin.* **5**:56–62.
70. Roussel, T. W., W. W. Culbertson, and N. S. Jaffe. 1987. Chronic postoperative endophthalmitis associated with propionibacterium acnes. *Arch. Ophthalmol.* **105**: 1199–1201.
70a. Schein, O. D., P. O. Beuhler, J. F. Stamler, D. D. Verdier, and J. Katz. 1994. The impact of overnight wear on the risk of contact lens-associated ulcerative keratitis. *Arch. Ophthalmol.* **112**:186–190.
71. Schein, O. D., R. J. Glynn, E. C. Poggio, J. M. Seddon, K. R. Kenyon, and the Microbial Keratitis Study Group. 1989. The relative risk of ulcerative keratitis among users of daily-wear and extended-wear soft contact lenses: a case-control study. *N. Engl. J. Med.* **321**:773–778.
72. Smolin, G., M. Okumoto, and R. A. Nozik. 1979. The microbial flora in extended wear soft contact lens wearers. *Am. J. Ophthalmol.* **88**:543–547.
73. Speaker, M. G., and J. A. Menikoff. 1991. Prophylaxis of endophthalmitis with topical povidone iodine. *Ophthalmology* **98**:1769–1775.
74. Stark, W. J., D. E. Whitney, J. W. Chandler, and D. M. Worthen. 1986. Trends in intraocular lens implantations in the United States. *Arch. Ophthalmol.* **104**:1769–1770.
75. Stark, W. J., D. M. Worthen, J. T. Holladay, P. E. Bath, M. E. Jacobs, G. C. Murry, E. T. McGhee, M. W. Talbot, M. D. Shipp, N. E. Thomas, R. W. Barnes, D. W. C. Brown, J. N. Buxton, R. D. Reinecke, C. S. Lao, and S. Fisher. 1984. The FDA report: intraocular lenses. *Aust. J. Ophthalmol.* **12**:61–69.
76. Stehr-Green, J. K., T. M. Failey, F. H. Brant, J. H. Carr, E. E. Bond, and G. S. Visvesvara. 1987. Acanthamoeba keratitis in soft contact lens wearers, a case control study. *JAMA* **258**:57–60.
77. Stern, C. A., and A. S. Zam. 1986. The pathogenesis of contact lens associated Pseudomonas aeruginosa corneal ulceration. 1. The effect of contact lens coatings on adherence of Pseudomonas aeruginosa to soft contact lenses. *Cornea* **5**:41–45.
78. Tabarra, K. E., F. Juffali, and R. M. Matossian. 1977. Bacillus laterosporus endophthalmitis. *Arch. Ophthalmol.* **95**:2187–2189.
79. Tennant, J. L. 1979. Removal of intraocular lenses. *Int. Ophthalmol. Clin.* **19**:195–209.
80. Verbraeken, H., A. Medoza, and R. Van Oye. 1983. Pseudophakic endophthalmitis. *Bull. Soc. Belge Ophtalmol.* **206**:55–59.
81. Weber, D. J., K. L. Hoffman, R. A. Thoft, and A. S. Baker. 1986. Endophthalmitis following intraocular lens implantation. *Rev. Infect. Dis.* **8**:12–20.
82. Wilson, L. A., and D. G. Ahearn. 1986. Association of fungi with extended wear contact lenses. *Am. J. Ophthalmol.* **101**:434–436.
83. Wilson, L. A., R. L. Schlitzer, and D. G. Ahearn. 1981. Pseudomonas corneal ulcers associated with soft contact lens wear. *Am. J. Ophthalmol.* **92**:546–554.
84. Worthen, D. M., J. A. Boucher, J. N. Buxton, S. S. Hayreh, G. Lowther, R. D. Reinecke, W. H. Spencer, M. Talbott, and D. F. Weeks. 1980. Interim FDS report on intraocular lenses. *Ophthalmology* **87**:267–271.
85. Wright, P., D. Warhurst, and B. R. Jones. 1985. Acanthamoeba keratitis successfully treated medically. *Br. J. Ophthalmol.* **69**:778–782.
86. Zaldman, G. W., and B. J. Mondino. 1982. Postoperative pseudophakic bacterial endophthalmitis. *Am. J. Ophthalmol.* **93**:218–233.

Infections Associated with Indwelling Medical Devices, 2nd ed.
Edited by Alan L. Bisno and Francis A. Waldvogel
© 1994 American Society for Microbiology, Washington, DC 20005

Chapter 7

Infections Associated with Endotracheal Intubation and Tracheostomy

Parvathi Tiruviluamala and Waldemar G. Johanson, Jr.

Nosocomial pneumonia is estimated to occur in 0.5 to 5.0% of hospitalized patients (67) and is the nosocomial infection most likely to cause death (36). Gram-negative bacilli (GNB) cause at least 60% of nosocomial pneumonias (52), and the case fatality rate is approximately 50% when these organisms are involved (33).

Most cases of nosocomial pneumonia occur in intensive care units (ICUs). However, the incidence of pneumonia varies markedly among different diagnostic groups. In one study, pneumonia developed in 12.2% of patients admitted to a medical ICU, including 24% of patients in respiratory failure but no patients admitted with suspected, but unproven, myocardial infarction (46). Potgieter et al. (70) found an overall nosocomial pneumonia infection rate of 23.6% among 250 patients admitted to a medical ICU. None of 56 patients without a tracheostomy or endotracheal tube developed a nosocomial infection, while infections occurred in 59 of 194 (30%) of those with an artificial airway; 51 of the 59 had pneumonia and 8 had sepsis. The Study of the Efficacy of Nosocomial Infection Control (SENIC) found that postoperative patients who required continuous ventilatory support were 21 times more likely to develop pneumonia than were postoperative patients who did not re-

Parvathi Tiruviluamala • Division of Pulmonary Diseases, Department of Medicine, MSB I-506, UMDNJ-New Jersey Medical School, 185 South Orange Avenue, Newark, New Jersey 09103.   **Waldemar G. Johanson, Jr.** • Department of Medicine, MSB I-506, UMDNJ-New Jersey Medical School, 185 South Orange Avenue, Newark, New Jersey 09103.

quire ventilatory support (37). These studies clearly show that patients in respiratory failure are at markedly increased risk of developing nosocomial pneumonia.

HOST DEFENSES

The normal lung is sterile distal to the central airways (54). In 1922 Bloomfield (7) recognized the sterility of the normal lung and described two mechanisms by which the lung maintained that state: "an anatomic structure which cuts off most of the organisms from the inspired air" and "a process which destroys or eliminates the few which do penetrate." This sophisticated concept is important to the understanding of infections associated with tracheostomies and endotracheal tubes, as these artificial airways tend to bypass the "anatomic structure" to which Bloomfield referred and may interfere with normal lung clearance mechanisms as well.

Inspired particles that exceed 10 to 15 μm in diameter are deposited by inertial impaction in the nose and pharynx because of sharp angulations at these sites (59). Smaller particles may reach respiratory bronchioles and even alveoli, while particles smaller than 1 μm behave like gas molecules and may be expired. Aspiration of liquids is prevented by reflex closure of the glottis following stimulation of receptors in the larynx and trachea and by the vigorous coughing that such stimulation evokes.

Particulates that are deposited in the airways are removed by the mucociliary system. Effective function of this complicated system requires that the thickness of the gel and sol layers of the mucous blanket be maintained at a constant depth so that ciliary action can propel it toward the mouth. Ciliary beat frequency, normally about 1,200/s, may be influenced by many factors, including environmental exposures such as high or low oxygen tensions, low humidity, and drugs. Effective function also requires that ciliary action proceed in wave-like fashion from the periphery toward the central airways, a phenomenon that requires cell-to-cell signaling by as yet unknown mechanisms.

Bacteria that are deposited in peripheral airways or alveoli are usually phagocytosed and killed in situ in the lungs (34). Species with limited virulence for the respiratory tract are phagocytosed and killed by resident alveolar macrophages. The lungs of animals exposed to aerosols of these bacteria, such as *Staphylococcus epidermidis*, show no inflammatory response despite the deposition of 10^5 or more bacteria in the lungs. Killing is accomplished swiftly, being essentially complete within a few hours.

In contrast, exposure of the lungs to aerosols of highly virulent bacteria, such as *Streptococcus pneumoniae* or *Pseudomonas aeruginosa*, elicits a prompt migration of polymorphonuclear leukocytes (PMNs) into the alveoli as well as mobilizing the resident alveolar macrophage population (75). These organisms are also cleared promptly under normal circumstances. However, if some factor unbalances this response, such as inhibition of PMN migration (diabetes, alveolar edema), or interferes with intracellular killing (hypoxia, acidosis), bacterial killing may occur more slowly than bacterial multiplication. The total bacterial population increases over time rather than diminishing, and tissue inflammation spreads. Morphologists recognize this tissue response (i.e., accumulation of PMNs, edema) as pneumonia; this histologic finding requires the presence of about 10^4 bacteria per g of lung tissue. Bacteria presented to the lung in a liquid bolus, such as contaminated upper airway secretions, are cleared more slowly than bacteria presented as a small-particle aerosol, presumably because of the greater local concentration of bacteria in the former and the possible protective effect of the fluid itself (38).

Several lung defense mechanisms may be impaired by the presence of a cuffed endotracheal tube. The act of coughing requires that the glottis be closed while the abdominal muscles contract to build up intrapulmonary pressure; the sudden opening of the glottis results in a rush of air through the trachea at high velocity, which tends to propel secretions and other foreign objects toward the airway opening. The presence of an endotracheal tube prevents the development of high intrathoracic pressures since glottic closure is not possible, thus reducing the effectiveness of cough.

Mucociliary transport is quickly impaired by cuffed endotracheal tubes. Sackner et al. (80) showed that the presence of an uninflated endotracheal tube had no effect on tracheal mucus velocity in anesthetized dogs, but inflation of the cuff led to significant decline in mucus velocity after only 1 h. Similarly, uninflated tracheostomy tubes caused no impairment in sheep, but minor manipulations of the airways, such as suctioning the trachea, reduced mucus clearance significantly (53). Forbes and Gamsu (31) demonstrated that mechanical ventilation alone reduced mucociliary function after controlling for the endotracheal tube. The cuffs on tracheostomy or endotracheal tubes produce measurable damage to the tracheal mucosa within a few days (26, 48, 50). Mucociliary transport is markedly diminished in areas of epithelial cell injury. Impairment of mucociliary function and mucus hypersecretion leads to pooling of secretions in the airways of intubated patients. Since bacteria, notably *P. aeruginosa*, adhere to receptors in respiratory mucus (72, 89), accumulation of secretions poses a risk for subsequent pneumonia.

COLONIZATION

The term "colonization" refers to the persistent presence of organisms at a particular site. Colonization of certain regions of the human body by certain species of bacteria is obviously normal. Colonization may be abnormal either when organisms are found at sites that are normally sterile or when organisms that are not normal inhabitants are found in a region.

Colonization of the Respiratory Tract

Johanson et al. (45) studied the oropharyngeal flora of normal subjects and patients with various illnesses and found that whereas only 6% of healthy subjects or patients on a psychiatry service were colonized by gram-negative bacilli (GNB), 35% of patients labeled "moderately ill" and 73% of "moribund" patients were colonized with GNB. A subsequent study of 213 patients admitted to a medical ICU reported GNB colonization in 45% (46).

The mechanism of GNB colonization appears to be an alteration in the surface characteristics of the upper respiratory epithelium. Bacteria that constitute the normal flora of a contaminated region demonstrate a propensity to bind to the surface of the regional epithelium; bacterial species that do not bind to the surface are swept away and fail to colonize. A change in cell binding properties may occur rapidly and can be studied in vitro (47). Buccal cell adherence of GNB in vitro was increased 24 h after major surgery, because of the loss of fibronectin from the epithelial cell surface (91). Leukocyte elastase appears to be at least one of the enzymes involved in this process (17). GNB appear to bind to cell surface receptors that are normally blocked by fibronectin. Certain members of the normal flora, on the other hand, bind to fibronectin and cannot bind to the cells if the latter protein is removed. These findings may underlie the shift in bacterial flora that is observed in ill patients (45). A recent report found fibronectin only on the basement membrane side of buccal cells, not on the luminal surface (57). These investigators propose that changes in the cell surface carbohydrates, rather than fibronectin, may be the critical alteration underlying increased susceptibility to colonization among ill patients. In either case, it is clear that the mucosal cells of seriously ill patients undergo a surface alteration that renders them susceptible to the adherence of bacteria that do not normally colonize the region.

Colonization is first found in the oropharynx, then in the trachea, and then in distal airways. Some organisms, notably *P. aeruginosa*, may colonize the trachea without a demonstrable initial presence in the oropharynx (61). This observation has been linked to the greater propensity of *P. aeruginosa* to adhere to tracheal epithelial cells than to buccal cells (62). Certain specialized respiratory pathogens, such as *Bordetella pertussis*, adhere only to specific cells in the tracheal epithelium (13). There is evidence to support a role for both pili (73, 92) and extracellular products (71) in promoting adherence. Ramphal et al. (74) found that *P. aeruginosa* adhered readily to damaged epithelium and exposed basement membrane but not to normal tracheal mucosa. Whether changes in adherence might underlie colonization of distal airways in chronically intubated patients remains unknown. An alternative explanation for the persistent presence of gram-negative bacilli in airway secretions might simply be repeated or continuous aspiration.

Aspiration of contaminated gastric contents may account for nosocomial pneumonia in the absence of demonstrable colonization of the oropharynx (4). Furthermore, it has been suggested that the prophylaxis for gastric stress ulcers may increase the risk of nosocomial pneumonias (24, 25). The bacterial population of the stomach rises as pH is increased under conditions of gastrointestinal tract stasis, an event that often follows serious illness. In studies of small numbers of patients, the incidence of nosocomial pneumonia has been higher in subjects receiving antacids and H_2-blocking agents than in those treated with mucosal-protecting agents (such as sucralfate) that do not alter pH (18). Some evidence suggests that sucralfate may possess direct antibacterial properties (88). However, a meta-analysis of a number of studies found that there was no consistent effect of prophylactic regimens that raise gastric pH (14). Overall, it seems that any putative effect of stress ulcer prophylaxis on the incidence of nosocomial pneumonia is so small that a large prospective study would be required to definitively answer this question.

Enteral feeding may be another risk factor for nosocomial pneumonia, although it is probably less of a hazard than total parenteral nutrition (68). Gastroduodenal dysfunction may be responsible for the overgrowth of GNB in the stomach (44); Inglis et al. (44) found a strong correlation between the presence of bilirubin, indicating reflux of duodenal fluid into the stomach, and the total bacterial count in gastric fluid.

Colonization of the Tracheostomy Stoma

Colonization of tracheostomy sites was examined by Lowbury et al. (56), who studied 63 patients with new tracheostomies who were admitted to an ICU; 21 (33%) became colonized, all with *P. aeruginosa*. Of the 21, 18 were colonized within the first week. Rogers and Osterhout (79) followed 83 patients undergoing tracheostomy. They noted the appearance of the nasopharyngeal flora at the tracheostomy site of nearly all patients, usually within 24 to 48 h. Todisco et al. (87), reviewing nine patients undergoing total laryngectomy for cancer, found that 100% of stomata became colonized, usually with gram-negative bacilli and usually within 24 to 48 h. Northey et al. (63) followed 14 patients receiving tracheostomies; colonization of the site occurred in 13 patients, usually within 2 days of the procedure.

Chronic tracheostomy sites are usually colonized as well. Niederman et al. (61) observed 15 patients with long-term tracheostomies (mean of 25 months) who were admitted to the hospital for at least 4 weeks and free of pneumonia upon admission. Three (20%) never had GNB isolated from the tracheostomy site. Seven (47%) were persistently colonized with *P. aeruginosa,* while the other five were transiently colonized with *P. aeruginosa* or another GNB. GNB were isolated more frequently from the tracheostomy site (76%) than from the oropharynx (37%). Repeated isolation of GNB was associated with the use of steroids, antibiotics, and mechanical ventilation. Three of the seven (43%) persistently colonized patients developed pneumonia, versus one of the other eight (12.4%). In 16 patients with long-term tracheostomies, aspirates from the level of the carina yielded an average of six isolates per specimen, mostly GNB, and there was no relationship to the oropharyngeal flora (6). These patients were stable, showing no signs of infection. Altogether, these studies indicate a very high rate of colonization in both fresh and chronic tracheostomies, usually with GNB. Antibiotic therapy is not useful in eradicating the organisms, and many patients tolerate this colonization without ill effect. The flora of a chronic tracheostomy appears to be distinct from that of the oropharynx, in contrast to that of the trachea associated with acute tracheostomy or endotracheal intubation.

Colonization of the Endotracheal Tube

Recently, it has been learned that certain bacteria aggregate with bacterial glycopolysaccharide or slime onto what has been termed a "biofilm" on contaminated surfaces (42, 44, 48, 85). These aggregations serve to promote colonization of surfaces in environments that might otherwise pose insurmountable obstacles to bacterial persistence, such as swiftly flowing currents of liquids or high-flow gas streams (15). Inglis et al. (43) found biofilms on 75% of endotracheal tubes examined after removal from the patients. There was no simple relation between the depth of biofilm and the duration of intubation. Cultures revealed significant bacterial growth in 33 of 45 (73%) tubes examined, with 29% of isolates being pseudomonads or members of the family *Enterobacteriaceae.*

Attempting to model what might happen in patients with contaminated tubes, these investigators also studied the aerosolization of organisms from the tube during a simulated ventilator breath. Bacteria were found to be projected up to 45 cm from the tip of the tube by a simulated tidal volume (42). Dislodgement of contaminated biofilm by suction catheters has been suggested by Sottile et al. (85) as another way in which the lungs may be inoculated. These investigators found that up to 84% of the internal surface area of endotracheal tubes removed from patients was covered by biofilm materials. Biofilm is particularly likely to form in areas of microscopic surface irregularities, which are most prominent near the tip and side-hole port (23). These bacterial microcolonies are protected from antibiotics by their location in the tube as well as by the glycocalyx surrounding them (60). Clearly, these tubes become contaminated by organisms that are already in the patients' respiratory tracts. However, it seems likely that the formation of biofilms in the tube provides another mechanism by which bacteria can persist in proximity to the lungs and by which the lungs are repetitively inoculated with bacteria.

BACTERIAL INOCULATION OF THE LUNGS

Contaminated Aerosols

Bacterial contamination of respiratory therapy equipment, especially nebulization devices, was responsible for many nosocomial outbreaks before this threat was recognized (5, 76). This equipment was most commonly contaminated with GNB, including *P. aeruginosa, Enterobacter aerogenes, Flavobacterium* spp., *Acinetobacter* spp., and many others. In recent years, the rate of contaminated respiratory therapy devices has become so low that routine monitoring is no longer justified, and it is now believed that organisms causing nosocomial pneumonia are rarely acquired from respiratory therapy equipment. When contamination is found, it usually proceeds from the patient to the equipment and not vice versa. The principal factor responsible for this dramatic change is the universal use of disposable equipment in this country. Excessive handling of ventilator circuits may also lead to contamination. Nosocomial pneumonias are less likely to occur when circuits are changed at 48 h than when they are changed every 24 h (49, 78). It has been proposed that changing ventilator circuits at all during prolonged ventilation is unnecessary, although most clinicians are unwilling to accept that recommendation without further study. It is important to keep the potential infection hazard posed by respiratory devices in mind. Outbreaks of respiratory infections have been associated with contamination of aerosol medications, mainstream nebulizers, and even bedside spirometers (16, 83). Continued vigilance is required to avoid a repeat of that history.

Aspiration

In 1937 Amberson (1) placed contrast medium in the mouths of sleeping patients and performed chest radiographs on the next morning. Traces of contrast were found as far down as the alveoli. Using a more sensitive radioisotopic technique, Huxley et al. (41) demonstrated nocturnal aspiration in 45% of normal subjects and 70% of individuals with impaired levels of consciousness. The presence of a cuffed endotracheal tube does not prevent aspiration. Low-pressure cuffs have largely replaced the older high-pressure, low-compliance cuffs because they produce less damage to the tracheal epithelium. Some studies of low-pressure, high-compliance endotracheal tube cuffs showed that all allowed aspiration, even when overinflated to 50 cm of H_2O (84). Other studies have found that aspiration was more likely to occur around the older styled cuffs. A study by Cameron et al. (11) with 61 patients with tracheostomies 1 to 28 days old demonstrated aspiration of dye placed in the mouth in 42 (69%), with an average latency of 7 h. Secretions accumulate in the trachea above the cuff. These secretions are milked around the cuff as it is moved during body movements or during cycles of the ventilator. In addition, folds have been noted in the inflated cuff itself, which facilitate the passage of secretions (11).

Bacterial inoculation of the lungs may occur prior to, or at the time of, placement of endotracheal tubes or tracheostomy, although the ensuing pneumonia is often attributed to the presence of the tube. The bacterial etiology of pneumonias that develop during the patient's initial 72 h differs from that of pneumonias developing later. Early pneumonias are caused predominantly by organisms that colonize the upper respiratory tracts of humans, such as streptococci, *Haemophilus* spp., and staphylococci, whereas later pneumonias are predominantly due to gram-negative bacilli (86). This observation suggests that these early pneumonias are caused by organisms that are aspirated into the lungs during the process of intubation and resuscitation.

PNEUMONIA

Nosocomial pneumonia is the principal infection associated with endotracheal tubes. It has become fashionable to refer to these infections as "ventilator-associated pneumonias." However, while endotracheal tubes are very important risk factors, at least 30% of nosocomial pneumonias occur in nonintubated patients. Tracheobronchitis probably is more common than pneumonia and is differentiated from pneumonia by the absence of new radiographic infiltrates. Uniform criteria for the diagnosis of tracheobronchitis have not been promulgated, whereas many investigators have contributed to the present state of knowledge about nosocomial pneumonia.

Diagnosis of Nosocomial Pneumonia

Most of the existing literature on nosocomial pneumonia utilizes diagnoses based on clinical criteria, usually fever, new radiographic infiltrates, leukocytosis, and purulent secretions. Using the presence of histologic findings of pneumonia to definitively diagnose pneumonia at autopsy, Andrews et al. (2) evaluated the accuracy of clinical findings in the setting of adult respiratory distress syndrome (ARDS). Approximately one-third of patients were misclassified by clinical criteria, with errors occurring equally in over- and underdiagnosis. The accuracy of clinical predictions and treatment plans was compared in living patients, using quantitative cultures obtained by the protected specimen brush (PSB) technique to definitively diagnose significant lung infections (28). Only one-third of the treatment plans developed on the basis of clinical information, including a Gram stain of tracheal secretions, were considered adequate. Errors included missed diagnoses of pneumonia, overdiagnoses of pneumonia, and selection of ineffective antibiotics. In some studies, the frequency of pneumonia among patients who meet all of the clinical criteria mentioned has been less than 40% (29). These data indicate that clinical criteria for the diagnosis of nosocomial pneumonia are inadequate and frequently misleading.

Bacterial pneumonia develops when a bacterial inoculum is not promptly cleared from the distal lung. Bronchopneumonia that is recognizable microscopically requires the presence of at least 10^4 bacteria per g of lung tissue. Clinically apparent community-acquired pneumonias are often associated with bacterial concentrations exceeding 10^6/ml in sputum. Both the PSB technique and bronchoalveolar lavage (BAL) provide specimens that accurately mirror the bacterial flora present in high concentrations in the lung (47). Since the PSB sample volume is about 0.001 ml, bacteria that are present in concentrations less than 10^3 to 10^4/ml are likely to be missed with this technique. Clinical experience with the PSB has shown that the presence of more than 10^3 bacteria/ml is highly predictive of pneumonia (27); this should not be surprising, since that value indicates the presence of at least 10^6/ml in the lung. The corresponding value for quantitative BAL specimens is 10^4/ml. These observations indicate that studies on the epidemiology, etiology, or treatment of nosocomial pneumonia that are based only on clinical criteria are seriously flawed, and much of the existing literature must be interpreted with caution because of this problem.

Recently, an International Consensus Conference (69) published criteria for diagnosing nosocomial pneumonias for use in subsequent studies (Table 1). The former clinical criteria have become indictors of patients at risk but are not considered diagnostic of pneumonia. "Definite pneumonias" require histologic evidence of pneumonia plus the presence of 10^4 or more bacteria per g or the presence of lung abscess with a positive aspiration culture. Relatively few patients will meet these criteria. "Probable pneumonias" utilize protected samples from the periphery of the lung; it is anticipated that with time and greater experience and validation, patients who meet these criteria will be moved into a "definite" category.

Table 1. Diagnostic criteria for nosocomial pneumonia[a,b]

Diagnosis	Criteria
Definite pneumonia	X-ray or CT evidence of cavitation plus positive needle aspirate from the abscess **or**
	Histologic pneumonia pluss tissue culture containing $\geq 10^4$ bacteria/g
Probable pneumonia	Positive[c] quantitative protected sample from distal lung **or**
	Bacteremia with same organism in lower respiratory tract secretions **or**
	Positive pleural fluid culture with same organism in lower respiratory tract secretions **or**
	Histologic findings of pneumonia
Definitive absence of pneumonia	Absence of pneumonia at autopsy within 3 days of sampling **or**
	Definite alternative diagnosis plus negative reliable culture **or**
	Cytologic identification of another lung process plus negative reliable culture
Probable absence of pneumonia	Definitive alternative diagnosis plus resolution without antibiotics of fever or radiographic infiltrate **or**
	Persistence of fever and infiltrate with a definitive other diagnosis established
False positive	Significant growth in a usually reliable specimen in patients meeting the criteria for definite or probable absence of pneumonia
False negative	Insignificant growth in a usually reliable specimen in patient who meets criteria for definitive or probable pneumonia
Inconclusive	Patients not classifiable by above

[a] From Pingleton et al. (69).
[b] All patients meet criteria of new or persistent radiographic infiltrate and purulent tracheal secretions.
[c] "Positive" was not defined because this value may change over time as new evidence is accumulated. Current understanding is $\geq 10^3$/ml for PSB and $\geq 10^4$/ml for BAL.

Incidence of Nosocomial Pneumonia

Despite the difficulties in diagnosis, available evidence indicates a significant risk of infection after placement of an artificial airway. One of the first studies to document infections associated with tracheostomies was performed in 1953 among 155 patients in long-term follow-up (19); 17 (11%) developed tracheobronchitis, 37 (24%) developed "atelectasis-pneumonia," and 8 (5%) developed wound infection. In 1961 Head (40) retrospectively examined 462 patients with tracheostomies and identified mediastinitis in 4 (<1%) and infection ("wound sepsis to severe pneumonia") in 80 (17%). Salata and coworkers (81) attempted to distinguish pneumonias from colonization in 51 medical ICU patients, all intubated for 4 days or more. Of these, 21 patients (42%) developed pneumonia, as diagnosed by rigorous clinical criteria; only 8 patients had neither pneumonia nor colonization. The duration of intubation of those with pneumonia was nearly twice as long as for those with colonization alone (mean of 19.5 versus 11.2 days). Cross and Roup (16) evaluated 108 episodes of nosocomial pneumonia that occurred in 13,086 hospital admissions. The risk of nosocomial pneumonia in the absence of any respiratory assistance device was 0.3%, versus 1.3% in those patients with an endotracheal tube alone and 3.7% in those with both an endotracheal tube and mechanical ventilation. The risk of nosocomial pneumonia increased significantly after day 5 of therapy, and no case occurred within the first 24 h of ventilation.

In later studies, Rogers and Osterhout (79) noted pneumonia in 17 (20.5%) of 83 patients, with 11 deaths (65% mortality versus 25.3% overall). The time of onset of pneumonia varied from 1 to 25 days, and the use of mechanical ventilation was not a risk factor. The same paper (79) retrospectively reviewed 509 patients with tracheostomies for 48 h or longer, yielding 77 cases (15%) of pneumonia. Bryant et al. (10) followed 101 patients with tracheotomies in place for 48 h on longer; 24 (24%) developed tracheobronchitis alone, while pneumonia was diagnosed in 44 (44%). The mean interval from surgery to the development of tracheobronchitis was 7.7 days, and the mean interval to pneumonia was 8.9 days. Although nearly all patients with tracheobronchitis received antibiotics, the lack of a bacteriologic improvement or the replacement with a resistant organism prompted a conclusion that antibiotics should not be given in the absence of true pneumonia. Northey et al. (63) examined 77 patients admitted to a surgical ICU, 14 of whom had a tracheostomy. Of the patients with a tracheostomy, 9 (64%) developed pneumonia (all with *P. aeruginosa*), versus 7 of 63 (11%) without a tracheostomy. Brook (8), following 27 pediatric patients requiring a tracheostomy and prolonged intubation (3 to 12 months), found that 24 of them developed both tracheobronchitis and pneumonia.

Some studies suggest a greater risk with tracheostomy than with endotracheal intubation. Cross and Roup (16) compared the frequency of nosocomial pneumonia in patients with and without mechanical ventilation. The endotracheal tube group had pneumonia rates of 1.3 and 3.7%, respectively, whereas the rates for the tracheostomy group were 25 and 66%, respectively. Pather et al. (65), evaluating 52 neonatal patients requiring paralysis for therapy of tetanus, randomized every other patient to receive either a nasal endotracheal tube or tracheostomy. Although the two groups otherwise seemed similar, pneumonia or sepsis developed in 14 (54%) of those with tracheostomies, versus 7 (27%) in those nasally intubated. This study implies an independent risk of infection in tracheostomies over that with endotracheal tubes; confirmation in adults is lacking. In aggregate, it appears that the risk of acquiring pneumonia after tracheostomy is even higher than that with endotracheal intubation. This is not surprising in view of the population that requires tracheostomy: these patients generally require the artificial airway for longer periods of time. In addition, the surgical procedure of tracheostomy itself adds a further risk of infection.

The bacterial agents responsible for nosocomial pneumonias are shown in Table 2. As discussed earlier, pneumonias that develop early in the patient's course tend to be caused by different organisms than those that cause later pneumonias, paralleling changes in colonization patterns. The pediatric population is somewhat different. In 27 patients

Table 2. Etiologic agents in nosocomial pneumonia[a]

Organism	NNIS data (%) (83a)	PBS samples (%) (79a)
Enteric GNB	50	75
P. aeruginosa	17	31
Enterobacter spp.	11	2
Klebsiella spp.	7	4
Others	15	50
Gram-positive cocci	17	45
Staphylococci	16	33
Streptococci	1	21
Anaerobes	N/A	2
Fungi	4	N/A
Haemophilus spp.	6	10

[a] Percentage of cultures containing specific organisms; many patients had more than one species isolated.

with long-term intubation and tracheostomies, the predominant organisms were *S. pneumoniae, Staphylococcus aureus,* and anaerobes (8). Harris et al. (39), studying neonates, found postintubation colonization with various organisms: most were gram-negative organisms, but many were streptococci and *S. aureus.*

Both endotracheal intubation and tracheostomy bypass major lung defense mechanisms and interfere with the effectiveness of others. The serious illnesses that require this form of care independently alter defense mechanisms and increase susceptibility of the respiratory tract to colonization and infection. It is not surprising that many intubated patients develop pneumonia; it is perhaps surprising that all do not!

MANAGEMENT

In a patient who meets criteria for being "at risk" of nosocomial pneumonia, the clinician must decide how far to go with the collection of samples before initiating therapy. Certainly, tracheal secretions should be obtained for Gram stain, and adequate samples (i.e., ≥25 PMNs and ≤10 squamous epithelial cells per low-power field) should be cultured. If the patient is not intubated, an expectorated specimen may suffice. If the patient cannot cooperate or cannot cough effectively, transnasal tracheal suction should be employed. As discussed earlier, only bronchoscopic BAL and PSB have been subjected to rigorous evaluation, and despite the frequent claims of experienced physicians to the contrary, clinical impressions and empiric therapy chosen on the basis of Gram stains of tracheal aspirates are often in error (28). Clinical judgment must weigh the advantages of a more precise bacteriologic diagnosis against the cost, delay, and rare complications of bronchoscopy. Factors that guide the choice of antimicrobial agents for empiric therapy include underlying disease, severity of illness, immune status, prior antibiotic therapy, previous isolates from respiratory tract secretions, antimicrobial resistance patterns of the institution, hospital incidence of legionellosis, and evidence of any recent outbreaks of viral infections in the hospital or the community (66). Traditional treatment has consisted of broad-spectrum antibiotics—aminoglycosides in combination with a beta-lactam agent. Increasing evidence suggests that monotherapy with an expanded-spectrum cephalosporin, imipenem, or ticarcillin-clavulanic acid is as effective as the traditional combination therapy in nonneutropenic patients (22). Since aztreonam and aminoglycosides are not efficacious against the gram-positive organisms that are increasingly isolated from patients with nosocomial pneumonia, they should not be used as single agents. Once antibiotic susceptibilities are known, therapy should be adjusted, taking into account the patient's response to initial therapy.

PROGNOSIS

Crude mortality rates for ventilator-associated nosocomial pneumonia range from 26 to 71% (32). Nosocomial pneumonia is estimated to be responsible for approximately 17,500 deaths in the United States each year (90). The major question has always been whether patients died prematurely of nosocomial pneumonia or whether this infection simply served as the mode of exit for a patient who would have died in any case. Gross et al. (36) were among the first to show that nosocomial pneumonia had a significant attributable mortality. In contrast, Bryan and Reynolds (9) found a mortality of 58% in 168 patients with bacteremic nosocomial pneumonia, but nearly all patients had severe, irreversible underlying diseases.

Two recent studies have addressed the issue of attributable mortality in nosocomial pneumonia. Leu et al. (55) studied 1,001 consecutive patients with nosocomial pneumonia and found an overall mortality of 30% and an attributable mortality of 33%. More recently, Fagon et al. (30) performed a prospective cohort study of mechanically ventilated patients. All patients with clinically suspected pneumonia underwent bronchoscopy with PSB and BAL; 48 patients met criteria for pneumonia. Controls were matched by age, severity of disease, indication for mechanical ventilation, and duration of exposure to risk. A successful match was achieved in 222 of 240 variables. Mortality among patients with pneumonia was 54%, compared with 27% in controls ($P < 0.01$). Attributable mortality was 27%, similar to 33% in the study by Leu et al. (55). The risk ratio for death was 2.0. When nosocomial pneumonia was due to *Pseudomonas* or *Acinetobacter* spp., mortality rate was 71%, attributable mortality was 43%, and risk ratio was 2.5%.

A very recent, provocative study addresses the adverse effect of prior antibiotic therapy on the prognosis of nosocomial pneumonia. Rello et al. (77) studied 129 consecutive episodes of ventilator-associated pneumonia prospectively; diagnosis of pneumonia was made by the PSB technique. Univariate and multivariate analyses were used to examine prognostic factors. Age over 45 years, corticosteroid use, presence of shock, antecedent chronic obstructive pulmonary disease, hospital days of pneumonia over 9 days, and prior antibiotic therapy were variables associated with mortality by univariate analysis. Stepwise logistic regression analysis, however, identified only prior antibiotic use as significantly influencing the risk of death. When the etiologic agent of pneumonia was included in the regression equation, prior antibiotic use entirely dropped out as a significant risk factor. Fagon et al. (30) had found a similar effect of prior antibiotic use; 83% of the 31 patients who received prior antibiotics died, compared with 48% of the patients without prior antibiotics. In an earlier study by Graybill et al. (33), high-dose or multiple-antibiotic therapy was associated with 55% mortality, compared with 8% mortality associated with low-dose or single-antibiotic therapy. Age and severe underlying diseases are well-documented factors that adversely affect prognosis in patients with nosocomial pneumonia. It appears that injudicious antibiotic use is also such a factor, probably by selection of resistant organisms that respond even less well to therapy.

SINUSITIS

Paranasal sinusitis has been recognized with increasing frequency. In one study, in which 111 patients were randomly assigned to either nasotracheal or orotracheal intubation, maxillary sinusitis was diagnosed by X ray in 2% of orally intubated and 43% of nasally intubated patients (82). Nasogastric suction catheters were also a significant risk factor for sinusitis. Removal of the offending tube failed to resolve the associated sinusitis in 5 of 17 patients in whom this was attempted as the primary therapy, leading to drainage procedures in each. Similar findings were reported by Michelson et al. (58). However, sonography was used in this study to detect sinus abnormalities, and the rate of abnormalities was much higher. Sixty percent of orally intubated and 95% of nasally intubated patients developed densities. Aspiration of the abnormal sinuses yielded bacteria in 22% of orally intubated and 54% of nasally intubated patients. Since the original description by Arens et al. (3) in 1974, there have been more than 75 reported cases (2, 6, 12, 13, 21, 26, 53, 65). Most have been simply sinusitis, responding to conservative measures, but there are several accounts of associated sepsis (51, 64). Causative organisms are often GNB (35), but a wide variety of microbes have been reported.

CONCLUSIONS

Bacterial infection of the respiratory tract is a common complication of intubation of the trachea whether performed by the oral, nasal, or tracheostomy route. These infections occur because normal antibacterial defenses are bypassed or impaired and because people with underlying diseases that impair host defenses are likely to require these procedures. Distinguishing the effects of intubation from those attributable to the underlying illness is not possible except for the risks that are directly due to the respiratory support devices. Contamination of respiratory therapy devices, especially mainstream nebulizers, has been largely relegated to history, because of the widespread use of disposable equipment. However, the formation of contaminated biofilms within endotracheal tubes appears to pose a significant risk of infection. Control of this factor might lead to further improvements in pneumonia prevention.

REFERENCES

1. **Amberson, J. B.** 1937. Aspiration bronchopneumonia. *Int. Anesthesiol. Clin.* **3**:126–138.
2. **Andrews, C. P., J. J. Coalson, J. D. Smith, and W. G. Johanson, Jr.** 1981. Diagnosis of nosocomial bacterial pneumonia in acute, diffuse lung injury. *Chest* **80**:254–258.
3. **Arens, J. F., F. E. LeJeune, Jr., and D. R. Webre.** 1974. Maxilliary sinusitis: a complication of nasotracheal intubation. *Anesthesiology* **40**:414–416.
4. **Atherton, S. T., and D. J. White.** 1978. Stomach as a source of bacteria colonizing respiratory tract during artificial ventilation. *Lancet* **ii**:968–969.
5. **Atik, M., and B. Hanson.** 1970. Gram-negative pneumonitis: a new postoperative menace. *Chest* **74**:635–639.
6. **Bartlett, J. G., L. J. Faling, and S. Willey.** 1978. Quantitative tracheal bacteriologic and cytologic studies in patients with long-term tracheostomies. *Chest* **74**:635–639.
7. **Bloomfield, A. L.** 1922. The mechanisms of elimination of bacteria from the respiratory tract. *Am. J. Med. Sci.* **164**:854–867.
8. **Brook, I.** 1979. Bacterial colonization, tracheobronchitis, and pneumonia following tracheostomy and long-term intubation in pediatric patients. *Chest* **76**:420–424.
9. **Bryan, C. S., and K. L. Reynolds.** 1984. Bacteremic nosocomial pneumonia. *Am. Rev. Respir. Dis.* **129**:668–671.
10. **Bryant, L. R., J. K. Trinkle, K. Mobin-Uddin, J. Baker, and W. O. J. Griffen.** 1972. Bacterial colonization profile with tracheal intubation and mechanical ventilation. *Arch. Surg.* **104**:647–651.
11. **Cameron, J. L., J. Reynolds, and G. D. Zuidema.** 1973. Aspiration in patients with tracheostomies. *Surg. Gynecol. Obstet.* **136**:68–70.
12. **Caplan, E. S.** 1982. Nosocomial sinusitis. *JAMA* **247**:639–641.
13. **Collier, A. M., L. P. Peterson, and J. B. Baseman.** 1977. Pathogenesis of infection with *Bordetella pertussis* in hamster tracheal organ culture. *J. Infect. Dis.* **136**:S196–S203.
14. **Cook, D. J., L. A. Laine, G. H. Guyatt, and T. A. Raffin.** 1991. Nosocomial pneumonia and the role of gastric pH: a meta-analysis. *Chest* **100**:7–13.
15. **Costerton, J. W., and R. T. Irwin.** 1981. The bacterial glycocalyx in nature and disease. *Annu. Rev. Microbiol.* **35**:299–324.
16. **Cross, A. S., and B. Roup.** 1981. Role of respiratory assistance devices in endemic nosocomial pneumonia. *Am. J. Med.* **70**:681–685.
17. **Dal Nogare, A. R., G. B. Toews, and A. K. Pierce.** 1987. Increased salivary elastase precedes gram-negative bacillary colonization in postoperative patients. *Am. Rev. Respir. Dis.* **134**:671–675.
18. **Daschner, F., I. Kappstein, I. Engels, K. Reuschenbach, J. Pfisterer, and P. Kreig.**

1988. Stress ulcer prophylaxis and ventilation pneumonia: prevention by antibacterial cytoprotective agents. *Control Hosp. Epidemiol.* **9:**59–65.

19. **Davis, H. S., H. E. Kretchmer, and R. Bryce-Smith.** 1953. Advantages and complications of tracheotomy. *JAMA* **153:**1156–1159.

20. **Deutschman, C. S., P. Wilton, J. Sinow, D. J. Dibbell, F. N. Konstantinides, and F. B. Cerra.** 1986. Paranasal sinusitis associated with nasotracheal intubation: a frequently unrecognized and treatable source of sepsis. *Crit. Care Med.* **14:**111–114.

21. **Deutschman, C. S., P. B. Wilton, J. Sinow, P. Thienprasit, F. N. Konstantinides, and F. B. Cerra.** 1985. Paranasal sinusitis: a common complication of nasotracheal intubation in neurosurgical patients. *Neurosurgery* **17:**296–299.

22. **Dever, L. L., and W. G. Johanson.** 1992. Nosocomial pneumonia, p. 1–28. *In* D. S. Simmons and D. E. Tierney (ed.), *Current Pulmonology,* 13th ed. Mosby-Year Book, Inc., St. Louis.

23. **Diaz-Blanco, J., R. C. Clawson, S. M. Roberson, C. B. Sanders, A. K. Pramanik, and J. J. Herbst.** 1989. Electron microscopic evaluation of bacterial adherence to polyvinyl chloride endotracheal tubes used in neonates. *Crit. Care Med.* **17:**1335–1340.

24. **Driks, M. R., D. E. Craven, B. R. Celli, M. Manning, R. A. Burke, G. M. Garvin, L. M. Kunches, H. W. Farber, S. A. Wedel, and W. R. McCabe.** 1987. Nosocomial pneumonia in intubated patients given sucralfate as compared with antacids or histamine type 2 blockers. *N. Engl. J. Med.* **317:**1376–1382.

25. **Du Moulin, G. C., D. G. Paterson, J. Hedley-Whyte, and A. Lisbon.** 1982. Aspiration of gastric bacteria in antacid-treated patients: a frequent cause of post operative colonization of the airway. *Lancet* **ii:**242–245.

26. **Dunn, C. R., D. L. Dunn, and K. M. Moser.** 1974. Determinants of tracheal injury by cuffed tracheostomy tubes. *Chest* **65:**128–135.

27. **Fagon, J., J. Chastre, Y. Domart, J. L. Troullet, J. Pierre, C. Darne, and C. Gibert.** 1989. Nosocomial pneumonia in patients receiving continuous mechanical ventilation. Prospective analysis of 52 episodes with use of a protected speciman brush and quantitative culture techniques. *Am. Rev. Respir. Dis.* **139:**877–884.

28. **Fagon, J., J. Chastre, A. J. Hance, Y. Domart, J. Trouillet, and C. Gibert.** 1993. Evaluation and clinical judgement in the identification and treatment of nosocomial pneumonia in ventilated patients. *Chest* **103:**547–553.

29. **Fagon, J., J. Chastre, A. J. Hance, M. Guiguet, J. Trouillet, Y. Domart, and C. Gibert.** 1988. Use of a protected specimen brush and quantitative culture techniques in 147 patients. *Am. Rev. Respir. Dis.* **138:**110–116.

30. **Fagon, J. Y., J. Chastre, A. J. Hance, P. Montravers, A. Novara, and C. Gibert.** 1993. Nosocomial pneumonia in ventilated patients: a cohort study evaluating attributable mortality and hospital stay. *Am. J. Med.* **94:**281–288.

31. **Forbes, A. R., and G. Gamsu.** 1979. Lung muciliary clearance after anesthesia with spontaneous and controlled ventilation. *Am. Rev. Respir. Dis.* **120:**857–862.

32. **George, D. L.** 1993. Epidemiology of nosocomial ventilator-associated pneumonia. *Infect. Control Hosp. Epidemiol.* **14:**163–169.

33. **Graybill, J. R., L. W. Marshall, P. Charache, C. K. Wallace, and V. B. Melvin.** 1973. Nosocomial pneumonia. *Am. Rev. Respir. Dis.* **108:**1130–1140.

34. **Green, G. M., G. J. Jakab, R. B. Low, and G. S. Davis.** 1977. Defense mechanisms of the respiratory membrane. *Am. Rev. Respir. Dis.* **115:**479–514.

35. **Grindlinger, G. A., I. Niehoff, S. L. Hughes, M. A. Humphrey, and G. Simpson.** 1987. Acute paranasal sinusitis related to nasotracheal intubation of head-injury patients. *Crit. Care Med.* **15:**214–217.

36. **Gross, P. A., H. C. Neu, P. Aswapokee, C. Van Antwerpen, and N. Aswapokee.**

1980. Deaths from nosocomial infections: experience in a community hospital. *Am. J. Med.* **68:**219–225.

37. **Haley, R. W., T. M. Hooton, D. H. Culver, R. C. Stanely, and T. G. Emori.** 1981. Nosocomial infections in U.S. hospitals, 1975–1976. *Am. J. Med.* **70:**947–959.

38. **Harris, G. D., D. E. Woods, R. Fine, and W. G. Johanson, Jr.** 1980. The effect of intraalveolar fluid on lung bacterial clearance. *Lung* **158:**91–100.

39. **Harris, H., D. Wirtschafter, and G. Cassady.** 1976. Endotracheal intubation and its relationship to bacterial colonization and systemic infection of newborn infants. *Pediatrics* **56:**816–823.

40. **Head, J. M.** 1961. Tracheostomy in the management of respiratory problems. *N. Engl. J. Med.* **264:**587–591.

41. **Huxley, E. J., J. Viroslav, W. R. Gray, and A. K. Pierce.** 1978. Pharyngeal aspiration in normal adults and patients with depressed consciousness. *Am. J. Med.* **64:**565–568.

42. **Inglis, T. J. J.** 1993. Evidence of dynamic phenomena in residual tracheal tube biofilm. *Br. J. Anaesth.* **70:**22–24.

43. **Inglis, T. J. J., M. R. Millar, J. G. Jones, and D. A. Robinson.** 1989. Tracheal tube biofilm as a source of bacterial colonization of the lung. *J. Clin. Microbiol.* **27:**2014–2018.

44. **Inglis, T. J. J., L. J. Sproat, M. J. Sherratt, P. N. Howkey, J. S. Gibson, and M. V. Shah.** 1992. Gastroduodenal dysfunction as a cause of gastric bacterial overgrowth in patients undergoing mechanical ventilation of the lungs. *Br. J. Anaesth.* **68:**499–502.

45. **Johanson, W. G., Jr., A. K. Pierce, and J. P. Sanford.** 1969. Changing pharyngeal bacterial flora of hospitalized patients. *N. Engl. J. Med.* **281:**1137–1140.

46. **Johanson, W. G., Jr., A. K. Pierce, J. P. Sanford, and G. D. Thomas.** 1972. Nosocomial respiratory infections with gram-negative bacilli. *Ann. Intern. Med.* **77:**701–706.

47. **Johanson, W. G., J. Seidenfeld, P. Gomez, R. Santos, and J. J. Coalson.** 1988. Bacteriologic diagnosis of nosocomial pneumonia following protracted mechanical ventilation. *Am. Rev. Respir. Dis.* **137:**259–264.

48. **Kastanos, N., R. E. Miro, A. M. Perez, A. X. Mir, and A. Agusti-Vidal.** 1983. Laryngotracheal injury due to endotracheal intubation: incidence, evolution, and predisposing factors. *Crit. Care Med.* **11:**362–367.

49. **Kingston, G. W., P. T. Phang, and M. J. Leathley.** 1991. Increased incidence of nosocomial pneumonia in mechanically ventilated patients with subclinical aspiration. *Am. J. Surg.* **161:**589–592.

50. **Klainer, A. S., H. Turndorf, W. H. Wu, H. Maewal, and P. Allender.** 1975. Surface alterations due to endotracheal intubation. *Am. J. Med.* **58:**674–683.

51. **Kronberg, F. G., and W. J. Goodwin, Jr.** 1985. Sinusitis in intensive care unit patients. *Laryngoscope* **95:**936–938.

52. **LaForce, F. M.** 1981. Hospital-acquired gram-negative rod pneumonias: an overview. *Am. J. Med.* **70:**664–669.

53. **Landa, J. F., M. A. Kwoka, G. A. Chapman, M. Brito, and M. A. Sackner.** 1980. Effects of suctioning on mucociliary transport. *Chest* **77:**202–207.

54. **Laurenzi, G. A., R. T. Potter, and E. H. Kass.** 1961. Bacteriologic flora of the lower respiratory tract. *N. Engl. J. Med.* **265:**1273–1278.

55. **Leu, H.-S., D. I. Kaiser, M. Mori, R. F. Woolson, and R. P. Wenzel.** 1989. Hospital-acquired pneumonia: attributable mortality and morbidity. *Am. J. Epidemiol.* **129:**1258–1267.

56. **Lowbury, E. J. L., B. T. Thom, H. A. Lilly, J. R. Babb, and K. Whittall.** 1970. Sources of infection with *Pseudomonas aeruginosa* in patients with tracheostomy. *J. Med. Microbiol.* **3:**39–56.

57. **Mason, C. M., R. E. Bawdon, A. K. Pierce, and A. R. Dal Nogare.** 1990. Fibronectin

is not detectable on the intact buccal epitherlial surface of normal rats or humans. *Am. J. Respir. Cell Mol. Biol.* **3**:563–570.

58. **Michelson, A., H. D. Kamp, and B. Schuster.** 1991. Sinusitis in long-term intubated intensive care patients: nasal versus oral intubation. *Anaesthetist* **40**:100–104.

59. **Newhouse, M., J. Sanchis, and J. Bienenstock.** 1976. Lung defense mechanisms. *N. Engl. J. Med.* **295**:990–998; 1045–1052.

60. **Nickel, J. C., I. Ruseka, J. B. Wright, and J. W. Costerton.** 1985. Tobramycin resistance of cells of *Pseudomonas aeruginosa* growing as a biofilm on urinary catheter material. *Antimicrob. Agents Chemother.* **27**:619–624.

61. **Niederman, M. S., R. D. Ferranti, A. Zeiger, W. W. Merril, and H. Y. Reynolds.** 1984. Respiratory infection complicating long-term tracheostomy. *Chest* **85**:39–44.

62. **Niederman, M. S., T. D. Rafferty, C. T. Sasaki, W. W. Merrill, R. A. Matthay, and H. Y. Reynolds.** 1983. Comparison of bacterial adherence to ciliated and squamous epithelial cells obtained from the human respiratory tract. *Am. Rev. Respir. Dis.* **127**: 85–90.

63. **Northey, D., M. L. Adess, J. M. Hartsuck, and E. R. Rhoades.** 1974. Microbial surveillance in a surgical intensive care unit. *Surg. Gynecol. Obstet.* **139**:321–325.

64. **O'Reilly, M. J., E. J. Reddick, W. Black, P. L. Carter, J. Erhardt, W. Fill, D. Maughn, A. Sado, and G. R. Klatt.** 1984. Sepsis from sinusitis in nasotracheally intubated patients *Am. J. Surg.* **147**:601–604.

65. **Pather, M., D. Hariparsad, and A. G. Wesley.** 1985. Nasotracheal intubation versus tracheostomy for intermittent positive pressure ventilation in neonatal tetanus. *Intensive Care Med.* **11**:30–32.

66. **Pennington, J. E.** 1989. Hospital-acquired pneumonia, p. 171–186. *In* J. E. Pennington (ed.), *Respiratory Infections: Diagnosis and Management.* Raven Press, New York.

67. **Pierce, A. J., J. P. Sanford, G. D. Thomas, and J. S. Leonard.** 1970. Long-term evaluation of decontamination of inhalation-therapy equipment and the occurrence of necrotizing pneumonia. *N. Engl. J. Med.* **282**:528–531.

68. **Pingleton, S. K.** 1989. Enteral nutrition as a risk factor for nosocomial pneumonia. *Eur. J. Clin. Microbiol. Infect. Dis.* **8**:51–55.

69. **Pingleton, S. K., J. Fagon, and K. V. Leeper.** 1993. Patient selection for clinical investigation of ventilator-associated pneumonia: criteria for evaluation diagnostic techniques. *Chest* **102**:553S–556S.

70. **Potgieter, P. D., D. M. Linton, S. Oliver, and A. A. Forder.** 1987. Nosocomial infections in a respiratory intensive care unit. *Crit. Care Med.* **14**:495–498.

71. **Ramphal, R., and G. B. Pier.** 1985. Role of *Pseudomonas aeruginosa* mucoid exopolysaccharide in adherence to tracheal cells. *Infect. Immun.* **47**:1–4.

72. **Ramphal, R., and M. Pyle.** 1983. Evidence for mucins and sialic acid as receptors for *Pseudomonas aeruginosa* in the lower respiratory tract. *Infect. Immun.* **41**:339–344.

73. **Ramphal, R., J. C. Sadoff, M. Pyle, and J. D. Silpigni.** 1984. Role of pili in the adherence of *Pseudomonas aeruginosa* to injured tracheal epithelium. *Infect. Immun.* **44**: 38–40.

74. **Ramphal, R., P. M. Small, J. W. Shands, Jr., W. Fischlschweiger, and P. A. Small, Jr.** 1980. Adherence of *Pseudomonas aeruginosa* to tracheal cells injured by influenza infection or by endotracheal intubation. *Infect. Immun.* **27**:614–619.

75. **Rehm, S. R., G. N. Gross, and A. K. Pierce.** 1980. Early bacterial clearance from murine lungs. Species-dependent phagocyte response. *J. Clin. Invest.* **66**:194–199.

76. **Reinarz, J. A., A. K. Pierce, B. B. Mays, and J. P. Sanford.** 1965. The potential role of inhalation therapy equipment in nosocomial pulmonary infection. *J. Clin. Invest.* **44**:831–839.

77. **Rello, J., E. Quintana, V. Ausina, J. Castella, M. Luquin, A. Net, and G. Prats.** 1991. Incidence, etiology, and outcome of nosocomial pneumonia in mechanically ventilated patients. *Chest* **100:**439–444.
78. **Rodriquez, J. L., K. J. Gibbons, L. G. Bitzer, D. E. Dechert, S. M. Steinberg, and L. M. Flint.** 1991. Pneumonia: incidence, risk factors, and outcome in injured patients. *J. Trauma* **31:**907–914.
79. **Rogers, L. A., and S. Osterhout.** 1970. Pneumonia following tracheostomy. *Am. Surg.* **36:**39–46.
79a. **Rouby, J. J., E. M. De Lassale, P. Poete, M. H. Nicholas, L. Bodin, V. Jarlier, Y. L. Carpentier, J. Grosset, and P. Viars.** 1992. Nosocomial bronchopneumonia in the critically ill: histologic and bacteriologic aspects. *Am. Rev. Respir. Dis.* **146:**1059–1066.
80. **Sackner, M. A., J. Hirsch, and S. Epstein.** 1975. Effect of cuffed endotracheal tubes on tracheal mucous velocity. *Chest* **68:**774–777.
81. **Salata, R. A., M. M. Lederman, D. M. Shlaes, M. R. Jacobs, E. Eckstein, D. Tweardy, A. Toossi, R. Chmielewski, J. Marino, C. H. King, R. C. Graham, and J. J. Ellner.** 1987. Diagnosis of nosocomial pneumonia in intubated intensive care unit patients. *Am. Rev. Respir. Dis.* **135:**426–432.
82. **Salord, F., P. Gaussorgues, J. Marti-Flich, M. Sirodot, C. Allimant, D. Lyonnet, and D. Robert.** 1990. Nosocomial maxillary sinusitis during mechanical ventilation: a prospective comparison of orotracheal versus nasotracheal route for intubation. *Intensive Care Med.* **16:**390–393.
83. **Sanders, C. V., Jr., J. P. Luby, W. G. Johanson, Jr., J. A. Barnett, and J. P. Sanford.** 1970. *Serratia marcescens* infections from inhalation therapy medications: nosocomial outbreak. *Ann. Intern. Med.* **73:**15–21.
83a. **Schaberg, D. R., D. H. Culver, and R. P. Gaynes.** 1991. Major trends in the microbial etiology of nosocomial infection. *Am. J. Med.* **Suppl. 3B:**72S–75S.
84. **Seegobin, R. D., and G. L. van Hasselt.** 1986. Aspiration beyond endotracheal cuffs. *Can. Anaesth. Soc. J.* **33:**273–279.
85. **Sottile, F. D., T. J. Marrie, D. S. Prough, C. D. Hobgood, D. J. Gower, L. X. Webb, J. W. Costerton, and A. G. Gristina.** 1986. Nosocomial pulmonary infection: possible etiologic significance of bacterial adhesion to endotracheal tubes. *Crit. Care Med.* **14:**265–270.
86. **Stoutenbeek, C. P., H. K. F. van Saene, D. R. Miranda, D. F. Zandstra, and B. Binnendijk.** 1984. The prevention of superinfection in trauma patients. *J. Antimicrob. Chemother.* **14(Suppl. B):**203–209.
87. **Todisco, T., M. Maurizi, G. Paludetti, M. Dottorini, and F. Merante.** 1984. Laryngeal cancer: long-term follow-up of respiratory functions after laryngectomy. *Respiration* **45:**303–315.
88. **Tryba, M., and F. Mantey-Stiers.** 1987. Antibacterial activity of sucralfate in human gastric juice. *Am. J. Med.* **83(Suppl. 3B):**125–127.
89. **Vishwanath, S., and R. Ramphal.** 1984. Adherence of *Pseudomonas aeruginosa* to human tracheobronchial mucin. *Infect. Immun.* **45:**197–202.
90. **Wenzel, R. P.** 1989. Hospital-acquired pneumonia: overview of the current state of the art for prevention and control. *Eur. J. Microbiol. Infect. Dis.* **8:**56–60.
91. **Woods, D. E., D. C. Straus, W. G. Johanson, Jr., and J. A. Bass.** 1981. Role of salivary protease activity in adherence of gram-negative bacilli to mammalian buccal epithelial cells in vitro. *J. Clin. Invest.* **68:**1435–1440.
92. **Woods, D. E., D. C. Straus, W. G. Johanson, Jr., V. K. Berry, and J. A. Bass.** 1980. Role of pili in adherence of *Pseudomonas aeruginosa* to mammalian buccal epithelial cells. *Infect. Immun.* **29:**1146–1151.

Infections Associated with Indwelling Medical Devices, 2nd ed.
Edited by Alan L. Bisno and Francis A. Waldvogel
© 1994 American Society for Microbiology, Washington, DC 20005

Chapter 8

Infections Caused by Intravascular Devices Used for Infusion Therapy: Pathogenesis, Prevention, and Management

Dennis G. Maki

> . . . *strong corruption inhabits our frail blood.*
> —William Shakespeare

Reliable vascular access for administration of fluids and electrolytes, blood products, drugs, and nutritional support and for hemodynamic monitoring is now one of the most essential features of modern medical care. Unfortunately, vascular access is associated with substantial and generally underappreciated potential for producing iatrogenic disease, particularly bloodstream infection originating from infection of the percutaneous device used for vascular access or from contamination of the infusate administered through the device (8). More than one half of all epidemics of nosocomial bacteremia or candidemia derive from vascular access in some form (129, 131). Nosocomial intravascular device-related bacteremia or candidemia in hospitalized patients is associated with two- to threefold increased attributable mortality (1, 114, 129, 242).

Intravascular device-related sepsis is largely preventable. The goal must not be simply to identify and treat device-related infections, but

Dennis G. Maki • Section of Infectious Diseases, Department of Medicine, University of Wisconsin Medical School, and Infection Control Department and Center for Trauma and Life Support, University of Wisconsin Hospital and Clinics, Madison, Wisconsin 53792.

rather to prevent them. Over the past decade, much has been learned about the pathogenesis and epidemiology of infections associated with intravascular devices. By drawing upon existent knowledge of pathogenesis and epidemiology, rational and effective guidelines for prevention can be formulated.

SOURCES AND FORMS OF INTRAVASCULAR DEVICE-RELATED SEPSIS

There are two major sources of bloodstream infection associated with any intravascular device: (i) colonization of the device itself and (ii) contamination of the fluid (infusate) administered through the device. Cannulas, which cause most endemic device-related infections, produce septicemia far more frequently than contaminated infusate, the source of most epidemics of infusion-associated sepsis (129). Cannula is a generic term that refers to all types of percutaneous devices used for vascular access, including small steel ("scalp-vein" or "butterfly") needles and plastic catheters of numerous forms and sizes.

Cannula-Related Infections

Between 5 and 25% of intravascular devices are colonized at the time of removal, as reflected by semiquantitative or quantitative cultures showing large numbers of organisms on the intravascular portion of the removed cannula or its tip. Surface colonization of the implanted portion of the cannula, which usually is asymptomatic, can be considered synonymous with local infection but forms the biologic setting for systemic infection to occur. Colonized cannulas are more likely than noncolonized ones to show local inflammation at the insertion site and are far more likely to cause cannula-related bacteremia or fungemia (7, 149, 187).

One of the most serious forms of intravascular device-related infection occurs when thrombus surrounding the cannula becomes infected, producing septic (suppurative) thrombophlebitis with peripheral intravenous (i.v.) cannulas (104, 197, 264) or septic thrombosis of a great central vein with centrally placed venous catheters (111, 197, 256, 273). With suppurative phlebitis, bloodstream infection characteristically persists after the cannula has been removed, producing a predictable clinical picture of overwhelming sepsis with high-grade bacteremia or fungemia. This syndrome is most often encountered in burned patients or other intensive care unit (ICU) patients who develop cannula-related infection that goes unrecognized, permitting microorganisms to proliferate to high levels within intravascular thrombus. The catheter insertion site is devoid of signs of inflammation more than half the time, and the clinical picture may not present until after the catheter has been removed. In any patient with an intravascular device who develops high-grade bacteremia or candidemia, persisting after an infected cannula has been removed, it is likely the patient has infected thrombus in the recently cannulated vein and may even have developed secondary endocarditis or seeding to other distant sites. Suppurative phlebitis of peripheral i.v. catheters is now rare, and the syndrome of intravenous suppuration is predominantly a complication of central venous catheters, typically catheters that have been left in place for many days in vulnerable ICU patients. The microorganisms most frequently implicated in suppurative phlebitis are the same organisms that cause uncomplicated cannula-related septicemia: *Staphylococcus aureus*, nosocomial aerobic gram-negative bacilli, and, especially in recent years, *Candida* spp.

Sepsis from Contaminated Infusate

It is also important to recognize that infusate—parenteral fluid, blood products, or i.v. medications—administered through an intravascular device can also become contaminated and produce device-related septicemia, which is more likely to culminate in septic shock than is cannula-related infection. Contaminated fluid is fortunately an infrequent cause of endemic infusion-related infection with most intravascular devices, with the exception of devices used for hemodynamic monitoring and surgically implanted cuffed Hickman or Broviac catheters. Most nosocomial epidemics of infusion-related septicemia, however, have been traced to contamination of infusate by gram-negative bacilli, introduced during its manufacture (intrinsic contamination) or during its preparation and administration in the hospital (extrinsic contamination) (129).

DIAGNOSIS OF INFUSION-RELATED SEPTICEMIA

Clinical Features

The general clinical features of infusion-related septicemia are nonspecific and indiscernible from bloodstream infections arising from any local infection, such as of the urinary tract or surgical wounds (Table 1). Infusion-related bacteremia or fungemia is usually identified by positive blood cultures but may be mistakenly ascribed to nosocomial pneumonia or to urinary tract or surgical wound infection or simply accepted as "cryptogenic" and treated.

Table 1. Clinical, epidemiologic, and microbiologic features of intravascular device-related sepsis[a]

Nonspecific
Fever
Chills, shaking rigors[b]
Hypotension, shock[b]
Hyperventilation, respiratory failure
Gastrointestinal[b]
Abdominal pain
Vomiting
Diarrhea
Neurologic[b]
Confusion
Seizures
Suggestive of device-related etiology
Patient unlikely candidate for sepsis (e.g., young, no underlying diseases)
Source of sepsis inapparent, no identifiable local infection
Intravascular device in place, especially central venous catheter
Inflammation or purulence at insertion site
Abrupt onset, associated with shock[b]
Septicemia caused by staphylococci (especially coagulase-negative staphylococci) or *Corynebacterium, Candida, Trichophyton, Fusarium,* or *Malassezia* species[c]
Very high-grade (>25 CFU per ml) candidemia
Cluster of cryptogenic infusion-associated bloodstream infections caused by *Enterobacter* species (especially *E. cloacae* or *E. agglomerans*) or *Serratia marcescens*
Sepsis refractory to antimicrobial therapy or dramatic improvement with removal of cannula and infusion[b]

[a] From D. G. Maki (132).
[b] Commonly seen in overwhelming gram-negative sepsis originating from contaminated infusate, peripheral suppurative phlebitis, or septic thrombosis of a central vein.
[c] Conversely, septicemia caused by streptococci, aerobic gram-negative bacilli, or anaerobes is unlikely to derive from an intravascular device.

Certain clinical, epidemiologic, and microbiologic findings point toward an intravascular device as the source (Table 1):

- A patient who is an unlikely candidate for sepsis, without underlying diseases (143, 165)
- No obvious local infection to account for the picture of sepsis (143, 165)
- An intravascular device, especially a central venous catheter, in place at the outset of sepsis (165)
- Local inflammation, especially purulence, at the insertion site (7, 12, 187)
- Abrupt onset, associated with fulminant shock, suggestive of heavily contaminated infusate (143)

- Nosocomial bloodstream infection caused by staphylococci (165), especially coagulase-negative staphylococci, *Corynebacterium* (especially *C. jeikeium*, or JK) or *Bacillus* species, or *Candida* (165), *Fusarium*, *Trichophyton*, or *Malassezia* species. In contrast, bacteremia caused by streptococci, aerobic gram-negative bacilli—especially *Pseudomonas aeruginosa*—or anaerobes is unlikely to have originated from infected intravascular device (165).
- High-grade (>25 CFU/ml) cryptogenic candidemia (257)
- Sepsis refractory to antimicrobial therapy or dramatic improvement with removal of the cannula and discontinuation of the infusion (143)

Blood Cultures

Blood cultures are essential to the diagnosis of device-related bloodstream infection, and in any patient suspected of infusion-related infection, two blood samples should be drawn for culture (275), ideally from peripheral veins, by separate venipunctures. Tincture of iodine is recommended for cutaneous antisepsis prior to each venipuncture on the basis of its superiority over 10% povidone-iodine in reducing the frequency of contaminated blood cultures (3.7 versus 6.2%, $P < 0.0001$) in a recent large prospective randomized trial (255). Every effort must be made to prevent introduced contamination when drawing blood for cultures, because a single contaminated blood culture has been shown to prolong hospitalization 4 days and increase the cost of hospitalization $4,400 (17).

The volume of blood cultured is essential to maximize the sensitivity of blood cultures for diagnosis of bacteremia or candidemia: in adults, obtaining at least 20 ml, ideally 30 ml, per drawing—each specimen containing 10 to 15 ml, inoculated into aerobic and anaerobic media—significantly improves the yield, compared with obtaining only 5 ml at each drawing and culturing a smaller total volume (161, 275). In adults, if at least 30 ml of blood is cultured, 99% of detectable bacteremias should be identified (278).

If the laboratory is prepared to do pour-plate blood cultures or has available an automated quantitative system for culturing blood, such as the Isolator lysis-centrifugation system (E. I. DuPont de Nemours & Co.), blood samples for quantitative culture drawn through the device and concomitantly by venipuncture from a peripheral vein can permit the diagnosis of central venous device-related bacteremia or fungemia to be made with sensitivity and specificity in the range of 90%, without removing the catheter (9, 19, 55, 74, 207, 267, 277). With infected catheters, cultures from the blood drawn through the catheter usually show a 10-fold or greater step-up in the concentration of organisms, contrasted with a quantitative culture of a blood sample drawn percutaneously through a peripheral vein. High-grade candidemia (>25 CFU/m) reflects an infected intravascular device 90% of the time (257). Quantitative cultures of catheter-drawn blood are most useful for diagnosis of infections of cuffed surgically implanted Hickman or Broviac catheters and subcutaneous central venous ports (19, 55, 74, 207, 277).

Recently, Rushforth et al. (221) have reported on the use of an acridine orange stain of a cytospin of lysed blood drawn through the central venous catheter as a rapid method for diagnosis of catheter-related sepsis. The novel technique was 87 and 94% specific, compared with quantitative cultures of catheter-drawn blood samples and semiquantitative samples from the catheter tip, respectively.

Microbiology of Device-Related Sepsis

As noted, the microbiologic profile of bloodstream infection (Table 2) usually points strongly toward an intravascular device as the source. Primary (cryptogenic) staphylococcal bacteremia, particularly with coagulase-negative staphylococci; bacteremia caused by *Enterococcus* or *Corynebacterium* species (especially JK) or *Bacillus* species; or fungemia caused by *Candida, Fusarium, Trichophyton,* or *Malassezia* spp. in a patient with a vascular catheter usually reflects catheter-related infection (129, 131, 165).

Bacteremias caused by members of the tribe *Klebsielleae (Enterobacter cloacae* or especially *Enterobacter agglomerans)* or by non-*P. aeruginosa* pseudomonads (particularly *Pseudomonas cepacia* or *Pseudomonas pickettii), Xanthomonas maltophilia,* or *Flavobacterium* or *Citrobacter* species, in the setting of infusion therapy, should prompt studies to rule out contaminated infusate (126) and may signal an epidemic. A cluster of cases mandates a full-scale investigation, which may include culturing in-use infusions and informing the local, state and federal public health authorities.

Primary nosocomial bacteremia caused by psychrophilic (cold-growing) organisms, such as non-*P. aeruginosa* pseudomonads or *Achromobacter, Flavobacterium, Enterobacter,* or *Serratia* species (25, 188), or by *Salmonella* (91, 212) or *Yersinia* species (35), with a picture of overwhelming sepsis, should raise suspicion of a contaminated blood product.

Cultures of Intravascular Devices

Too many laboratories still culture vascular catheters qualitatively, in liquid media. Unfortunately, a positive culture by this diagnostic technique has poor specificity. Studies in many centers have shown that culturing catheter segment semiquantitatively on solid media (38, 43, 45, 75, 149, 243) or quantitatively in liquid media—removing organisms by

Table 2. Microorganisms most frequently encountered in various forms of intravascular device-related infection

Source	Pathogens
Catheter-related	
Peripheral i.v. catheter	*Staphylococcus aureus*
	Coagulase-negative staphylococci
	Candida spp.
Central venous catheters	Coagulase-negative staphylococci
	S. aureus
	Candida spp.
	Corynebacterium spp. (especially JK-1)
	Klebsiella and *Enterobacter* spp.
	Mycobacterium spp.
	Trichophyton beiglii
	Fusarium spp.
	Malassezia spp.[a]
Contaminated i.v. infusate	Tribe *Klebsielleae*
	Enterobacter cloacae
	Enterobacter agglomerans
	Serratia marcescens
	Klebsiella spp.
	Pseudomonas cepacia, P. acidivorans, P. pickettii
	Xanthomonas maltophilia
	Citrobacter freundii
	Flavobacterium spp.
	Candida tropicalis
Contaminated blood products	*E. cloacae*
	S. marcescens
	Achromobacter spp.
	Flavobacterium spp.
	Pseudomonas spp.
	Salmonella spp.
	Yersinia spp.

[a] Also seen with peripheral i.v. catheters used for the administration of lipid emulsion.

sonication (29, 204, 232)—provides superior sensitivity and specificity for diagnosis of catheter-related infection, with a strong correlation between high colony counts and catheter-related bloodstream infection. Direct Gram stains (45) or acridine orange stains (286) of intravascular segments of removed catheters also show excellent correlation with quantitative techniques for culturing catheters and can permit rapid diagnosis of catheter-related infection.

A novel culture-brush, which is passed down the lumen and out the end of an implanted catheter to pick up lumenal biofilm and colonized fibrin and thrombus around the tip, has been developed to diagnose infections of central venous catheters without having to remove the catheter. Preliminary studies suggest it provides sensitivity and specificity comparable to that of semiquantitative culture of the catheter tip (152).

Diagnosis of infection caused by contaminated infusate requires a sample of fluid to be aspirated from the line and cultured quantitatively (126). Anaerobic culture techniques are not necessary unless blood or another biologic product is involved.

Definitions for Infusion-Related Infection

Using the results of semiquantitative or quantitative culture of the catheter and cultures of the hub of the catheter and infusate aspirated from the line, with concomitant blood cultures, it is possible to formulate rigorous definitions for intravascular device-related infection.

Local catheter-related infection. A positive semiquantitative (or quantitative) culture of the catheter, considered synonymous with colonization of the catheter

Catheter-related septicemia. (i) Semiquantitative (or quantitative) catheter culture and blood cultures positive for the same species, with a negative culture of infusate; (ii) clinical and microbiologic data disclose no other clear-cut source for the septicemia

Septicemia due to a contaminated hub. (i) Isolation of the same species from the catheter hub and from cultures of separate percutaneously drawn blood, with semiquantitative (or quantitative) culture of the catheter negative for the infecting organism; (ii) no other identifiable source for the septicemia

Septicemia due to contaminated infusate. (i) Isolation of the same species from infusate and from cultures of separate, percutaneously drawn blood with semiquantitative (or quantitative) culture of the catheter negative for the infecting organism; (ii) no other identifiable source for the septicemia

These definitions have served well for research purposes (134–137, 139, 142, 143–149, 150) but may be too rigorous for routine clinical use or nosocomial surveillance. The Centers for Disease Control (CDC) has used the following definitions for intravascular device-related infection for the purposes of nosocomial infection surveillance (84). (i) Organism isolated from culture of artery or vein (of access site) removed during surgery. (ii) Evidence of infection at involved (vascular access) site seen during surgery or by histopathologic examination. (iii) One of the following: fever (>38°C) or pain, erythema, or heat at involved vascular (access) site and more than 15 colonies cultured from intravascular cannula tip, using semiquantitative culture method, with or without recognized pathogen isolated from blood culture and pathogen is not related to (local) infection at another (extravascular) site. (iv) One of the following: fever (>38°C), chills, or hypotension and any of the following: (a) common skin contaminant isolated from two blood cultures drawn on separate occasions AND organism is not related to infection at another site; (b) common skin contaminant isolated from blood cultures from patient with intravascular access device and physician institutes appropriate antimicrobial therapy. OR (v) Patient less than 12 months of age has one of the following: fever (>38°C), hypothermia (>37°C), apnea, or bradycardia and any of the following: (a) common skin contaminant isolated from cultures of two blood samples drawn on separate occasions and organism is not related to infection another site; (b) common skin contaminant isolated from blood cultures from patient with extravascular device and physician institutes appropriate antimicrobial therapy.

CANNULA-ASSOCIATED INFECTION

Incidence of Cannula-Related Septicemia

The true incidence of vascular cannula-related bloodstream infection is underestimated in most centers because a cannula is often not suspected as the source of a patient's clinical picture of nosocomial sepsis and is not cultured. Prospective studies in which devices are routinely cultured at the time of removal show that every type of intravascular device carries some risk of causing bloodstream infection but that the magnitude of risk varies greatly, depending on its type. Table 3 shows representative rates of infection for various types of intravascular devices.

Peripheral venous catheters

Small Teflon or polyurethane catheters and scalp-vein or butterfly steel needles inserted peripherally are now associated with a very low risk of infection, less than one bacteremia per 500 devices placed (47, 118, 135, 144, 146, 265, 280). Two large comparative trials have shown that if they are inserted under conditions of scrupulous asepsis, small peripheral i.v. catheters probably pose no greater risk of causing bacteremia than do steel needles (265, 280). The small Teflon and polyurethane catheters now used for peripheral i.v. therapy appear to be far safer with

Table 3. Approximate risks of bloodstream infection (BSI) associated with various types of devices for intravascular access[a]

Type of device	Representative rate	Range
Temporary short-term access (no. BSIs per 100 devices)		
Peripheral i.v. cannulas		
Winged steel needles	<0.2	0–1
Peripheral i.v. catheters		
Percutaneously inserted	0.2	0–1
Cutdown	6	1–6
Arterial catheters	1	0–2
Central venous catheters (noncuffed)		
All-purpose, multilumen	3	1–7
Swan-Ganz	1	0–5
Hemodialysis	5	3–18
Long-term or permanent access (no. BSIs per 100 device-days)		
Peripherally inserted central venous catheters (PICCs)	0.20	—[b]
Cuffed central catheters (Hickman, Broviac)	0.20	0.10–0.53
Subcutaneous central venous ports (Infusaport, Port-a-Cath)	0.04	0–0.10

[a] Based on data from recent prospective studies.
[b] —, Insufficient data to provide range.

regard to infection than the larger polyvinyl chloride or polyethylene catheters used 15 to 20 years ago and to be associated with a 2 to 5% risk of bacteremia if left in place for more than 48 h (138). Peripheral catheters inserted by surgical cutdown are now rarely used, which is probably desirable, because older studies reported prohibitively high rates of complicating septicemia, in the range of 6% (170).

Arterial catheters for hemodynamic monitoring

Recent prospective studies of arterial catheters used for hemodynamic monitoring have found rates of infusion-related bacteremia in the range of 1% (82, 145, 235, 259).

Umbilical catheters

Catheterization of the umbilical artery or vein is used near-universally for vascular access in neonates, especially very-low-birth-weight infants who require prolonged support in a neonatal ICU. The only prospective study in recent years found a 5% rate of umbilical catheter-related bacteremia (117).

Central venous catheters

The device that poses the greatest risk of device-related bloodstream infection today is the central venous catheter in its many forms (Table 3). Notably, central venous catheters have been shown to be the most important risk factor for nosocomial candidemia, rivaling antimicrobial therapy and serious underlying disease (27, 114, 279). Prospective studies of short-term, noncuffed, single- or multilumen catheters inserted percutaneously into the subclavian or internal jugular vein have found rates of catheter-related septicemia in the range of 3 to 5%, with rates of 7 to 10% in some hospitals (6, 7, 23, 38, 45, 73, 134, 137, 142, 148–150, 178, 214, 241, 243). Percutaneously inserted, noncuffed central venous catheters used for hemodialysis have been associated with the highest rates of bacteremia, in the range of 10% (40, 185, 230). Swan-Ganz pulmonary-artery catheters used for hemodynamic monitoring have been associated with rates of infection in the range of 1 to 3% (162, 163). Recent studies suggest that peripherally inserted central venous catheters (PICCs) may pose much lower risks of catheter-related bloodstream infection (87) and bear closer study.

The lowest rates of infection with central venous devices have been with surgically implanted Hickman or Broviac catheters with a subcutaneous Dacron cuff, which have been associated with rates of infection in the range of 0.2 bacteremias per 100 catheter-days (81, 195, 282), and surgically implanted subcutaneous central venous ports, associated with rates of bacteremia in the range of 0.04 per 100 device-days (28, 39, 122).

The best data indicate that at the present time, 80 to 90% of intravascular device-related bloodstream infections originate from central venous catheters of various types (131, 178, 214). Data from the CDC's National Nosocomial Infection Surveillance study show that the incidence of secondary bloodstream infections, stemming from local infections of the urinary tract, postoperative surgical wounds, or pneumonias, has remained stable over the past decade; in contrast, the incidence of primary nosocomial bloodstream infections, the largest proportion of which derive from intravascular devices, has increased more than twofold over this same period (15, 131), reflecting the great increase in the use of infusion therapy and especially, the use of central venous devices of all types. It seems clear that the greatest hope for reducing the risk of intravascular device-related sepsis will come from better understanding of the epidemiology and pathogenesis of infection with central venous catheters.

Epidemiology

Strategies for prevention of central venous catheter-related bloodstream infection should be guided by an understanding of pathogenesis,

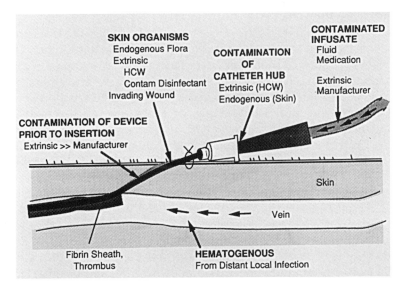

Figure 1. Sources of infection of a percutaneous intravascular device. The major sources are the skin flora, contamination of the catheter hub, contamination of infusate, and hematogenous colonization of the intravascular device and its fibronectin-fibrin sheath from distant, unrelated sites of infection (from D. G. Maki [132]).

particularly the major source or sources of microorganisms that colonize catheters. Short-term, noncuffed, central venous catheters become infected from multiple potential sources (Fig. 1) including contaminants in infusate that gain access intralumenally, microorganisms that contaminate the catheter hub where the administration set attaches to the catheter, organisms carried hematogenously from remote sources of local infection, or microorganisms of cutaneous origin that invade the percutaneous tract extralumenally at the time the catheter is inserted or in the days following insertion—probably facilitated by capillary action (46). Considerable evidence suggests that the largest proportion of catheter-related bacteremias derive in some fashion from the cutaneous microflora of the insertion site.

- Coagulase-negative staphylococci, the predominant aerobic species on the human skin (125), are now the most common agent of catheter-related bacteremia (Table 2) (6, 7, 23, 38, 45, 73, 134, 137, 142, 148–150, 178, 214, 241, 243).
- Prospective studies have shown strong concordance between organisms present on skin surrounding the catheter wound and organisms

recovered from central venous catheters producing septicemia (23, 40, 73, 75, 137, 142, 148, 243).

- Heavy colonization of the insertion site has been shown to have strong predictive value for the occurrence of catheter-related bacteremia (23, 150, 157, 244).
- Cutaneous colonization by *S. aureus* is associated with a sixfold higher risk of vascular access-related bacteremia in patients on hemodialysis (284).
- Use of recombinant interleukin-2 with or without lymphokine-activated killer cells for cancer immunotherapy, which produces dermatotoxicity (desquamation) and heavy cutaneous colonization by *S. aureus*, has been associated with a very high incidence of i.v. catheter-related *S. aureus* bacteremia (246).
- Numerous outbreaks of intravascular catheter-related bacteremia have been caused by contaminated cutaneous disinfectants (101, 129, 131).
- High counts of microorganisms on semiquantitative culture of the external surface of a removed catheter are strongly associated with bacteremia caused by the catheter (38, 43, 45, 75, 149, 243).
- Microscopic examination of infected central venous catheters has shown organisms primarily on the external surface (45).
- Use of a more effective cutaneous disinfectant, 2% chlorhexidine rather than 10% povidone-iodine or alcohol, for disinfection of the insertion site at the time of catheter insertion and in follow-up care of the catheter was shown in a recent study to reduce the risk of device-related septicemia sixfold (134).
- A prospective trial has shown that applying povidone-iodine ointment to the insertion site of central venous catheters used for hemodialysis reduces the risk of catheter-related bacteremia fourfold (120).
- Surgically implanted Broviac or Hickman catheters, with a subcutaneous Dacron cuff that becomes ingrown by tissue and poses a mechanical barrier against invasion of the tract by skin organisms, have been associated with lower rates of catheter-related bacteremia (approximately 0.20 cases per 100 catheter days) than have short-term, noncuffed central venous catheters (approximately 0.6 to 1.0 per 100 catheter days) (Table 3).
- Clinical trials of a subcutaneous silver-impregnated silver cuff that can be attached to a short-term central venous catheter at the time of insertion have shown that the cuff significantly reduces the risk of catheter-related septicemia (73, 137).
- Studies have shown that coating central venous catheters at the bedside with an antibiotic before insertion (109) or impregnating the exter-

nal surface with an antiseptic at the time of manufacture (148) greatly reduces the risk of catheter-related bloodstream infection.
• Pulmonary-artery catheters that have heparin bonded to the external surface exhibit surface antimicrobial activity and appear to be associated with a lower incidence of catheter-related bloodstream infection in clinical practice (164).

Sitges-Serra and his coworkers have shown that hubs of central venous catheters often become contaminated, particularly by coagulase-negative staphylococci, and can also cause catheter-related bacteremia (121, 239, 240), but contaminated hubs do not appear to be as important in the pathogenesis of intravascular device-related sepsis with most short-term, noncuffed venous catheters as are microorganisms from the skin that invade the intracutaneous catheter tract (Table 4) (38, 40, 75, 137, 163). However, with surgically implanted cuffed Hickman or Broviac catheters, microorganisms colonizing the hub and lumen may be the most important source of bloodstream infection deriving from these long-term central venous devices (74, 277). Central venous and arterial catheters can also become colonized hematogenously, from remote unrelated sites of infection (23, 139, 151), but the evidence suggests that this is an uncommon cause of bloodstream infection (23, 134, 137, 147, 148, 151, 163) (Table 4).

Whereas infusate not infrequently becomes contaminated by small numbers of organisms, mainly by skin commensals such as coagulase-

Table 4. Sources of central venous catheter-related infection, based on a prospective study of 234 central venous catheters[a]

Potential source	No. of catheter-related infections associated with the source[b]	
	Local (>15 CFU) (n = 40)	With bacteremia (n = 6)
Colonization of skin of insertion site	36	6
Contamination of catheter hub	4	2
Contaminated i.v. fluid	1	1
Hematogenous colonization from remote site of infection	4	0
Unknown	1	0

[a] From Maki et al. (137).
[b] Based on finding bacteriologic concordance between the potential source (or sources) and the colonized catheter (>15 CFU on semiquantitative culture). There were six catheters with more than one source of the organisms causing catheter-related infection: skin and hub, 3 (including 1 bacteremia); skin, hub, and fluid, 1 (including 1 bacteremia); skin and hematogenous, 2.

negative staphylococci, with the exception of arterial and pulmonary-artery catheters used for hemodynamic monitoring (145, 147, 163), endemic bacteremic infections originating from contaminated infusate are infrequent and appear to be linked to guidewire exchanges and hub contamination (134, 137, 148). In contrast, as noted, contaminated infusate is the single most common cause of epidemic nosocomial bacteremia (129, 131).

In a prospective study of the mechanisms of catheter-related infection of 234 central venous catheters inserted in patients in three hospitals' ICUs (Table 4), it was found that the most common source of organisms colonizing 40 catheters and accounting for all six catheter-related bacteremias was skin of the insertion site. Four colonized catheters were also associated with concordant contamination of the hub and two were associated with concordant bacteremias. However, with both bacteremias, skin of the insertion site, and with one, i.v. fluid as well, were also concordantly colonized; four catheters exposed to bacteremia or candidemia from a distant and unrelated site of infection became hematogenously colonized, although none later produced septicemia, probably because the catheter had been removed after bloodstream infection had been identified (137).

To identify most rigorously the source of microorganisms causing vascular catheter-related bloodstream infection in prospective studies, it is necessary to culture all potential sources at the time of catheter removal (Fig. 1). If the results of these cultures appear to link a bloodstream infection with microorganisms isolated from one or more portions of the device, efforts then need to be made to conclusively establish concordance, beyond speciation and antimicrobial susceptibility pattern, using one or more molecular subtyping systems, such as multilocus enzyme analysis, plasmid profile, or restriction enzyme analysis of chromosomal DNA (102).

Recent studies of the pathogenesis and epidemiology of catheter-related infection with Swan-Ganz pulmonary-artery catheters (147, 163) and multilumen central venous catheters used in ICU patients (148) utilized molecular subtyping by plasmid profile or restriction fragment polymorphism (102) to rigorously establish epidemiologic relatedness of blood and catheter isolates (Fig. 2). Approximately one half of the infected catheters showed concordance with organisms cultured from skin of the insertion site and the remainder showed concordance with a contaminated hub or contamination of infusate; nearly all bacteremic catheters that appeared to have an intralumenal source of infection were second catheters placed in an old site over a guidewire. These data indicate that for maximal benefit, strategies for prevention of infection with cen-

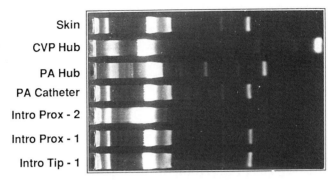

Skin
CVP Hub
PA Hub
PA Catheter
Intro Prox - 2
Intro Prox - 1
Intro Tip - 1

Figure 2. Plasmid profiles of seven isolates of coagulase-negative staphylococci from potential sources of infection with an infected Swan-Ganz catheter that caused bacteremia. Intro Prox-1 and Intro Prox-2, isolates 1 and 2 from proximal introducer segment; Intro Tip-1, isolate from introducer tip; CVP Hub, isolate from hub of the central venous lumen of the PA catheter; PA Hub, isolate from hub of PA lumen of the PA catheter. Isolate 1 from the proximal segment and tip of the introducer (and blood) shows concordance (three plasmids) with isolates from skin of the insertion site and from the infected PA catheter. The second isolate from the introducer and the strains isolated from the PA catheter hub and the CVP hub differ from the infecting strain. Presumed pathogenesis: skin → introducer [→ PA catheter] → blood (from Mermel et al. [163]).

tral venous catheters must be multifaceted, designed to block microbial invasion from all possible sources.

Risk factors predisposing to vascular catheter-related infection have been analyzed by stepwise logistic regression analysis of data from large, prospective studies done in one university center of peripheral i.v. catheters (144), arterial catheters used for hemodynamic monitoring (145), multilumen central venous catheters used in ICU patients (150), and Swan-Ganz, pulmonary-artery, balloon-flotation catheters (147). These studies show that heavy cutaneous colonization of the insertion site is the single most important predictor of catheter-related infection with all types of short-term, percutaneously-inserted catheters (Table 5). With central venous catheters in ICU patients, exposure to bacteremia or fungemia from a remote source and catheterizations exceeding 4 days were also shown to be independent risk factors (150). With Swan-Ganz catheters, insertion into an internal jugular vein rather than the subclavian vein, catheterization exceeding 3 days, and insertion with less stringent barrier precautions were each associated with significantly increased risk of catheter-related infection (147). Associated active urinary tract infections (116) or lower respiratory tract colonization or infection (62) also increase the risk of bacteremic infections of central venous catheters.

Table 5. Risk factors for intravascular catheter-related infection based on multivariate analysis of data from four large prospective studies in University of Wisconsin Hospital and Clinics

Type of catheter (reference)	No. of catheters studied	Risk factors	Approximate magnitude of increased risk[a]
Peripheral i.v. (144)	2,050	Cutaneous colonization of site, $>10^2$ CFU	3.9
		Contamination of catheter hub	3.8
		Moisture on site, under dressing	2.5
		Placement, >3 days	1.8
		Systemic antimicrobial therapy	0.5
Arterial (145)	491	Cutaneous colonization of site, $>10^2$ CFU	10.0
		Second catheter in site, placed over guidewire	. . .[b]
Central venous in an ICU (150)	345	Exposure of catheter to unrelated bacteremia	9.4
		Cutaneous colonization of site, $>10^2$ CFU	9.2
		Placement, >4 days	. . .
Swan-Ganz pulmonary artery (163)	297	Cutaneous colonization of site, $>10^3$ CFU	5.5
		Internal jugular vein cannulation	4.3
		Duration, >3 days	3.1
		Placement in operating room under less stringent barrier precautions	2.1

[a] Relative risk or odds ratio (all $P < 0.05$, most $P < 0.01$).
[b] Indeterminate (e.g., zero incidence).

Pathogenesis

Foreign body infections derive from a complex interaction between the microsurface of the foreign body, the host, and the pathogen (89). Examination of an infected intravascular device by scanning electron microscopy characteristically shows the surface covered by a biofilm, composed of host proteins and microcolonies of the infecting organism encased in a thick matrix of glycocalyx (slime) (76, 153) (Fig. 3). Studies have shown considerable differences in the capacity of microorganisms to adhere to various foreign materials in vitro and in vivo. In vitro, catheters made of Teflon or polyurethane are more resistant to bacterial adherence, especially by staphylococci, than are catheters made of polyethylene, polyvinyl chloride, or silicone (10, 16, 220, 234); these differences diminish, however, if the experiments are done with implanted catheters (16) or catheters precoated with specific plasma proteins (183, 270).

Adherence appears to be promoted by protease-sensitive adhesins (260, 261), surface exoglycocalyx (41, 53, 68, 115, 219, 225, 269, 271) and hydrophobicity (10, 183, 225) of the infecting strain; however, the impor-

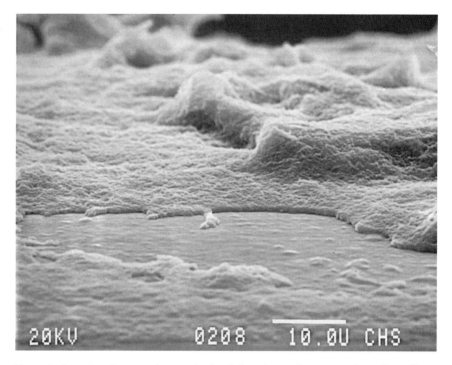

Figure 3. Scanning electron micrograph of an infected central venous catheter (magnification, ×2,000). The amorphous matrix encasing the microcolonies of *Staphylococcus epidermidis* is glycocalyx (slime).

tance of glycocalyx in mediating adherence (68) or contributing materially to pathogenicity (115) is not yet completely resolved.

Host factors also play an important role in modulating microbial adherence to foreign bodies: following insertion, the surface becomes coated by platelets and plasma and tissue proteins, such as albumin, fibrinogen-fibrin, fibronectin, laminin, thrombospondin, collagen, and immunoglobulins (270). Albumin inhibits adherence whereas fibronectin—to a lesser degree fibrinogen-fibrin and laminin—promotes adherence in vivo (93, 222, 269–271). Thrombosis on the catheter surface also appears to promote adherence and catheter-associated infection (70, 202, 253).

Whereas subtherapeutic levels of antibiotics reduce microbial adherence (183, 225), once microorganisms such as coagulase-negative staphylococci colonize a prosthetic surface, host defenses become impaired and are unable to eradicate the infection (56, 88, 268). Moreover, once associated with a foreign surface, microorganisms exhibit increased resistance to antimicrobial agents (66, 89, 233). It should be no surprise that many infections of vascular catheters cannot be cured with antimicrobial therapy alone and that the infected catheter needs to be removed. In general, if a short-term, noncuffed catheter is strongly suspected of being infected or has been shown to be infected, it should be removed.

SEPSIS FROM CONTAMINATED INFUSATE

Whereas most intravascular device-related bloodstream infections originate from infection of the percutaneous catheter tract or contamination of the catheter hub, contamination of infusate is the most common cause of epidemic device-related bloodstream infection (129). From 1965 to 1978, 28 (85%) of 30 epidemics of intravascular device-related bacteremia were traced to contaminated infusate, organisms introduced during its manufacture (intrinsic contamination, 7 epidemics) or during its preparation, and administration in the hospital (extrinsic contamination, 21 epidemics) (129).

Growth Properties of Microorganisms in Parenteral Fluids

The pathogens implicated in septicemias linked to contamined infusate have with rare exceptions been aerobic gram-negative bacilli capable of rapid growth at room temperature (25°C) in the solution implicated (126, 129, 131): vis-a-vis, certain members of the family *Enterobacteriaceae* in dextrose-containing solutions and pseudomonads or *Serratia* spp. in distilled water. It must be emphasized that microbial growth in most parenteral solutions—the exception being lipid emulsion—is quite limited.

Studies of the growth properties of microorganisms in various commercial parenteral products show (126) rapid multiplication in 5% dextrose in water limited mainly by the tribe *Klebsielleae* and *P. cepacia;* in distilled water by *P. aeruginosa, P. cepacia,* and *Acinetobacter* and *Serratia* spp.; and in lactated Ringer's solution by *P. aeruginosa, Enterobacter* spp., and *Serratia* spp. Normal (0.9%) sodium chloride solution allows growth of most bacteria while supporting the growth of *Candida* spp. rather poorly. *Candida* species grow in the synthetic amino acid-hypertonic glucose solutions used for total parenteral nutrition, but rather slowly; most bacteria are inhibited. Nearly all microorganisms grow rapidly in commercial 10% lipid emulsion for infusion (Intralipid) (48).

The growth properties of microorganisms in commercial parenteral admixtures and the aggregate experience with epidemics and endemic bloodstream infections traced to contaminated infusate have shown that the identity of an organism causing nosocomial bloodstream infection usually points toward contaminated fluids as a suspect source: *Enterobacter* species, particularly *E. agglomerans* or *E. cloacae, Serratia marcescens, P. cepacia,* or *Citrobacter* spp. cultured from the blood of a patient receiving infusion therapy should prompt strong suspicion of contaminated infusate—a parenteral admixture or an i.v. drug (Table 2). Conversely, recovery of organisms such as *Escherichia coli, Proteus* spp., *Acinetobacter* spp., or staphylococci, all of which grow poorly in parenteral admixtures, indicates that the bacteremia is very unlikely to be due to contaminated infusate (141).

Mechanisms of Fluid Contamination

Whereas most nosocomial bloodstream infections traced to contaminated infusate and reported in the literature occurred in an epidemic setting (129, 131), parenteral fluids commonly become contaminated during administration in the hospital. Culture surveys of in-use i.v. fluids in the hospital have shown contamination rates in the range of 1 to 2% (13, 32, 85, 107, 136, 245); however, most of the time the organisms recovered from positive cultures are skin commensals that grow poorly in the parenteral admixture, and the level of contamination (<10 CFU/ml) is usually too low to produce clinical illness, even in the most compromised host. However, when contamination occurs with gram-negative bacilli able to grow rapidly to concentrations exceeding 10^2 to 10^3 CFU/ml, the risk of bacteremia and even septic shock becomes substantial.

The likelihood of fluid becoming contaminated during use is generally related to the duration of uninterrupted infusion through the same administration set and the frequency with which the set is manipulated. Microorganisms gain access from air entering bottles as they evacuate; during injections into the line or withdrawal of blood specimens from the catheter; or at the junction between the administration set and the catheter hub. Microorganisms capable of growth in fluid, once introduced into a running infusion, may persist in an administration set for days despite replacements of the container and high rates of flow (143, 168).

A filmy cloud within a glass i.v. bottle usually denotes contamination by a filamentous fungus, such as *Penicillium* or *Aspergillus* spp., which has gained access through a microscopic crack before the bottle was hung for use. Fortunately, fungus balls in i.v. bottles have rarely resulted in fungemia in patients receiving a mold-contaminated infusion (51).

The incidence of endemic nosocomial bacteremia caused by extrinsically contaminated i.v. fluid is not precisely known, but from studies of the pathogenesis of catheter-related infection it is probably 3- to 10-fold lower than the incidence of endemic cannula-related septicemia. Moreover, prospective studies of the best intervals for periodic replacement of administration sets (13, 32, 85, 107, 136, 245), which involved cultures of infusate from thousands of in-use infusions, have shown low rates of contamination and an infinitesimal risk of related septicemia. In five studies encompassing more than 9,000 infusions, no bacteremias caused by contamination of infusate were identified.

Recent studies have shown that approximately one half of the septicemias caused by arterial infusions used for hemodynamic monitoring originate from contamination of infusate within the administration set (139, 145), perhaps because these infusions consist of a stagnant column of fluid subjected to frequent manipulations, especially entries for drawing blood specimens. Over the past 20 years, there have been more than 30 epidemics of nosocomial bloodstream infection traced to contaminated fluid within arterial infusions used for hemodynamic monitoring (101, 160). Nearly all of these epidemics have involved gram-negative bacilli, particularly *S. marcescens*, pseudomonads, or *Enterobacter* species that multiply rapidly within the 0.9% NaCl solution used in these infusions.

Between less than 1% and 6% of blood units contain small numbers of microorganisms (99, 281), yet endemic bacteremias deriving from contaminated blood products have been rare, presumably because most blood products are refrigerated before use and because of universal awareness that blood products should be administered immediately after removal from refrigeration. Bacteremia from contaminated blood is characteristically associated with overwhelming septic shock and high mortality because of the huge numbers of psychrophilic (cold-growing) organisms such as *Serratia* spp., pseumonads other than *P. aeruginosa,* and other uncommon nonfermentative gram-negative bacilli, such as *Flavobacterium* species, in the contaminated unit (25, 188).

The most important measures to prevent rare sporadic septicemias from contaminated in-use fluid are stringent asepsis during the preparation and compounding of admixtures in the hospital central pharmacy or on individual patient care units and good aseptic technique when infusions are handled during use, such as during injections of medications or changing bags or bottles of fluids. Replacing the administration set at periodic intervals can prevent the buildup of dangerous introduced contaminants and further reduce the risk of related septicemia (136, 143).

EPIDEMIC INFUSION-RELATED SEPTICEMIAS

Whereas only 10 to 20% of endemic nosocomial bloodstream infections in U.S. hospitals are considered to be infusion related, more than one half of all epidemics of hospital-acquired bacteremia derive from infusion therapy in some form (129, 131). The proportion of outbreaks investigated by the CDC that were device, procedure, or product related increased more than 50% between 1986 and 1990 (101).

Outbreaks Due to Intrinsic Contamination

Since 1970, there have been more than a dozen reported epidemics of infusion-related bacteremia caused by intrinsically contaminated infusate (34, 36, 37, 101, 108, 126, 143, 155, 159, 182, 186, 212, 216, 237, 251, 252)—blood products, i.v. fluid, or drugs administered intravenously or Vacutainer tubes that became contaminated during their manufacture (Table 6). Many involved multiple hospitals and were of national scope. The frequency and size of outbreaks, fortunately, have declined in recent years (131), suggesting improved quality control during the manufacturing process.

Outbreaks of pyrogenic reactions (251) and epidemic *Pseudomonas* species septicemia (252) have been traced to intrinsically contaminated normal serum albumin, and epidemics of *E. cloacae* (30), *Salmonella* (91, 212), and *Yersinia* (35) septicemia have been traced to organisms from intrinsically contaminated platelet concentrates (which are maintained at 25°C to enhance viability). Most notably, during the past decade, outbreaks of *Pseudomonas* infection have been traced to intrinsic contamination of 10% povidone-iodine (36, 101, 182), the most widely used chemical antiseptic in North American hospitals.

All of these outbreaks illustrate how subtle and insidious the factors that influence sterility can be. In many instances, there was no documented failure of the sterilization process. Instead, seemingly minor alterations in the manufacturing process resulted in contamination of individual units in the manufacturing plant after the sterilization stage (124). Although intrinsic contamination is, fortunately, exceedingly rare, its potential for producing harm is great because of the large numbers of patients in multiple hospitals who may be affected. Also, contamination of infusate at the manufacturing level permits contaminants to proliferate to dangerously high concentrations.

If intrinsic contamination of a commercially distributed product is identified, or even suspected, especially if clinical infections have occurred as a consequence, the local, state, and federal (CDC and FDA) public health authorities must be immediately contacted. Unopened samples of the suspect lot or lots should be quarantined and saved for their analysis.

Table 6. Reported causes of epidemic intravascular device-related bloodstream infections[a]

Extrinsic contamination
  Antiseptics or disinfectants
  Arterial pressure monitoring infusate
    Disinfectants
    Failed decontamination of transducers
    Aneroid pressure-calibration device
    Retrograde syringes in manifold
    Heparin
    Ice for chilling blood-gas syringes
    Flush solutions
    Arterial blood gas analyzer
    Hand carriage by medical personnel
  Hemodialysis-related
    Failed decontamination of dialyzer coils
    Contaminated dialysate water
    Contaminated disinfectants
  Parenteral crystalloid solutions
  Lipid emulsion
  Hyperalimentation solutions compounded in pharmacy
  i.v. medications, multidose vials
  Theft of fentanyl and replacement by (contaminated) distilled water
  Blood products
    Whole blood
    Platelet packs
    Lymphokine-activated killer cells
    Blood donor with silent transient bacteremia
  i.v. radiologic contrast media
  Sclerosing solution for injecting esophageal varices
  Use of same i.v. infusion with multiple consecutive patients
  Central venous catheter hubs
  Leaking catheter hub-administration set connections
  Adhesive tape used in i.v. site dressings
  Warming bath for blood products
  Heart-lung machine
  Intra-aortic balloon pump
  Green soap
  Hand carriage by medical personnel
  Inordinately prolonged intravascular catheterization in ICU patients
Intrinsic contamination (during manufacture)
  Commercial i.v. crystalloid solutions, closures for i.v. bottles
  Blood products
    Platelet packs
    Human albumin
    Plasma protein fraction
  i.v. drugs
  Vacutainer tubes

[a] From D. G. Maki (132).

Outbreaks Due to Extrinsic Contamination

Even when commercially manufactured products are sterile on arrival in the hospital, circumstances of hospital use can compromise that initial sterility. As noted, most sporadic infections deriving from infusion therapy, whether due to the cannula or contaminated infusate, are of extrinsic origin. Most reported epidemics have originated from exposure of multiple patients' infusions to a common source of contamination in the hospital (101, 127, 129, 131).

Investigations of more than 100 epidemics over the past two decades have documented contamination of in-use infusate or cannula insertion sites, deriving from a myriad of extrinsic sources within the hospital (Table 6), illustrating the potential for contamination of parenteral drugs or admixtures and the extraordinary range of possible mechanisms of such contamination. Numerous outbreaks have stemmed from use of unreliable chemical antiseptics or disinfectants, such as aqueous benzalkonium or aqueous chlorhexidine, for cutaneous disinfection or for decontaminating transducer components used in hemodynamic monitoring (160). One third of all outbreaks of nosocomial bacteremia investigated by the CDC between 1977 and 1987 were traced to contaminated infusions used for arterial pressure monitoring (18, 101). Outbreaks of bacteremia or candidemia have been traced to contamination of hyperalimentation solutions during compounding in the hospital's pharmacy (60, 190, 250). In one extraordinary outbreak, *P. pickettii* bacteremias following open heart surgery were traced to theft of fentanyl from predrawn syringes, with replacement by distilled water that unfortunately was contaminated (140). In many outbreaks, especially with *Candida* spp., the hospital reservoir of the epidemic pathogen and the mode of transmission were not elucidated, but the microorganism was found in large numbers on the hands of health care providers caring for the patients receiving i.v. therapy and handling their infusions (31, 190, 208, 231, 249, 250).

Manipulations of the delivery system, especially the administration set, appear to provide an effective means for introduction of contaminants, as illustrated by a spate of outbreaks across the U.S. traced to in-use contamination of a newly released intravenous anesthetic, propofol (Diprivan), a solution that has been found to be a rich medium for microbial proliferation of nearly all species of bacteria and fungi. Outbreaks of primary bacteremia or surgical wound infection with skin organisms, especially *S. aureus,* have resulted from in-use contamination of propofol during compounding or administration (37, 50).

Approach to an Epidemic

If an epidemic is suspected, the epidemiologic approach must be methodical and thorough, yet expeditious, directed toward establishing the bona fide nature of the putative epidemic infections (i.e., ruling out "pseudoinfections") (128) and confirming the existence of an epidemic (i.e., ruling out a "pseudoepidemic") (128); defining the reservoirs and modes of transmission of the epidemic pathogens; and, most importantly, controlling the epidemic, quickly and completely. Control measures are predicated upon accurate delineation of the epidemiology of the epidemic pathogen. The essential steps in dealing with a suspected nosocomial outbreak have recently been reviewed (132).

STRATEGIES FOR PREVENTION

It must be reaffirmed that measures for prevention of any nosocomial infection should, whenever possible, be based on an understanding of pathophysiology and epidemiology—reservoirs, modes of transmission, and risk factors—and controlled clinical trials.

Aseptic Technique

Barrier precautions

Vigorous handwashing, ideally with an antiseptic-containing preparation, must always precede the insertion of a peripheral i.v. cannula and should also precede later handling of the device or the administration set (130). Sterile gloves should be used during the insertion of peripheral i.v. cannulas in high-risk patients, such as leukemics. Sterile gloves are strongly recommended for placement of all other types of intravascular devices that are associated with a 1% or higher risk of associated bacteremia—specifically arterial and central venous catheters. Although there has been considerable controversy as to the level of barrier precautions necessary during insertion of a central venous catheter, recent studies (163, 201) have shown that the use of maximal precautions, including a long-sleeved, sterile surgical gown, mask, cap, and large sterile drape, as well as sterile gloves, significantly reduces the risk of central venous catheter-related bacteremia (Table 7). The use of maximal barriers has further been shown to be highly cost-effective (201). Considering that of all intravascular devices, central venous catheters are most likely to produce nosocomial bloodstream infection, a strong case can be made for mandating maximal barrier precautions during the insertion of such devices.

Table 7. Prospective randomized study of maximal barrier precautions during insertion of central venous catheters[a]

Parameter	Minimal precautions	Maximal precautions
Nature of precautions	Sterile gloves Small drape	Sterile gloves Large drape Long-sleeved sterile gown Mask Cap
No. of catheters studied	167	176
No. of catheter-related bacteremias (%)	6 (3.5)	1 (0.6)
Catheter-related bacteremias per 1,000 catheter-days	0.5	0.08[b]

[a] From Raad et al. (201).
[b] $P < 0.02$

i.v. teams

Aseptic technique is also very important. Studies have shown that the use of special i.v. therapy teams, consisting of trained nurses or technicians who can ensure a consistent and high level of asepsis during catheter insertion and in follow-up care of the catheter, have been associated with substantially lower rates of catheter-related infection (21, 71, 78, 113, 175, 176, 223, 248, 263] (Table 8). Tomford and Hershey have shown that an i.v. team is highly cost-effective, reducing the costs of complications of infusion therapy nearly tenfold (262). Even if an institution does not have an i.v. team, it can greatly reduce its rate of intravascular device-related sepsis by intensive training of nurses and physicians and stringent adherence to catheter-care protocols (198, 266).

Cutaneous Antisepsis

Given the evidence for the importance of cutaneous microorganisms in the pathogenesis of intravascular device-related infections, measures to reduce colonization of the insertion site would seem of the highest priority, particularly the choice of chemical antiseptics for disinfection of the site. In the United States, iodophors such as 10% povidone-iodine are used most widely. In the only large, prospective trial of cutaneous antiseptics for vascular access (Table 9), 668 patients' central venous and arterial catheters in a surgical ICU were randomized to have 10% povidone-iodine, 70% alcohol, or 2% aqueous chlorhexidine used for disinfecting the insertion site (134). Fourteen device-related bacteremias were

Table 8. Impact of a dedicated i.v. team on the rate of catheter-related septicemia[a]

Type of study and authors (reference)	Type of catheter[b]	Care given by:	No. of catheters	Incidence of septicemia (per 100 catheters)
Concurrent but not randomized				
Bentley and Lepper (21)	PIV	House officers	4,270	0.40
		i.v. team	470	0.04
Freeman et al. (78)	CVC-TPN	Ward nurses	33	21.2
		i.v. nurses	78	2.3
Nehme and Trigger (175)	CVC-TPN	Ward nurses	391	26.2
		i.v. team	284	1.3
Faubion et al. (71)	CVC-TPN	Ward nurses	179	24.0
		i.v. team	377	3.5
Nelson et al. (176)	CVC-TPN	House officers	45	28.8
		i.v. nurses	30	3.3
Historical controls				
Sanders and Sheldon (223)	CVC-TPN	Ward nurses	335	28.6
		i.v. team	172	4.7
Keohane et al. (113)	CVC-TPN	Ward nurses	51	33.0
		i.v. nurses	48	4.0
Randomized, concurrent controls				
Tomford et al. (263)	PIV	House officers	427	2.1
		i.v. team	433	0.2
Soifer et al. (248)	PIV	House officers	453	1.5
		i.v. team	412	0.02

[a] From D. G. Maki (132).
[b] PIV, peripheral i.v. catheter; CVC, central venous catheter; TPN, total parenteral nutrition.

Table 9. Results of a prospective randomized trial of three cutaneous antiseptics for prevention of intravascular device-related septicemia[a]

Source of septicemia	10% Povidone-iodine ($n = 227$)	70% Alcohol ($n = 227$)	2% Chlorhexidine ($n = 214$)
Catheter-related	6	3	1
Contaminated:			
Infusate	. . .	3[b]	. . .
Hub	1[b]	. . .	. . .
All sources (%)	7 (3.1)	6 (2.6)	1 (0.5)[c]

[a] From Maki et al. (134).
[b] All four bacteremias derived from catheters placed in an old site over a guidewire.
[c] Compared with the other two groups combined; odds ratio, 0.16; $P = 0.04$.

identified during the study, one in the chlorhexidine group and 13 in the other two groups (odds ratio, 0.16; $P = 0.04$). This study suggests that the use of 2% chlorhexidine, rather than 10% povidone-iodine or 70% alcohol, for cutaneous disinfection before insertion of an intravascular device and in postinsertion site care will substantially reduce the incidence of device-related infection. A recent smaller but similar trial also found that cutaneous disinfection with 2% chlorhexidine was superior to that with povidone-iodine for reducing colonization of catheters in an ICU (229).

In an historical analysis of the impact on the incidence of catheter-related sepsis of using different antiseptics for site care and disinfecting tubing connections in a home nutritional support program, Rannem et al. reported a rate of 0.58 cases per catheter-year during the use of 10% povidone-iodine, contrasted with 0.26 to 0.28 cases per catheter-year during use of tincture of iodine or tincture of chlorhexidine (206). Also, as previously noted, the use of 2% iodine tincture, compared with 10% povidone-iodine, was associated with a twofold reduction in contaminated blood cultures in a recent large prospective trial (255).

Iodophors can certainly be considered acceptable for cutaneous disinfection in clinical practice; however, 1 to 2% tincture of iodine is highly effective, inexpensive, and well tolerated by patients and is recommended at the present time, until a 2% chlorhexidine solution becomes available commercially in the U.S. For patients with rare iodine allergy, 70% alcohol is acceptable. Whatever agent is used should be scrubbed on for a least 1 min and allowed to dry before inserting the catheter (72).

"Defatting" the skin with acetone is yet practiced in many centers as an adjunctive measure for disinfecting central venous catheter sites. However, it was found to be of no benefit whatsoever in a prospective randomized trial (142). The use of acetone, paradoxically, was associated with increased inflammation of insertion sites and discomfort.

Topical Antimicrobial Ointments

In theory, application of a topical antimicrobial agent to the catheter insertion site should confer some protection against microbial invasion. Clinical trials of a topical combination antibacterial ointment containing polymyxin, neomycin, and bacitracin on peripheral i.v. catheters have shown marginal benefit (135, 177, 285), but the use of polyantibiotic ointments was associated with an increased frequency of *Candida* infections (73, 135). Study of a new topical antibacterial, mupirocin, which is active primarily against gram-positive organisms, has shown significant reduction in colonization of internal jugular catheters without colonization by *Candida* spp. (94). Emerging resistance of *S. aureus* to mupiricin may diminish the promise of this new topical agent (11).

There have been two prospective studies of topical povidone-iodine ointment applied to central venous catheter sites; one large randomized trial in a surgical ICU showed no benefit (194), but a recent comparative trial with subclavian hemodialysis catheters showed a fourfold reduction in the incidence of catheter-related bacteremia (120). If a topical agent is to be used, an iodophor may be most desirable.

Dressings

The importance of the cutaneous microflora in the pathogenesis of device-related infection suggests that the dressing applied to the catheter insertion site could have considerable influence on the incidence of catheter-related infection. However, few studies examined the specific aspects of site care of intravascular catheter sites until transparent polyurethane films for dressing vascular catheters became available 15 years ago. When used on vascular catheters, polyurethane dressings permit continuous inspection of the site, secure the device reliably, and are generally more comfortable than gauze and tape. Moreover, they permit patients to bathe and shower without saturating the dressing. Although polyurethane dressings are semipermeable and studies in volunteers have shown little effect on the cutaneous microflora (199, 211), reports have raised concern that these dressings could increase cutaneous colonization and the risk of catheter-related infection (54, 97, 110, 166).

Peripheral i.v. catheters

The reported trials of polyurethane dressings compared with gauze and tape on peripheral venous catheters have ranged in size from 77 to 2,088 catheters (5, 47, 83, 98, 106, 112, 144, 213). Small trials (5, 106, 112) found significantly higher rates of local catheter-related infection with transparent dressings left on indefinitely. Other larger studies, however, did not find significant differences (47, 83, 98, 144, 213). Rates of local catheter-related infection in all of these trials were low with all dressings, in the range of 1.6 to 8.5%. Only 3 catheter-related bacteremias were identified among the nearly 4,000 catheters studied in all of the reported trials.

In the largest prospective randomized trial of polyurethane dressings (2,088 peripheral i.v. catheters) (144), the polyurethane dressing left on for the lifetime of the catheter was not associated with increased cutaneous colonization under the dressing or an increased rate of catheter-related infection, compared with control gauze and tape dressings;

no catheter caused bacteremia. Logistic regression showed cutaneous colonization of the insertion site (relative risk of infection, 3.9) and moisture under the dressing (relative risk, 2.5) were significant risk factors for catheter-related infection. This study indicates that it is not cost-effective to redress peripheral i.v. catheters at periodic intervals and that for most patients, either sterile gauze or a high-quality polyurethane transparent dressing can be used and left on until the catheter is removed.

Central venous catheters

Studies of polyurethane dressings on short-term, noncuffed central venous catheters have yielded conflicting results (44, 147, 151, 156, 175, 181, 192, 193, 213, 228, 283), in part reflecting differences in study protocols and different dressings studied. A small trial by Conly et al. (44) found a much higher rate of catheter-related septicemia with catheters dressed with polyurethane than with catheters dressed with gauze and tape. A similar and much larger trial, except that it was done in ICU patients, found that the polyurethane dressing studied adhered well and that there were no significant differences between catheter-related infection with polyurethane dressings and gauze dressings when the transparent dressing was changed every 2 days (151).

A recent meta-analysis suggests that the risk of central venous catheter-related infection associated with the use of polyurethane dressings is increased, compared with the risk if conventional sterile gauze and tape dressings are used (98). This meta-analysis is flawed by the inclusion of studies in which the dressing groups were not comparable and also by the failure to include the results of recent large, comparative trials. It must be pointed out that most of the randomized trials of polyurethane dressings on central venous catheters, which in aggregate studied hundreds of central venous catheters in high-risk patients, many of whom were receiving total parenteral nutrition through the catheter, did not find an increased risk of catheter-related bloodstream infection associated with leaving transparent dressing on for up to 7 days, compared with gauze and tape replaced every second or third day (147, 151, 156, 175, 181, 193, 213, 228, 283).

In a recent large trial of barrier precautions during insertion of central venous catheters in patients with cancer (201), polyurethane dressings placed over gauze were used on most of the catheters—the "island dressing"—probably a less permeable dressing than either gauze or a polyurethane dressing alone. Use of polyurethane-gauze dressings in this study was associated with a very low risk of infection when maximal barrier precautions were used during catheter insertion (Table 7). No dressing can be considered fail-safe if aseptic technique is less than optimal.

Whereas many still question the safety of polyurethane dressings on central venous catheters, the largest randomized trials have not shown an increased risk.

Hickman catheters

There have been only two reported randomized studies of the use of transparent dressings on surgically implanted Hickman catheters in which microbiologic data were provided (151, 236); in both trials, one in renal transplant patients (151) and the other in bone marrow transplant recipients (236), the polyurethane dressings studied provided satisfactory cover, even when left on for for up to 5 to 7 days, and were not associated with an increased risk of exit site or tunnel infection or of catheter-related bacteremia.

Arterial catheters

There have also been only two reported studies of polyurethane dressings with arterial catheters (151, 213). In a prospective study with arterial catheters used for hemodynamic monitoring in a surgical ICU, the use of a polyurethane dressing, even replaced every other day, was associated with a greatly increased incidence of catheter-related bacteremia, compared with that with gauze and tape (151). Polyurethane dressings should probably not be used on arterial catheters until future studies confirm their safety.

Duration of Catheterization

With every type of intravascular device, the longer the device is left in place, the higher the cumulative (actuarial) risk of device-related bacteremia.

Peripheral i.v. cannulas

With peripheral i.v. cannulas, the risk of catheter-related infection is very low for the first 48 to 72 h and then begins to rise (47, 83, 98, 135, 138, 144, 146). The most frequent complication of peripheral i.v. cannulas is now infusion phlebitis. Users should strive to rotate sites for peripheral i.v. access every 48 to 72 h to minimize phlebitis; this practice should also hold the incidence of catheter-related bacteremia at less than 1 per 500 catheters (<1 per 1,000 catheter days) (146).

Arterial catheters

In a recent large prospective study of infections caused by arterial catheters used for hemodynamic monitoring it was found that the actuarial risk of catheter-related bacteremia with first catheters in a site was low, reaching 1% only after the seventh day; in contrast, catheters placed in an old site over a guidewire were associated with a risk of bacteremia exceeding 6% by day 7 (145). These data indicate that it should be safe in patients needing long-term arterial monitoring to allow catheters placed in a new site to remain in place for up to a week or longer, with good site care, but that it may not be desirable to exchange arterial catheters over a guidewire unless there are compelling indications.

Central venous catheters

The cumulative risk of central venous catheter-related infection also rises continuously the longer a catheter is in place. In many centers the length of time that noncuffed central venous catheters are allowed to remain in place in ICU patients is arbitrarily limited to 3 to 7 days, replacing the catheter with a new one placed in a new site—which increases the risk of pneumothorax and other mechanical complications—or exchanging the old catheter with a new one in the same site, over a guidewire (6, 86, 95, 180, 191, 241). Recent prospective trials in ICU populations have not been able to show that routine site rotations or periodic catheter exchange over a guidewire are of benefit (42, 67, 184, 247); however, these studies had limited statistical power.

Prospective studies of central venous catheters using multivariate analysis (6, 150, 163, 210, 214) have found a strong association between prolonged catheterization and an increased risk of catheter colonization or bacteremia (Table 5). To better understand the relationship between catheter-related bloodstream infection and duration of catheterization for Swan-Ganz catheters used in patients in an ICU, data from four large prospective studies of Swan-Ganz catheters, in which complete information was available in all cases, were combined (162). Figure 4 shows that the actuarial risk of Swan-Ganz catheter-related bloodstream infection is very low for the first 4 days but rises sharply thereafter—whether expressed per 100 catheters or per 100 catheter-days. This analysis indicates that efforts should be made to limit the length of time a Swan-Ganz catheter or other central venous catheter in an ICU patient remains in place to no longer than 4 days.

If it is considered essential to continue the use of a short-term central venous catheter in an ICU patient beyond 4 days, the clinician has three options: (i) leave the catheter in place, accepting that the risk will begin

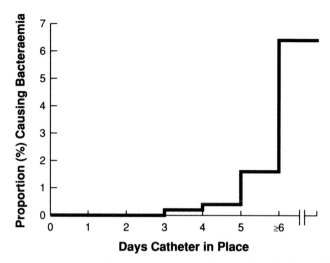

Figure 4. Relationship between the duration of Swan-Ganz catheterization and the actuarial risk of catheter-related bloodstream infection, based on pooled data (988 catheters) from four prospective studies (from Mermel and Maki [162]).

to rise after 4 days; (ii) remove the catheter, place a new catheter in a new site, gaining another 4 days of low risk; or (iii) replace the old catheter over a guidewire, using the protocol described (162), which includes culturing the old catheter and, if it is shown to be infected, removing the new catheter from the infected site. If the old catheter is not found to be infected, the new catheter can be left in the site safely for another 4 days, with a low risk of infection.

The use of novel technologies that prevent catheter colonization and, in the process, device-related bacteremia should allow central venous catheters in the future to remain in place safely for greatly extended periods.

Measures Aimed at the Delivery System

Replacing the delivery system

Whereas most infusion-related bacteremias are caused by infection of the device used for vascular access, infusate can become contaminated and cause occasional endemic bacteremias (40, 145, 147, 148, 163, 169). If an infusion runs continuously for an extended period, the cumulative risk of contamination increases, and there is further risk that contaminants can grow to concentrations that could produce bacteremia in the recipient of the fluid. For more than 20 years, most U.S. hospitals have routinely replaced the entire delivery system of patients' i.v. infusions at 24- or 48-h intervals (138) to reduce the risk of sepsis from extrinsically contaminated fluid. Recent studies indicate that i.v. delivery systems do not need to be replaced more frequently than every 72 h, including infusions used for total parenteral nutrition or any infusions in ICU patients (13, 32, 85, 107, 136, 245); extending the duration of use permits considerable cost savings to hospitals (136). Unless a hospital detects frequent contamination of intramurally compounded solutions for total parenteral nutrition or experiences a high rate of cryptogenic primary bacteremia associated with total parenteral nutrition, there seems little basis for changing the delivery sets of infusions for parenteral nutrition more frequently than every 72 h (78, 136, 224).

Four clinical settings might be regarded as exceptions to using 72 h as an interval for routine set change (136): (i) administration of blood products; (ii) administration of lipid emulsion; (iii) arterial pressure monitoring; or (iv) a suspected epidemic of infusion-related septicemia. In these circumstances, it may be most prudent to change administration sets routinely at 24- or 48-h intervals.

Minute amounts of blood buffer acidic solutions and provide organic nutrients that greatly enhance the ability of most microorganisms to grow in parenteral fluids (141, 209). Moreover, most hospital pathogens, including coagulase-negative staphylococci, grow rapidly in commercial lipid emulsion (48), and sporadic epidemic septicemias and outbreaks have been traced to contaminated lipid emulsion (100, 158). A recent case-control analysis found that infants in a neonatal ICU given lipid emulsion as part of a peripherally administered parenteral nutrition formula were 3.5 times more likely to develop primary nosocomial bacteremia with coagulase-negative staphylococci (77).

Arterial infusions used for hemodynamic monitoring appear to be more vulnerable to becoming contaminated during use and producing endemic (139, 145) or epidemic (160) septicemia caused by gram-negative bacilli. If the infusion for hemodynamic monitoring is set up so that the fluid flows continuously through the chamber dome—eliminating a blind stagnant column of fluid—extrinsic contamination appears to be greatly reduced, and this may even eliminate the need to replace the administration set, chamber dome, and other components of the system at frequent intervals (123, 179, 189, 235). If disposable transducers and chamber domes are used, there appears to be no need to replace the transducer assembly and other components of the delivery system more frequently than every 4 days (123), and it may be safe to replace them even less frequently (179, 189, 235).

If infusion-related septicemias occur in epidemic numbers, especially caused by *Enterobacter, Serratia,* or *Pseudomonas* spp., contaminated infusate must be suspected, and it may be prudent to reduce the interval for routine set change to every 24 or 48 h.

In-line filters

Terminal in-use membrane filters have been advocated as a means of reducing the hazard of contaminated infusate. However, filters must be changed at periodic intervals and can become blocked, leading to added manipulations of the system and, paradoxically, greater potential for contamination (78, 169). Moreover, filters are expensive amd must be replaced at periodic intervals, and their use adds substantially to the costs of infusion therapy. Controlled clinical trials that establish their cost-effectiveness are needed before the routine use of in-line filters can be advocated (80, 238), especially as a control measure for prevention of septicemias deriving from extrinsic contamination of infusate.

Innovative Technology

The development and application of novel technology holds the greatest promise for a quantum reduction in the incidence of nosocomial infection in general, including bloodstream infections from devices used for intravascular access. Innovations in the design or construction of the infusion apparatus or device that deny access of microorganisms into the system or that prevent organisms that might gain access from proliferating to high concentrations or colonizing the implanted device can obviate poor aseptic technique or undue patient vulnerability.

Dressings

Studies of incorporating an antiseptic, namely povidone-iodine, into a transparent catheter dressing have been disappointing (144). However, considering the superiority of chlorhexidine over povidone-iodine for cutaneous disinfection of vascular catheter sites (134), incorporation of chlorhexidine into a dressing might prove more effective.

Cannulas

The surgically implanted Hickman or Broviac catheter, which incorporates a Dacron cuff that is rapidly ingrown by host tissue, creates a mechanical barrier against infection of the tract by skin organisms. Rates of bloodstream infection with these catheters, approximately 0.20 cases per 1,000 catheter-days, are far lower than those with short-term percutaneously inserted, noncuffed central venous catheters inserted in the ICU

(Table 1). Cuffed, surgically implanted central catheters can thus be considered a quantum advance for safer vascular access. The use of Dacron cuffs on central venous catheters used for temporary hemodialysis has greatly reduced the risk of catheter-related bacteremias with short-term access for dialysis (33, 57).

A tissue-interface barrier (VitaCuff, Vitaphore Corporation) incorporates the technology of Hickman and Broviac catheters with an attachable cuff made of biodegradable collagen to which silver ion is chelated (Fig. 5). The cuff can be attached to any short-term central venous catheter or Swan-Ganz introducer at the time of insertion. After insertion, subcutaneous tissue grows into the collagenous matrix, anchoring the catheter and creating a barrier against invasion of microorganisms from the skin. The silver ion provides an additional chemical barrier against introduced contamination. In prospective, randomized trials (Table 10), catheters inserted with the cuff were less likely to be colonized on removal than

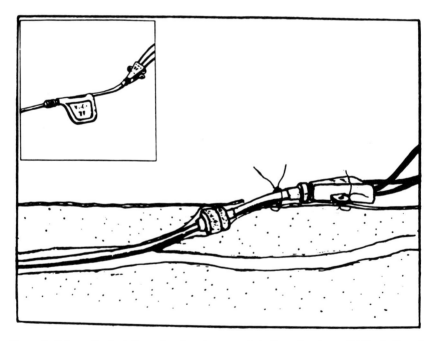

Figure 5. Schematic depiction of a silver-impregnated, tissue-barrier cuff (VitaCuff) and the cuff attached to a central venous catheter in situ. It is important for the cuff to be positioned at least 0.5 to 1.0 cm below the surface of the skin and for the catheter to be well immobilized, preferably with a skin suture, to prevent extrusion (from Maki et al. [137]).

Table 10. Multicenter randomized trial of a silver-impregnated cuff for prevention of infection with short-term central venous catheters[a]

Condition	Controls ($n = 135$)	Cuffed catheters ($n = 99$)
Catheter-related infection, no. (%):		
Local (≥15 CFU)	33 (28.9)	7 (9.1)[b]
With bacteremia	5 (3.7)	1 (1.0)
Infecting organisms, no. (bacteremia):		
Coagulase-negative staphylococci	23	5
Staphylococcus aureus	. . .	1
Enterococci	2	. . .
Gram-negative bacilli	8 (3)	2 (1)
Candida species	4 (2)	. . .

[a] From Maki et al. (137).
[b] $P = 0.002$, compared with control catheters.

were control catheters and were less likely to produce bacteremia (73, 137). Adverse effects from the cuff were not seen. Use of the cuff permitted high-risk short-term central venous catheters to be left in place safely for considerably longer periods (137).

Given the multiplicity of potential sources for infection of an intravascular device and the importance of adherence of microorganisms to the catheter surface in the pathogenesis of infection, the best strategy for prevention might be to develop a catheter material implicitly resistant to colonization. Coating the catheter surface with a nontoxic antiseptic or antimicrobial agent or incorporating such a substance into the catheter material itself might prove to be the ultimate technologic innovation for prevention of device-related infection.

Heparin is now commonly bonded to the external surface of pulmonary-artery Swan-Ganz catheters during their manufacture to reduce thrombosis on the catheter surface after insertion (96). Because the surfactant used to bind the heparin, benzalkonium chloride, has antimicrobial activity against a broad range of microbial pathogens, including *Candida* spp., heparin-bonded catheters exhibit considerable surface antimicrobial activity in vitro (164). Although no prospective clinical trial has examined the efficacy of heparin bonding in preventing catheter-related bacteremia, an analysis of prospective studies of Swan-Ganz catheters suggests that heparin bonding reduces the risk of infection (164).

In a randomized clinical trial with central venous and arterial catheters in a surgical ICU, catheters coated with cefazolin bonded to the surface with a cationic surfactant were associated with a sevenfold reduction in colonization; however, there were no catheter-related bacteremias identified in the study (109). Potential drawbacks of using antibiotics for coating percutaneous intravascular catheters are the ineffectiveness of antibiotics against antibiotic-resistant nosocomial bacteria and yeasts, the risk of bacterial resistance emerging during long-term use, and the potential for patient hypersensitization.

A novel central venous catheter made of polyurethane impregnated with minute quantities of silver sulfadiazine and chlorhexidine (ArrowGard, Arrow International) has recently become available. In a randomized, comparative trial in 402 patients in a surgical ICU, antiseptic catheters were fivefold less likely to produce bacteremia (148). Adverse effects from the novel catheter were not seen.

Catheter hubs

A novel catheter hub, engineered to reduce the risk of hub contamination, was shown by Stotter et al. to significantly reduce the rate of central venous catheter-related bacteremia (254) but is not yet available commercially.

Infusate

A novel closed system, which utilizes a diaphragm rather than a stopcock for obtaining blood specimens from arterial lines, was recently studied clinically in a comparative trial: the diaphragm was associated with a sixfold lower rate of contamination of fluid in the line than use of standard stopcocks; however, no infusion-related bacteremias were identified during the study (49).

The addition of a nontoxic, biodegradable antiseptic to i.v. fluid (79) might eliminate the hazard of fluid contamination altogether and further reduce the risk of hub contamination, obviating the need for periodic replacement of the delivery system. This approach might be most useful for long-term Hickman and Broviac catheters and subcutaneous ports. Use of EDTA, which has intrinsic antimicrobial activity (217), rather than heparin in the flush solutions for these devices might significantly reduce the risk of associated bacteremia and should be studied clinically.

Surveillance

Because bacteremia connotes unimpeachable laboratory confirmation of infection, surveillance data on nosocomial bacteremias are highly reliable epidemiologically and provide an accurate barometer of a hospital's problem with nosocomial infection in general (129). Whereas the value of comprehensive surveillance of all nosocomial infections as a control measure remains unclear, surveillance of all bacteremias, especially intravascular device-related bacteremias, is much simpler, far less expensive, and clearly worthwhile. However, for maximal benefit it is imperative that (i) blood isolates are routinely identified through species, (ii) antimicrobial susceptibility testing using standardized methods is performed routinely because the susceptibility pattern (antibiogram) may be of value as an epidemiologic marker and allows surveillance of antibiotic resistance, and (iii) an isolate from each bacteremia is routinely saved for at least 24 months for future study, should an epidemic occur.

The Joint Commission on Accreditation of Hospitals now strongly recommends surveillance of catheter-related bloodstream infections per 1,000 central venous catheter-days, especially within ICUs.

TREATMENT OF INFECTION

Management of the Device

If a short-term, noncuffed intravascular catheter is suspected of being infected because the patient has no obvious other source of infection to explain fever, there is inflammation at the insertion site, or cryptogenic staphylococcal bacteremia or candidemia has been documented (Table 1), the catheter and the administration set should be removed, and the catheter should be cultured. Whereas many infected central venous catheters, especially those infected with coagulase-negative staphylococci, can be successfully treated without removing the catheter, the risk of recurrent bacteremia is approximately 20% (200). Failure to remove an infected catheter puts the patient at increased risk of developing septic thrombophlebitis of a peripheral vein with peripheral i.v. catheters (104, 264), septic thrombosis of a great central vein with central devices (111, 256, 273), or even endocarditis (63, 258, 276). Continued access, if necessary, can be established with a new catheter inserted in a new site. A new catheter should never be placed in an old site over a guidewire if the first catheter is suspected of being infected, especially if there is purulence at the site.

Bloodstream infections that might originate from a surgically implanted cuffed Hickman or Broviac catheter, on the other hand, do not automatically mandate removal of the device unless there has been persistent exit site infection; the tunnel is obviously infected (195); there is evidence of complicating endocarditis or septic thrombosis of the cannulated vein (195); the infecting pathogen is *Corynebacterium* JK (215), *S. aureus* (58), a *Bacillus* species (14), a *Xanthomonas* species (64), a filamentrous fungus or *Malessezia* species (52), or a mycobacterial species (205); or bacteremia or candidemia persists for more than 3 days (195). Approximately two thirds of uncomplicated Hickman or other implanted catheter-related bacteremias can be cured with antibiotics given through the device for 7 to 10 days (33, 90, 103, 195, 196, 227, 274). Bacteremias, particularly with coagulase-negative staphylococci, can often be cured by simply "locking" a highly concentrated solution of antibiotic within the lumen of the catheter for 12 h a day, for 2 weeks (55, 167). The use of thrombolytic agents, such as streptokinase or urokinase, has been advocated as adjunctive therapy for infected implanted catheters (105, 227) but has not been studied in a randomized trial.

Infection of a subcutaneous central port, on the other hand, associated with bacteremia or fungemia is rarely curable without removing the device, and if the device itself is clearly infected (e.g., an aspirate from the port shows heavy growth), it is best removed (28, 39, 122).

Anti-Infective Therapy

The decision to treat suspected catheter-related bloodstream infection before microbiologic confirmation, i.e., empirically, comes down to clinical judgment, weighing the evidence suggesting bacteremia and the risks of delayed treatment of occult bloodstream infection—e.g., the patient has a prosthetic heart valve. Nosocomial bacteremia occurring in a patient with a prosthetic heart valve was found in a recent prospective multicenter study to result in endocarditis in 16% of cases; an infected intravascular device was the source of one third of all cases of nosocomial prosthetic valve endocarditis identified (69).

If empiric therapy is deemed essential, after cultures have been obtained, the combination of i.v. vancomycin (for staphylococci and enterococci) with an aminoglycoside or a quinolone (for aerobic gram-negative bacilli) should prove effective against the bacterial pathogens likely to be encountered with an infected intravascular device (Tables 1 and 2). Definitive therapy should be based on the microbiologic identification and susceptibility of the infecting organism.

How long to treat catheter-related bloodstream infection will be influenced by whether the patient has underlying valvular heart disease, already has evidence of endocarditis or septic thrombosis, or shows evidence of metastatic infection. If endocarditis is suspected, transesophageal echocardiography offers superior sensitivity and discrimination for detecting vegetations, compared with that of transthoracic echocardiography (65, 172). In patients with high-grade bacteremia or fungemia, but without clinical or echocardiographic evidence of endocarditis, septic thrombosis should be suspected. Central venous thrombosis can be diagnosed by venography (111, 256, 273), ultrasonography (2), computed tomography (2, 26, 171), or magnetic resonance imaging (26).

With uncomplicated device-related bloodstream infection—the bacteremia or candidemia clears rapidly and the patient does not have un- derlying valvular heart disease or clinical evidence of endocarditis, septic thrombosis, or metastatic infection—parenteral antimicrobial therapy given for 7 to 14 days will be adequate in the majority of cases. With uncomplicated catheter-related *S. aureus* bacteremia, 14 days of paren- teral antimicrobial therapy has been shown to have a very high cure rate (24, 61, 173, 203) and can be considered acceptable if the patient defervesces completely within 3 days (203). Similarly, nosocomial entero- coccal bacteremia deriving from an intravascular device is rarely associ- ated with endocarditis, and unless there is clinical or endocardiographic evidence of endocarditis, treatment with i.v. ampicillin or vancomycin alone for 7 to 14 days should suffice (133).

Bacterial endocarditis originating from an intravascular device, while rare, should be treated similarly to endocarditis unrelated to a catheter, with prolonged, bactericidal antimicrobial therapy given paren- terally, using a dosage regimen appropriate for endocarditis (226, 258). Catheter-related septic thrombosis of a great central vein, which charac- teristically produces high-grade bacteremia or candidemia, can be relia- bly cured in most cases without surgical intervention, with 4 to 6 weeks of parenteral antimicrobial therapy (111, 256, 273). Candida can be cured with i.v. amphotericin B in a daily dose of 0.7 mg/kg and a total dose of approximately 20 mg/kg (256). Unless there are contraindications, the patient should also be anticoagulated with heparin (111, 256, 273).

All patients with catheter-related candidemia should be treated, even if the patient becomes afebrile and blood cultures spontaneously revert to negative following removal of the catheter without antifungal therapy (22, 59, 119, 218). Catheter-related candidemia that responds rapidly to removal of the catheter and institution of i.v. amphotericin B can be reliably treated with a daily dose of 0.3 to 0.5 mg/kg and a total dose of 3 to 5 mg/kg (59, 119, 154, 218). Fluconazole (2 to 800 mg/day) shows promise as an alternative, less-toxic drug for treatment of deep candida infections (3, 4, 20, 272).

All patients with device-related bloodstream infection must be moni- tored closely for at least 6 weeks after completing therapy, especially if they have had high-grade bacteremia or candidemia, to detect late- appearing endocarditis (218, 258, 273), retinitis (92, 218), or other meta- static infection, such as vertebral osteomyelitis.

THE FUTURE

Much has been learned about the epidemiology and pathogenesis of infection caused by intravascular devices over the past decade, with studies showing reduced rates of infection with the use of more stringent barrier precautions during insertion of central venous catheters (Table 7) (201), with i.v. teams (Table 8), with the use of more effective cutaneous antiseptics (134, 206) (Table 9), with the use of topical povidone-iodine (120) or mupiricin (94) on central venous catheter insertion sites, and with innovative technologies, such as contamination-resistant hubs (254), attachable cuffs (Table 10) (73, 138), and catheters with colonization-resistant surfaces (109, 148, 164).

Future research must strive to better understand the biologic forces governing cutaneous colonization in order to develop more effective strategies to suppress it with new antiseptics that exhibit much higher and more prolonged levels of surface activity; to delineate fully the molecular mechanisms of microbial adherence to prosthetic surfaces in order to develop new materials intrinsically resistant to colonization; to design devices that intrinsically deny microbial access; to identify new technologies to allow rapid detection of contamination of infusate, device colonization, and bloodstream infection; and to devise more cost-effective programs for care of intravascular devices.

Scientia est potentia

Acknowledgments. I wish to acknowledge the contributions of my colleagues in many of the studies cited from the University of Wisconsin-Madison, particularly Carla Alvarado, Jeffrey Band, Carol Hassemer, Rita McCormick, Leonard Mermel, Marilyn Ringer, Sue Stolz, Lazaro Velez, Susan Wheeler, and Lorna Will, and to express my deep appreciation to my wife, Gail, who provided invaluable assistance in the preparation of this manuscript.

REFERENCES

1. **Ada, N., L. Quintana, R. Mera, C. Lopez, and R. B. Van Dyke.** 1991. One-year historic prospective series of central venous catheter infections in a children's hospital (abstract). *Clin. Res.* **39**:842A.
2. **Albertyn, L. E., and M. K. Alcock.** 1987. Diagnosis of internal jugular vein thrombosis. *Radiology* **162**:505–508.
3. **Anaisse, E., H. Pinczowski, L. Elting, D. Kontoyiannis, S. Vartivarian, and G. P. Bodey.** 1992. Response of fluconazole-treated cancer patients with candidemia compared with patients treated with amphotericin B. A prospective matched pairs study, abstr. 630. *Program Abstr. 32nd Intersci. Conf. Antimicrob. Agents Chemother.* American Society for Microbiology, Washington, D.C.
4. **Anaissie, E. J., R. Darwiche, J. Mera, L. Gentry, D. Abi-Said, and G. P. Bodey.** 1993. A prospective randomized multicenter study comparing fluconazole to amphotericin B for nosocomial candidiasis, abstr. 808. *Program Abstr. 33rd Intersci. Conf. Antimicrob. Agents Chemother.* American Society for Microbiology, Washington, D.C.
5. **Andersen, P. T., P. Herlevsen, and H. Schaumburg.** 1986. A comparative study of 'Op-site' and 'Nobecutan gauze' dressings for central venous line care. *J. Hosp. Infect.* **7**:161–168.

6. **Armstrong, C. W., G. Mayhall, K. B. Miller, H. H. Newsome, Jr., H. J. Sugerman, H. P. Dalton, G. O. Hall, and C. Gennings.** 1986. Prospective study of catheter replacement and other risk factors for infection of hyperalimentation catheters. *J. Infect. Dis.* **154:**808–816.

7. **Armstrong, C. W., C. G. Mayhall, K. B. Miller, H. H. Newsome, Jr., H. J. Sugerman, H. P. Dalton, G. O. Hall, and S. Hunsberger.** 1990. Clinical predictors of infection of central venous catheters used for total parenteral nutrition. *Infect. Control Hosp. Epidemiol.* **11:**71–78.

8. **Arnow, P. M., E. M. Quimosing, and M. Beach.** 1993. Consequences of intravascular catheter sepsis. *Clin. Infect. Dis.* **16:**778–784.

9. **Ascher, D. P., B. A. Shoupe, M. Robb, D. A. Maybee, and G. W. Fischer.** 1992. Comparison of standard and quantitative blood cultures in the evaluation of children with suspected central venous line sepsis. *Diagn. Microbiol. Infect. Dis.* **15:**499–503.

10. **Ashkenazi, S., E. Weiss, and M. M. Drucker.** 1986. Bacterial adherence to intravenous catheters and needles and its influence by cannula type and bacterial surface hydrophobicity. *J. Lab. Clin. Med.* **107:**136–140.

11. **Baird, D., and J. Cola.** 1987. Mupiricin-resistance *Staphylococcus aureus. Lancet* **ii:** 387–388.

12. **Band, J. D., and D. G. Maki.** 1979. Infections caused by indwelling arterial catheters for hemodynamic monitoring. *Am. J. Med.* **67:**735–742.

13. **Band, J. D., and D. G. Maki.** 1979. Safety of changing intravenous delivery systems at longer than 24-hour intervals. *Ann. Intern. Med.* **91:**173–178.

14. **Banerjee, C., C. I. Bustamante, R. Wharton, E. Talley, and J. C. Wade.** 1988. Bacillus infections in patients with cancer. *Arch. Intern. Med.* **148:**1769–1774.

15. **Banerjee, S. N., G. Emori, D. H. Culver, R. P. Gaynes, W. R. Jarvis, T. Horan, J. R. Edwards, J. Tolson, T. Henderson, W. J. Martone, and National Nosocomial Infections Surveillance System.** 1991. Secular trends in nosocomial primary bloodstream infections in the United States, 1980–1989. *Am. J. Med.* **91**(Suppl. 3B):86S–89S.

16. **Barrett, S. P.** 1988. Bacterial adhesion to intravenous cannulae: influence of implantation in the rabbit and of enzyme treatments. *Epidemiol. Infect.* **100:**91–100.

17. **Bates, D. W., L. Goldman, and T. H. Lee.** 1991. Contaminant blood cultures and resource utilization. *JAMA* **265:**365–369.

18. **Beck-Sague, C. M., and W. R. Jarvis.** 1989. Epidemic bloodstream infections associated with pressure transducers: a persistent problem. *Infect. Control Hosp. Epidemiol.* **10:**54–59.

19. **Benezra, D, T. Kiehn, J. W. M. Gold, A. E. Brown, A. D. M. Turnbull, and D. Armstrong.** 1988. Prospective study of infections in indwelling central venous catheters using quantitative blood cultures. *Am. J. Med.* **85:**495–498.

20. **Bennett, J. E., A. M. Sugar, P. V. Pappas, C. M. Van Der Horst, J. E. Edwards, R. G. Washburn, W. M. Scheld, A. W. Karchmer, H. C. Neu, J. J. Stern, C. U. Tauzon, A. P. Dine, M. J. Levenstein, C. D. Webb, and NIAID MSG, Candidemia Study Group.** 1993. Fluconazole (FLU) vs amphotericin B (AMB) for treatment of candidemia: results of a randomized, multicenter trial, abstr. 805. *Program Abstr. 33rd Intersci. Conf. Antimicrob. Agents Chemother.* American Society for Microbiology, Washington, D.C.

21. **Bentley, D. W., and M. H. Lepper.** 1968. Septicemia related to indwelling venous catheter. *JAMA* **206:**1749–1752.

22. **Beutler, S. M., L. S. Young, L. B. Linquist, J. Z. Montomerie, and J. E. Edwards, Jr.** 1982. Delayed complications of candidemia, abstr. 496. *Program Abstr. 22nd Intersci. Conf. Antimicrob. Agents Chemother.* American Society for Microbiology, Washington, D.C.

23. Bjornson, H. S., R. Colley, R. H. Bower, V. P. Duty, J. T. Schwartz-Fulton, and J. E. Fischer. 1982. Association between microorganism growth at the catheter site and colonization of the catheter in patients receiving total parenteral nutrition. *Surgery* **92**:720–772.

24. Bowler, I, C. Conlon, D. Crook, and K. T. Peto. 1992. Optimum duration of therapy for catheter related *Staphylococcus aureus* bacteremia: a cohort study of 75 patients, abstr. 833. *Program Abstr. 32nd Intersci. Conf. Antimicrob. Agents Chemother.* American Society for Microbiology, Washington, D.C.

25. Braude, A. I., F. J. Carey, and J. Siemienski. 1955. Studies of bacterial transfusion reactions from refrigerated blood: the properties of cold-growing bacteria. *J. Clin. Invest.* **34**:311–325.

26. Braun, I. F., J. C. Haffman, J. A. Malko, R. I. Petigrew, W. Danniels, and P. C. Davis. 1985. Jugular venous thrombosis: MR imaging. *Radiology* **157**:357–360.

27. Bross, J., G. H. Talbot, G. Maislin, and S. Hurwitz. 1989. Risk factors for nosocomial candidemia: a case-control study in adults without leukemia. *Am. J. Med.* **87**:614–620.

28. Brothers, T. E., L. K. Von Moll, J. I. Niederhuber, J. A. Roberts, and W. D. Ensminger. 1988. Experience with subcutaneous infusion ports in three hundred patients. *Surg. Gynecol. Obstet.* **166**:295–301.

29. Brun-Buisson, C., F. Abrouk, P. Legrand, Y. Huet, S. Larabi, and M. Rapin. 1987. Diagnosis of central venous catheter-related sepsis. Critical level of quantitative tip cultures. *Arch. Intern. Med.* **147**:873–877.

30. Buchholz, D. H., V. M. Young, N. R. Friedman, J. A. Reilly, and M. R. Mardiney, Jr. 1971. Bacterial proliferation in platelet products stored at room temperature. Transfusion-induced Enterobacter sepsis. *N. Engl. J. Med.* **285**:429–433.

31. Burnie, J. P., F. C. Odds, W. Lee, C. Webster, and J. D. Williams. 1985. Outbreak of systemic *Candida albicans* in an intensive care unit caused by cross infection. *Br. Med. J.* **290**:746–748.

32. Buxton, A. E., A. K. Highsmith, J. S. Garner, et al. 1979. Contamination of intravenous fluid: effects of changing administration sets. *Ann. Intern. Med.* **90**:764–768.

33. Cappello, M., L. De Pauw, G. Bastin, F. Prospert, D. Delcour, C. Thaysse, M. Dhaene, J. L. Vanherweghem, and P. Kinnaert. 1989. Central venous access for haemodialysis using the Hickman catheter. *Nephrol. Dial. Transplant* **4**:988–992.

34. Center for Disease Control. 1973. Septicemias associated with contaminated intravenous fluids. *Morbid. Mortal. Weekly Rep.* **22**:99, 114, 124.

35. Centers for Disease Control. 1988. *Yersinia enterocolitica* bacteremia and endotoxin shock associated with red blood cell transfusion. *Morbid. Mortal. Weekly Rep.* **37**: 577–578.

36. Centers for Disease Control. 1989. Contaminated povidone-iodine solution—Texas. *Morbid. Mortal. Weekly Rep.* **38**:133–135.

37. Centers for Disease Control. 1990. Postsurgical infections associated with an extrinsically contaminated intravenous anesthetic agent—California, Illinois, Maine, and Michigan, 1990. *Morbid. Mortal. Weekly Rep.* **39**:426–433.

38. Cercenado, E., J. Ena, M. Rodriguez-Creixems, I. Romero, and E. Bouza. 1990. A conservative procedure for the diagnosis of catheter-related infections. *Arch. Intern. Med.* **150**:1417–1420.

39. Champault, G. 1986. Totally implanted catheters for cancer chemotherapy: French experience on 325 cases. *Cancer Drug Delivery* **3**:131–137.

40. Cheesbrough, J. S., R. G. Finch, and R. P. Burden. 1986. A prospective study of the mechanisms of infection associated with hemodialysis catheters. *J. Infect. Dis.* **154**:579–589.

41. **Christensen, G. D., W. A. Simpson, J. J. Younger, L. M. Baddour, F. F. Barrett, D. M. Melton, and E. H. Beachey.** 1985. Adherence of coagulase-negative staphylococci to plastic tissue culture plates: a quantitative model for the adherence of staphylococci to medical devices. *J. Clin. Microbiol.* **22:**996–1006.

42. **Cobb, D. K., K. P. High, R. G. Sawyer, C. A. Sable, R. B. Adams, D. A. Lindley, T. L. Pruett, K. J. Schwartzer, and B. M. Earr.** 1992. A controlled trial of scheduled replacement of central venous and pulmonary-artery catheters. *N. Engl. J. Med.* **327:** 1062–1068.

43. **Collignon, P. J., N. Soni, and I. Y. Pearson.** 1986. Is semiquantitative culture of central vein catheter tips useful in the diagnosis of catheter-associated bacteremia? *J. Clin. Microbiol.* **24:**532–535.

44. **Conly, J. M., K. Grieves, and B. Peters.** 1989. A prospective, randomized study comparing transparent and dry gauze dressings for central venous catheters. *J. Infect. Dis.* **159:**310–319.

45. **Cooper, G. L., and C. C. Hopkins.** 1985. Rapid diagnosis of intravascular catheter-associated infection by direct gram staining of catheter segments. *N. Engl. J. Med.* **318:**1142–1150.

46. **Cooper, G. L., A. L. Schiller, and C. C. Hopkins.** 1988. Possible role of capillary action in pathogenesis of experimental catheter-associated dermal tunnel infections. *J. Clin. Microbiol.* **26:**8–12.

47. **Craven, D. E., A. Lichtenberg, L. M. Kunches, A. T. McDonough, M. I. Gonzalez, T. C. Heeren, and W. R. McCabe.** 1985. A randomized study comparing a transparent polyurethane dressing to a dry gauze dressing for peripheral intravenous catheter sites. *Infect. Control.* **6:**361–366.

48. **Crocker, K. S., R. Noga, D. J. Filibeck, et al.** 1984. Microbial growth comparisons of five commercial parenteral lipid emulsions. *J. Parenter. Enteral Nutr.* **8:**391–394.

49. **Crow, S., S. A. Conrad, K. Chaney-Rowell, and J. W. King.** 1989. Microbial contamination of arterial infusions used for hemodynamic monitoring: a randomized trial of contamination with sampling through conventional stopcocks versus a novel closed system. *Infect. Control Hosp. Epidemiol.* **10:**557–561.

50. **Dailey, M. J., J. B. Dickey, and K. H. Packo.** 1991. Endogenous *Candida* endophthalmitis after intravenous anesthesia with propofol. *Arch. Ophthalmol.* **109:**1081–1084.

51. **Daisy, J. A., E. A. Abrutyn, and R. R. MacGregor.** 1979. Inadvertent administration of intravenous fluids contaminated with fungus. *Ann. Intern. Med.* 563–565.

52. **Danker, W. M., S. A. Spector, J. Fierrer, and C. E. Davis.** 1987. Malassezia fungemia in neonates and adults: complication of hyperalimentation. *Rev Infect Dis* **9:**743–753.

53. **Davenport, D. S., R. M. Massanari, M. A. Pfaller, M. J. Bale, S. A. Streed, and W. J. Hierholzer, Jr.** 1986. Usefulness of a test for slime production as a marker for clinically significant infections with coagulase-negative staphylococci. *J. Infect. Dis.* **153:**332–339.

54. **Dickerson, N., P. Horton, S. Smith, and R. Rose III.** 1989. Clinically significant central venous catheter infections in a community hospital: association with type of dressing. *J. Infect. Dis.* **160:**720–721.

55. **Douard, M. C., G. Leverger, R. Paulien, C. Waintrop, E. Clementi, B. Eurin, and G. Schaison.** 1991. Quantitative blood cultures for diagnosis and management of catheter-related sepsis in pediatric hematology and oncology patients. *Intensive Care Med.* **17:**30–35.

56. **Dougherty, S. I. I.** 1988. Pathobiology of infection in prosthetic devices. *Rev. Infect. Dis.* **10:**1102–1117.

57. **Dryden, M. S., A. Samson, H. A. Ludlam, A. J. Wing and I. Phillips.** 1991. Infective

complications associated with the use of the Quinton "Permcath" for long-term central vascular access in haemodialysis. *J. Hosp. Infect.* **19**:257–262.

58. **Dugdale, D. A., and P. G. Ramsey.** 1990. *Staphylococcus aureus* bacteremia in patients with Hickman catheters. *Am. J. Med.* **89**:137–141.

59. **Edwards, J. E.** 1992. Editorial response: Should all patients with candidemia be treated with antifungal agents? *Clin. Infect. Dis.* **15**:422–423.

60. **Edwards, K. E., J. R. Allen, M. J. Miller, R. Ylgev, P. C. Hoffman, R. Klotz, S. Marubio, E. Burkholder, T. Williams, and A. T. Davis.** 1978. *Enterobacter aerogenes* primary bacteremia in pediatric patients. *Pediatrics* **62**:304–308.

61. **Ehni, W. F., and L. B. Reller.** 1989. Short-course therapy for catheter-associated *Staphylococcus aureus* bacteremia. *Arch. Intern. Med.* **149**:533–536.

62. **Ehrenkranz, N. J., D. G. Eckert, and P. M. Phillips.** 1989. Sporadic bacteremia complicating central venous catheter use in a community hospital: a model to predict frequency and aid in decision-making for initiation of investigation. *Am. J. Infect. Control* **17**:69–76.

63. **Ehrie, M., A. P. Morgan, F. D. Moore, and N. E. O'Connor.** 1978. Endocarditis with the indwelling balloon-tipped pulmonary artery catheter in burn patients. *J. Trauma* **18**:664–666.

64. **Elting, L. S., and G. P. Bodey.** 1990. Septicemia due to *Xanthomonas* species and non-Aeruginosa *Pseudomonas* species: increasing incidence of catheter-related infections. *Medicine* **69**:296–306.

65. **Erbel, R., S., Rohmann, M. Drexler, S. Mohr-Kahaly, C. D. Gerharz, S. Iversen, H. Oebert, and J. Meyer.** 1988. Improved diagnostic value of echocardiography in patients with infective endocarditis by transesophageal approach. A prospective study. *Eur. Heart J.* **9**:43–53.

66. **Evans, R. C., and C. J. Holmes.** 1987. Effect of vancomycin hydrochloride on *Staphylococcus epidermidis* biofilm associated with silicone elastomer. *Antimicrob. Agents Chemother.* **31**:889–894.

67. **Eyer, S., C. Brummitt, K. Crossley, R. Siegel, and F. Cerra.** 1990. Catheter-related sepsis: prospective, randomized study of three methods of long-term catheter maintenance. *Crit. Care Med.* **18**:1073–1079.

68. **Falcieri, E., P. Vaudaux, E. Huggler, D. Lew, and F. Waldvogel.** 1987. Role of bacterial expolymers and host factors on adherence and phagocytosis of *Staphylococcus aureus* in foreign body infection. *J. Infect. Dis.* **155**:524–531.

69. **Fang, G., T. F. Keys, L. O. Gentry, A. A. Harris, N. Rivera, K. Getz, P. C. Fuchs, M. Gustafson, E. S. Wong, A. Goetz, M. M. Wagener, and V. L. Yu.** 1993. Prosthetic valve endocarditis resulting from nosocomial bacteremia. A prospective, multicenter study. *Ann. Intern. Med.* **119**:560–567.

70. **Farkas, J.-C., J.-F. Timsit, J.-M. Boyer, J.-B. Martin, F. Bismut, S. Chevret, and J. Carlet.** 1994. Does catheter-related thrombosis (CRT) increase the risk of catheter-related sepsis (CRS) in ICU patients? abstr. 52 *Proceedings and Abstracts of the Third International Congress on Prevention of Infection.* Nice, France.

71. **Faubion, W. C., J. R. Wesley, N. Khalidi, and J. Silva.** 1986. Total parenteral nutrition catheter sepsis: impact of the team approach. *J. Parenter. Enteral Nutr.* **10**:642–645.

72. **Fauerbach, L. L., M. J. Schoppman, V. R. Singh, L. S. Netardus, D. L. Pickett, and J. W. Shands.** 1991. A comparison of the efficacy of different antiseptics for intravascular site preparation, abstr. 1269. *Program Abstr. 31st Intersci. Conf. Antimicrob. Agents Chemotherapy.* American Society for Microbiology, Washington, D.C.

73. **Flowers, R. H., III, K. J. Schwenzer, R. J. Kopel, M. J. Fisch, S. I. Tucker, and B. M. Farr.** 1989. Efficacy of an attachable subcutaneous cuff for the prevention of intravascular catheter-related infection. *JAMA* **261**:878–883.

74. **Flynn, P. M., J. L. Shencp, D. C. Stokes, and F. F. Barrett.** 1987. *In situ* management of confirmed central venous catheter-related bacteremia. *Pediatr. Infect. Dis. J.* **6:** 729–734.

75. **Franceschi, D., R. L. Gerding, G. Phillips, and R. B. Gratianne.** 1989. Risk factors associated with intravascular catheter infections in burned patients: a prospective, randomized study. *J. Trauma* **29:**811–816.

76. **Franson, T. R., N. K. Sheth, H. D. Rose, and P. G. Sohnle.** 1987. Scanning electron microscopy of bacteria adherent to intravascular catheters. *J. Clin. Microbiol.* **20:** 500–505.

77. **Freeman, J., D. A. Goldmann, N. E. Smith, D. G. Sidebottom, M. F. Epstein, and R. Platt.** 1990. Association of intravenous lipid emulsion and coagulase-negative staphylococcal bacteremia in neonatal intensive care units. *N. Engl. J. Med.* **323:** 301–308.

78. **Freeman, J. B., A. Lemire, and L. D. MacLean.** 1972. Intravenous alimentation and septicemia. *Surg. Gynecol. Obstet.* **135:**708–712.

79. **Freeman, R., M. P. Holden, R. Lyon, et al.** 1982. Addition of sodium metabisulfite to left atrial catheter infusate as a means of preventing bacterial colonization of the catheter tip. *Thorax* **37:**142–144.

80. **Friedland, G.** 1985. Infusion-related phlebitis—is the in-line filter the solution? (Editorial). *N. Engl. J. Med.* **312:**113–115.

81. **Fuchs, P. C., M. E. Gustafson, J. T. King, and P. T. Goodall.** 1984. Assessment of catheter-associated infection risk with the Hickman right atrial catheter. *Infect. Control* **5:**226–230.

82. **Furfaro, S., M. Gauthier, J. Lacroix, D. Nadeau, L. Lafleur, and S. Mathews.** 1991. Arterial catheter-related infections in children. *Am. J. Dis. Child.* **145:**1037–1042.

83. **Gantz, N. M., G. M. Presswood, R. Goldberg, and G. Doern.** 1984. Effects of dressing type and change interval on intravenous therapy complication rates. *Diagn. Microbiol. Infect. Dis.* **2:**325–332.

84. **Garner, J. S., W. R. Jarvis, T. G. Emori, T. C. Horan, and J. M. Hughes.** 1988. CDC definitions for nosocomial infections. *Am. J. Infect. Control* **16:**128–140.

85. **Gorbea, H. F., D. R. Snydman, A. Delaney, et al.** 1984. Intravenous tubing with burettes can be safely changed at 48-hour intervals. *JAMA* **251:**2112–2115.

86. **Graeve, A. H., C. M. Carpenter, and W. R. Schiller.** 1981. Management of central venous catheters using a wire introducer. *Am. J. Surg.* **142:**752–755.

87. **Graham, D. R., M. M. Keldermans, L. W. Klemm, N. J. Semenza, and M. L. Shafer.** 1991. Infectious complications among patients receiving home intravenous therapy with peripheral, central, or peripherally placed central venous catheters. *Am. J. Med.* **91**(Suppl. 3B):95S–100S.

88. **Gristina, A. G.** 1987. Biomaterial-centered infection: microbial adhesion versus tissue integration. *Science* **237:**1588–1595.

89. **Gristina, A. G., R. A. Jennings, P. T. Naylor, Q. N. Myrvik, and L. X. Webb.** 1989. Comparative in vitro antibiotic resistance of surface-colonizing coagulase-negative staphylococci. *Antimicrob. Agents Chemother.* **33:**813–816.

90. **Hartman, G. E., and S. J. Shochat.** 1987. Management of septic complications associated with Silastic catheters in childhood malignancy. *Pediatr. Infect. Dis. J.* **6:** 1042–1047.

91. **Heal, J. M., M. E. Jones, A. Chaudry, and R. L. Stricop.** 1987. Fatal *Salmonella* septicemia after platelet transfusion. *Transfusion* **27:**2–5.

92. **Henderson, D. K., J. E. Edwards, and J. Z. Montgomerie.** 1981. Hematogenous Candida endophthalmitis in patients receiving parenteral hyperalimentation fluids. *J. Infect. Dis.* **143:**655–661.

93. Herrmann, M., P. E. Vaudaux, D. Pittet, R. Auckenthaler, P. D. Lew, F. Schumacher-Perdreau, G. Peters, and F. A. Waldvogel. 1988. Fibronectin, fibinogen, and laminin act as mediators of adherence of clinical staphylococcal isolates to foreign material. *J. Infect. Dis.* **158**:693–701.

94. Hill, R. L. R., A. P. Fisher, R. J. Ware, S. Wilson, and M. W. Casewell. 1990. Mupirocin for the reduction of colonization of internal jugular cannulae—a randomized controlled trial. *J. Hosp. Infect.* **15**:311–321.

95. Hilton, F., T. M. Haslett, M. T. Borenstein, V. Tucci, H. D. Isenberg, and C. Singer. 1988. Central catheter infections: single- versus triple-lumen catheters. Influence of guide wires on infection rates when used for replacement of catheters. *Am. J. Med.* **84**:667–672.

96. Hoar, P. F., R. M. Wilson, D. T. Mangano, G. J. Avery, R. J. Szarnicki, and J. D. Hill. 1981. Heparin bonding reduces thrombogenicity of pulmonary artery catheters. *N. Engl. J. Med.* **305**:993–995.

97. Hoffman, K. K., D. J. Weber, G. P. Samsa, and W. A. Rutala. 1992. Transparent polyurethane film as an intravenous catheter dressing. A meta-analysis of infection rates. *JAMA* **267**:2072–2076.

98. Hoffman, K. K., S. A. Western, D. L. Kaiser, R. P. Wenzel, and D. H. Groschel. 1988. Bacterial colonization and phlebitis-associated risk with transparent polyurethane film for peripheral intravenous site dressings. *Am. J. Infect. Control* **16**:101–106.

99. James, J. D. 1959. Bacterial contamination of reserved blood. *Vox Sang.* **4**:177–181.

100. Jarvis, W. R., A. K. Highsmith, J. R. Allen, et al. 1983. Polymicrobial bacteremia associated with use of lipid emulsion in a neonatal intensive care unit. *Pediatr. Infect. Dis.* **2**:203–209.

101. Jarvis, W. R., et al. 1991. Nosocomial outbreaks: The Centers for Disease Controls; Hospital Infections Program experience, 1980–1991. *Am. J. Med.* **91**(Suppl. 3B): 101S–106S.

102. John, J. F., Jr. 1989. Molecular analysis of nosocomial epidemics. *Infect. Dis. Clin. North Am.* **3**:683–700.

103. Johnson, P. R., M. D. Decker, K. M. Edwards, W. Schaffner, and P. F. Wright. 1986. Frequency of Broviac catheter infections in pediatric oncology patients. *J. Infect. Dis.* **154**:570–578.

104. Johnson, R. A., R. A. Zajac, and M. E. Evans. 1986. Suppurative thrombophlebitis: correlation between pathogen and underlying disease. *Infect. Control* **7**:582–585.

105. Jones, G. R., G. K. Konsler, R. P. Dunaway, S. R. Lacey, and R. G. Azizkhan. 1993. Prospective analysis of urokinase in the treatment of catheter sepsis in pediatric hematology-oncology patients. *J. Pediatr. Surg.* **28**:350–357.

106. Joseph, P., and J. Marzouk. 1985. Transparent vs. dry gauze dressings for peripheral IV sites. *Program Abstr. Annu. Meet. Am. Soc. Microbiol.* 1985. American Society for Microbiology, Washington, D.C., abstr. 378.

107. Josephson, A., M. E. Gombert, M. F. Sierra, L. V. Karanfil, and G. F. Tansino. 1985. The relationship between intravenous fluid contamination and the frequency of tubing replacement. *Infect. Control* **6**:367–370.

108. Kahan, A., A. Philippon, G. Paul, S. Weber, C. Richard, G. Hazebroucq, and M. Degeorges. 1983. Nosocomial infections by chlorhexidine solution contaminated with *Pseudomonas pickettii* (biovar VA-I). *J. Infect.* **7**:256–263.

109. Kamal, G. D., M. A. Pfaller, L. E. Rempe, and P. J. R. Jebson. 1991. Reduced intravascular catheter infection by antibiotic bonding. *JAMA* **265**:2364–2368.

110. Katich, M., and J. Band. 1985. Local infection of the intravenous-cannulae wound associated with transparent dressings. *J. Infect. Dis.* **151**:971–972.

111. **Kaufman, J., C. Demas, K. Stark, and L. Flancbaum.** 1986. Catheter-related septic central venous thrombosis—current therapeutic options. *West. J. Med.* **145:**200–203.
112. **Kelsey, M. C., and M. Gosling.** 1984. A comparison of the morbidity associated with occlusive and non-occlusive dressings applied to peripheral intravenous devices. *J. Hosp. Infect.* **5:**313–321.
113. **Keohane, P. P., B. J. M. Jones, H. Attrill, A. Cribb, J. Northover, P. Frost, and D. B. A. Silk.** 1983. Effect of catheter tunnelling and a nutrition nurse on catheter sepsis during parenteral nutrition. A controlled trial. *Lancet* **ii:**1388–1390.
114. **Komshian, S. V., A. K. Uwaydah, J. D. Sobel, and L. R. Crane.** 1989. Fungemia caused by *Candida* species and *Torulopsis glabrata* in the hospitalized patient: frequency, characteristics, and evaluation of factors influencing outcome. *Rev. Infect. Dis.* **3:**379–390.
115. **Kotilainen, P.** 1990. Association of coagulase-negative staphylococcal slime production and adherence with the development and outcome of adult septicemias. *J. Clin. Microbiol.* **28:**2779–2785.
116. **Kovacevich, D. S., W. C. Faubion, J. M. Bender, D. R. Schaberg, and J. R. Wesley.** 1986. Association of parenteral nutrition catheter sepsis with urinary tract infections. *J. Parenter. Enteral Nutr.* **10:**639–641.
117. **Landers, S., A. A. Moise, J. K. Fraley, E. O. Smith, and C. J. Baker.** 1991. Factors associated with umbilical catheter-related sepsis in neonates. *Am. J. Dis. Child.* **145:** 657–680.
118. **Larson, E., and C. Hargiss.** 1984. A decentralized approach to maintenance of intravenous therapy. *Am. J. Infect. Control* **12:**177–186.
119. **Leccoines, J. A., J. W. Lee, E. E. Navarro, F. G. Witebsky, D. Marshall, S. M. Steinberg, P. A. Pizzo, and T. J. Walsh.** 1992. Vascular catheter-associated fungemia in patients with cancer: analysis of 155 episodes. *Clin. Infect. Dis.* **14:**875–883.
120. **Levin, A., A. J. Mason, K. K. Jindal, I. W. Fong, and M. B. Goldstein.** 1991. Prevention of hemodialysis subclavian vein catheter infections by topical povidone-iodine. *Kidney Int.* **40:**934–938.
121. **Linares, J., A. Sitges-Serra, J. Garau, et al.** 1985. Pathogenesis of catheter sepsis: a prospective study with quantitative and semiquantitative cultures of catheter hub and segments. *J. Clin. Microbiol.* **21:**357–360.
122. **Lokich, J. J., A. Bothe, P. Benotti, et al.** 1985. Complications and management of implanted venous access catheters. *J. Clin. Oncol.* **3:**710–717.
123. **Luskin, R. L., R. A. Weinstein, C. Nathan, et al.** 1986. Extended use of disposable pressure transducers: a bacteriologic evaluation. *JAMA* **255:**916–920.
124. **Mackel, D. C., D. G. Maki, R. L. Anderson, F. S. Rhame, and J. V. Bennett.** 1975. Nationwide epidemic of septicemia caused by contaminated intravenous products: mechanisms of intrinsic contamination. *J. Clin. Microbiol.* **2:**486–497.
125. **Maibach, H. I., and G. Hildick-Smith.** 1965. *Skin Bacteria and Their Role in Infection.* McGraw-Hill Book Co., New York.
126. **Maki, D. G.** 1977. Growth properties of microorganisms in infusion fluid and methods of detection, p. 13–47. *In* I. Phillips (ed.) *Microbiologic Hazards of Intravenous Therapy.* MTP Press Ltd., Lancaster, England.
127. **Maki, D. G.** 1977. Sepsis arising from extrinsic contamination of the infusion and measure for control, p. 99–141. *In* I. Phillips (ed.), *Microbiologic Hazards of Infusion Therapy.* MTP Press, Ltd., Lancaster, England.
128. **Maki, D. G.** 1980. Through a glass darkly. Nosocomial pseudoepidemics and pseudo-bacteremias. *Arch. Intern. Med.* **140:**26–28. (Editorial.)
129. **Maki, D. G.** 1981. Nosocomial bacteremia. *Am. J. Med.* **70:**183–196.

130. **Maki, D. G.** 1989. The use of antiseptics for handwashing by medical personnel. *J. Chemother.* **1**(Suppl. 1):3–11.
131. **Maki, D. G.** 1990. The epidemiology and prevention of nosocomial bloodstream infections, abstr. 3. *Program Abstr. Third Int. Conf. Nosocomial Infections.* Atlanta, Centers for Disease Control, The National Foundation for Infectious Diseases, and the American Society for Microbiology.
132. **Maki, D. G.** 1992. Infections due to infusion therapy, p. 849–898. *In* J. V. Bennett and P. S. Brachman (ed.), *Hospital Infections.* Little, Brown & Co., Boston.
133. **Maki, D. G., and W. A. Agger.** 1988. Enterococcal bacteremia. Natural history, the risk of endocarditis, and management. *Medicine* **67**:248–269.
134. **Maki, D. G., C. J. Alvarado, and M. Ringer.** 1991. A prospective, randomized trial of povidone-iodine, alcohol and chlorhexidine for prevention of infection with central venous and arterial catheters. *Lancet* **338**:339–343.
135. **Maki, D. G., and J. D. Band.** 1981. A comparative study of polyantibiotic and iodophor ointments in prevention of catheter-related infection. *Am. J. Med.* **70**:739–744.
136. **Maki, D. G., J. T. Botticelli, M. L. LeRoy, and T. S. Thielke.** 1987. Prospective study of replacing administration sets for intravenous therapy at 48- vs 72-hour intervals. *JAMA* **258**:1777–1781.
137. **Maki, D. G., L. Cobb, J. K. Garman, J. Shapiro, M. Ringer, and R. B. Helgerson.** 1988. An attachable silver-impregnated cuff for prevention of infection with central venous catheters. A prospective randomized multi-center trial. *Am. J. Med.* **85**:307–314.
138. **Maki, D. G., D. A. Goldmann, and F. S. Rhame.** 1973. Infection control in intravenous therapy. *Ann. Intern. Med.* **79**:867–887.
139. **Maki, D. G., and C. H. Hassemer.** 1981. Endemic rate of fluid contamination and related septicemia in arterial pressure monitoring. *Am. J. Med.* **70**:733–738.
140. **Maki, D. G., B. S. Klein, R. D. McCormick, C. J. Alvarado, M. A. Zilz, S. M. Stolz, C. A. Hassemer, J. Gould, and A. R. Liegel.** 1991. Nosocomial *Pseudomonas pickettii* bacteremias traced to narcotic tampering. A case for selective drug screening of health care personnel. *JAMA* **265**:981–986.
141. **Maki, D. G., and W. T. Martin.** 1975. Nationwide epidemic of septicemia caused by contaminated infusion products. IV. Growth of microbial pathogens in fluids for intravenous infusion. *J. Infect. Dis.* **131**:267–272.
142. **Maki, D. G., and K. N. McCormack.** 1987. Defatting catheter insertion sites in total parenteral nutrition is of no value as an infection control measure. *Am. J. Med.* **83**:833–840.
143. **Maki, D. G., F. S. Rhame, D. C. Mackel, and J. V. Bennett.** 1976. Nationwide epidemic of septicemia caused by contaminated intravenous products. *Am. J. Med.* **60**:471–485.
144. **Maki, D. G., and M. Ringer.** 1987. Evaluation of dressing regimens for prevention of infection with peripheral intravenous catheters. *JAMA* **258**:2396–2403.
145. **Maki, D. G., and M. Ringer.** 1989. Prospective study of arterial catheter-related infection: incidence, sources of infection and risk factors, abstr. 1075. *Program Abstr. 29th Intersci. Conf. Antimicrob. Agents Chemother.* American Society for Microbiology, Washington, D.C.
146. **Maki, D. G., and M. Ringer.** 1991. Risk factors for infusion-related phlebitis with small peripheral venous catheters. *Ann. Intern. Med.* **114**:845–854.
147. **Maki, D. G., S. M. Stolz, S. J. Wheeler, and L. A. Mermel.** A prospective, randomized, three-way clinical comparison of novel highly permeable polyurethane dressing with 442 Swan-Ganz catheters. *Crit. Care Med.*, in press.

148. **Maki, D. G., S. J. Wheeler, S. M. and L. A. Mermel.** 1991. Clinical trial of a novel antiseptic central venous catheter, abstr. 461. *Program Abstr. 31st Intersci. Conf. Antimicrob. Agents Chemother.* American Society for Microbiology, Washington, D.C.

149. **Maki, D. G., C. E. Weise, and H. W. Sarafin.** 1977. A semiquantitative culture method for identifying intravenous-catheter-related infection. *N. Engl. J. Med.* **296:** 1305–1309.

150. **Maki, D. G., and L. Will.** 1990. Risk factors for central venous catheter-related infection with an ICU. A prospective study of 345 catheters. *Program Abstr. 30th Intersci. Conf. Antimicrob. Agents Chemother.* American Society for Microbiology, Washington, D.C.

151. **Maki, D. G., and L. Will.** 1984. Colonization and infection associated with transparent dressings for central venous, arterial, and Hickman catheters: a comparative trial, abstr. 991. *Program Abstr. 24th Intersci. Conf. Antimicrob. Agents Chemother.* American Society for Microbiology, Washington, D.C.

152. **Markus, S., and S. Buday.** 1989. Culturing indwelling central venous catheters in situ. *Infect. Surg.* 157–162.

153. **Marrie, T. J., and J. W. Costerton.** 1984. Scanning and transmission electron microscopy of in situ bacterial colonization of intravenous and intraarterial catheters. *J. Clin. Microbiol.* **19:**687–693.

154. **Marsh, P. K., F. P. Tally, J. Kellum, A. Callow, and S. L. Gorbach.** 1993. Candida infections in surgical patients. *Ann. Surg.* **198:**42–47.

155. **Matsaniotis, N. S., V. P. Syriopolou, M. C. Theodoridou, K. G. Tzanetou, and G. I. Mostrou.** 1984. Enterobacter sepsis in infants and children due to contaminated intravenous fluids. *Infect. Control* **5:**471–477.

156. **McCredie, K. B., M. Lawson, K. Marts, and J. Stern.** 1984. A comparative evaluation of transparent dressings and gauze dressings for central venous catheters. Abstr. *J. Parenter. Enteral Nutr.* **8:**96.

157. **McGeer, A., and J. Righter.** 1987. Improving our ability to diagnose infections associated with central venous catheters: value of Gram's staining and culture of entry site swabs. *Can. Med. Assoc. J.* **137:**1009–1021.

158. **McKee, K. T., M. A. Melly, H. H. Greene, et al.** 1979. Gram-negative bacillary sepsis associated with use of lipid emulsion in parenteral nutrition. *Am. J. Dis. Child.* **133:** 649–650.

159. **Meers, P. D., M. W. Calder, M. M. Maxhar, and G. M. Lawrie.** 1973. Intravenous infusion of contaminated dextrose solution: the Devonport incident. *Lancet* **ii:**1189.

160. **Mermel, L. A., and D. G. Maki.** 1989. Epidemic bloodstream infections from hemodynamic pressure monitoring: signs of the times. *Infect. Control Hosp. Epidemiol.* **10:** 47–53.

161. **Mermel, L. A., and D. G. Maki.** 1993. Detection of bacteremia in adults: consequences of culturing an inadequate volume of blood. *Ann. Intern. Med.* **119:**270–272.

162. **Mermel, L. A., and D. G. Maki.** 1994. Infectious complications of Swan-Ganz pulmonary artery catheters. Pathogenesis, epidemiology, prevention and management. *Am. J. Respir. Crit. Care Med.* **149:**1020–1036.

163. **Mermel, L., S. Stolz, and D. G. Maki.** 1991. Epidemiology and pathogenesis of infection with Swan-Ganz catheters. A prospective study using molecular epidmiology. *Am. J. Med.* **91**(3B):197–295S.

164. **Mermel, L. A., S. M. Stolz, and D. G. Maki.** 1993. Surface antimicrobial activity of heparin-bonded and antiseptic-impregnated vascular catheters. *J. Infect. Dis.* **167:** 920–924.

165. **Mermel, L. A., L. A. Velez, M. A. Zilz, and D. G. Maki.** 1991. Epidemiologic and microbiologic features of nosocomial bloodstream infection (NBSI) implicating a vascular catheter source: a case-control study of 85 vascular catheter-related and 101 secondary NBSIs, abstr. 454. *Program Abstr. 31st Intersci. Conf. Antimicrob. Agents Chemother.* American Society for Microbiology, Washington, D.C.

166. **Mertz, P. M., and W. H. Eaglestein.** 1984. The effect of a semiocclusive dressing on the microbial population in superficial wounds. *Arch. Surg.* **119:**287–289.

167. **Messing, B., S. Peitra-Cohen, A. Debure, M. Beliah, and J.-J. Bernier.** 1988. Antibiotic-lock technique: a new approach to optimal therapy for catheter-related sepsis in home-parenteral nutrition patients. *J. Parenter. Enteral Nutr.* **12:**185–189.

168. **Michaels, L., and B. Ruebner.** 1953. Growth of bacteria in intravenous infusion fluids. *Lancet* **i:**722–774.

169. **Miller, R. C., and J. B. Grogan.** 1973. Incidence and source of contamination of intravenous nutritional infusion systems. *J. Pediatr. Surg.* **8:**185–190.

170. **Moran, J. M., R. P. Atwood, and M. I. Rowe.** 1965. A clinical bacteriologic study of infections associated with venous cut downs. *N. Engl. J. Med.* **272:**554–560.

171. **Mori, H., T. Fukua I. Isomoto, H. Maeda, and K. Hayashi.** 1990. CT diagnosis of catheter-induced septic thrombus of vena cava. *J. Comput. Assist. Tomogr.* **14:**236–238.

172. **Mügge, A., W. G. Daniel, G. Frank, and P. R. Lichtlen.** 1989. Echocardiography in infective endocarditis: reassessment of prognostic implications of vegetation size determined by the transthoracic and the transesophageal approach. *J. Am. Coll. Cardiol.* **14:**631–638.

173. **Mylotte, J. M., and C. McDermott.** 1987. *Staphylococcus aureus* bacteremia caused by infected intravenous catheters. *Am. J. Infect. Control* **15:**1–6.

174. **Nehme, A. E.** 1980. Nutritional support of the hospital patients: the team concept. *JAMA* **243:**1906–1908.

175. **Nehme, A. E., and J. A. Trigger.** 1984. Catheter dressings in central parenteral nutrition: a prospective randomized comparative study. *Nutr. Support Serv.* **4:**42–43.

176. **Nelson, D. B., C. L. Kien, B. Mohr, S. Frank, and S. D. Davis.** 1986. Dressing changes by specialized personnel reduce infection rates in patients receiving central venous parenteral nutrition. *J. Parenter. Enteral Nutr.* **10:**220–222.

177. **Norden, C. W.** 1969. Application of antibiotic ointment to the site of venous catheterization—a controlled trial. *J. Infect. Dis.* **120:**611–615.

178. **Nystrom, B., S. Olesen Larsen, J. Dankert, F. Daschner, D. Greco, P. Gronroos, O. B. Jepsen, A. Lystad, P. D. Meers, and M. Rotter.** 1983. Bacteraemia in surgical patients with intravenous devices: a European multicentre incidence study. *J. Hosp. Infect.* **4:**338–349.

179. **O'Malley, M. K., J. Chen, S. Cameron, B. A. Juni, A. J. Streifel, R. C. McComb, F. B. Cerra, D. Ursley, and F. S. Rhame.** 1990. Study of long duration placement of pressure monitoring systems, abstr. 84. *Program Abstr. 3rd Int. Conf. Nosocomial Infect.* Centers for Disease Control, The National Foundation for Infectious Diseases.

180. **Padberg, F. T., Jr., J. Ruggiero, G. L. Blackburn, and B. R. Bistrian.** 1981. Central venous catheterization for parenteral nutrition. *Ann. Surg.* **193:**264–270.

181. **Palidar, P. J., D. A. Simonowitz, M. R. Oreskovich, E. P. Dellinger, W. A. Edwards, S. Adams, and J. Karkeck.** 1982. Use of Op-Site as an occlusive dressing for total parenteral nutrition catheters. *J. Parenter. Enteral Nutr.* **6:**150–151.

182. **Parrott, P. L., P. M. Terry, E. N. Whitworth, L. W. Frawley, R. S. Coble, I. K. Wachsmuth, and J. E. McGowan, Jr.** 1982. *Pseudomonas aeruginosa* peritonitis associated with contaminated poloxamer-iodine solution. *Lancet* **ii:**683–685.

183. **Pascual, A., A. Fleer, N. A. C. Westerdaal, and J. Verhoef.** 1986. Modulation of adherence of coagulase-negative staphylococci to Teflon catheters in vitro. *Eur. J. Clin. Microbiol.* **5:**518–522.

184. **Pettigrew, R. A., S. D. R. Lang, D. A. Haydock, B. R. Parry, D. A. Bremmer, and G. L. Hill.** 1985. Catheter-related sepsis in patients on intravenous nutrition: a prospective study of quantitative catheter cultures and guidewire changes for suspected sepsis. *Br. J. Surg.* **72:**52–55.

185. **Pezzarossi, H. E., S. Ponce de León, J. J. Calva, S. A. Lazo de la Vega, and G. M. Ruiz-Palacios.** 1986. High incidence of subclavian dialysis catheter-related bacteremias. *Infect. Control* **7:**596–599.

186. **Phillips, I., and S. Eykyn.** 1971. *Pseudomonas cepacia* (multivorans) septicaemia in an intensive care unit. *Lancet* **i:**375–377.

187. **Pittet, D., C. Churad, A. C. Rae, and R. Auckenthaler.** 1991. Clinical diagnosis of central venous catheter line infections: a difficult job, abstr. 453. *Program Abstr. 31st Intersci. Conf. Antimicrob. Agents Chemother.* American Society for Microbiology, Washington, D.C.

188. **Pittman, M.** 1953. A study of bacteria implicated in transfusion reactions and of bacteria isolated from blood products. *J. Lab. Clin. Med.* **42:**273.

189. **Platzner, N., J. A. Marino, F. B. Cerra, et al.** 1982. Eliminating the cul-de-sac from pressure cone infusion systems reduces fluid contamination, abstr. 931. *Proc. 22nd Intersci. Conf. Antimicrob. Agents Chemother.*

190. **Plouffe, J. F., D. G. Brown, J. Silva, R. Eck, R. L. Stricof, and F. R. Fekery, Jr.** 1977. Nosocomial outbreak of *Candida parapsilosis* fungemia related to intravenous infusions. *Arch. Intern. Med.* **137:**1686–1689.

191. **Porter, K. A., B. R. Bistrian, and G. L. Blackburn.** 1988. Guidewire catheter exchange with triple culture technique in the management of catheter sepsis. *J. Parenter. Enteral Nutr.* **12:**628–632.

192. **Powell, C., C. Regan, P. J. Fabri, and R. L. Ruberg.** 1982. Evaluation of opsite catheter dressings for parenteral nutrition: a prospective, randomized study. *J. Parenter. Enteral Nutr.* **6:**43–46.

193. **Powell, C. R., M. J. Traetow, P. J. Fabri, K. A. Kudsk, and R. L. Ruberg.** 1985. Op-site dressing study: a prospective randomized study evaluating povidone iodine ointment and extension set changes with 7-day op-site dressings applied to total parenteral nutrition subclavian sites. *J. Parenter. Enteral Nutr.* **9:**443–446.

194. **Prager, R. L., and J. Silva.** 1984. Colonization of central venous catheters. *South. Med. J.* **77:**458–461.

195. **Press, O. W., P. G. Ramsey, E. B. Larson, A. Fefer, and R. O. Hickman.** 1984. Hickman catheter infections in patients with malignancies. *Medicine* **63:**189–200.

196. **Prince, A., B. Heller, J. Jevy, and W. C. Heird.** 1986. Management of fever in patients with central vein catheters. *Pediatr. Infect. Dis. J.* **5:**20–24.

197. **Pruitt, B. A., Jr., W. F. McManus, S. H. Kim, and R. C. Treat.** 1980. Diagnosis and treatment of cannula-related intravenous sepsis in burn patients. *Ann. Surg.* **191:**546–554.

198. **Puntis, J. W. L., C. E. Holden, S. Smallman, Y. Finkel, R. H. George, and I. W. Booth.** 1990. Staff training: a key factor in reducing intravascular catheter sepsis. *Arch. Dis. Child.* **65:**335–337.

199. **Quinlan, A.** 1990. *In vivo* assessment of microbial proliferation under OpSite IV 3000, Tegaderm and Tegaderm Plus, with and without serum (abstract no. P12/22). *Proc. Abstr. Third Int. Meet. Hosp. Infect. Soc.* Hospital Infection Society, London.

200. **Raad, I., S. Davis, A. Khan, J. Tarrand, L. Elting, and G. P. Bodey.** 1992. Impact

of central venous catheter removal on the recurrence of catheter-related coagulase-negative staphylococcal bacteremia. *Infect. Control Hosp. Epidemiol.* **13**:215–221.

201. **Raad, I. I., D. C. Hohn, B. J. Gilbreath, N. Suleiman, L. A. Hill, P. A. Bruso, K. Marts, P. F. Mansfield, and G. P. Bodey.** 1994. Prevention of central venous catheter-related infections by using maximal sterile barrier precautions during insertion. *Infect. Control. Hosp. Epidemiol.* **15**:231–238.

202. **Raad, I. I., M. Luna, S.-A. M. Khalil, J. W. Costerton, C. Lam, and G. P. Bodey.** 1994. The relationship between the thrombotic and infectious complications of central venous catheters. *JAMA* **271**:1014–1016.

203. **Raad, I. I., and M. F. Sabbagh.** 1992. Optimal duration of therapy for catheter-related *Staphylococcus aureus* bacteremia: a study of 55 cases and review. *Clin. Infect. Dis.* **14:** 75–82.

204. **Raad, I. I., M. F. Sabbagh, K. H. Rand, and R. J. Sherertz.** 1992. Quantitative tip culture methods and the diagnosis of central venous catheter-related infections. *Diagn. Microbiol. Infect. Dis.* **15**:13–20.

205. **Raad, I. I., S. Vartivarian, A. Khan, and G. P. Bodey.** 1991. Catheter-related infections caused by the *Mycobacterium fortuitum* complex: 15 cases and review. *Rev. Infect. Dis.* **13**:1120–1125.

206. **Rannem, T., K. Ladefoged, J. Hegnhoj, E. Hylander Moller, B. Bruun, and S. Jarnum.** 1990. Catheter-related sepsis in long-term parenteral nutrition with Broviac catheters. An evaluation of different disinfections. *Clin. Nutr.* **9**:131–136.

207. **Raucher, H. S., A. C. Hyatt, A. Barzilai, M. B. Harris, M. A. Weiner, N. S. LeLeiko, and D. S. Hodes.** 1984. Quantitative blood cultures in the evaluation of septicemia in children with Broviac catheters. *J. Pediatr.* **104**:29–33.

208. **Reagan, D. R., M. A. Pfaller, R. J. Hollis, and R. P. Wenzel.** 1990. Characterization of the sequence of colonization and nosocomial candidemia using DNA fingerprinting and a DNA probe. *J. Clin. Microbiol.* **28**:2733–2738.

209. **Reier, D., F. S. Rhame, and D. Vesley.** 1984. Growth of microorgahisms in IV solutions containing blood. (Abstr.) *Am. J. Infect. Control* **12**:346.

210. **Rello, J., P. Coll, M. Ricart, A. Net, and G. Prats.** 1993. Infection of pulmonary artery catheters. Epidemiologic characteristics and multivariate analysis of risk factors. *Chest* **103**:132–136.

211. **Rhame, F. S., J. F. Feist, C. L. Mueller, K. J. Steere, and S. Cameron.** 1983. Transparent adherent dressings (TADs) do not promote abnormal skin flora. (Abstr.) *Am. J. Infect. Control* **11**:152.

212. **Rhame, F. S., R. K. Root, S. D. MacLowry, T. A. Dadisman, and J. V. Bennett.** 1973. Salmonella septicemia from platelet transfusions. Study of an outbreak traced to a hematogenous carrier of *Salmonella cholerae-suis. Ann. Intern. Med.* **78**:633–641.

213. **Ricard, P., R. Martin, and J. A. Marcoux.** 1985. Protection of indwelling vascular catheters: incidence of bacterial contamination and catheter-related sepsis. *Crit. Care Med.* **13**:541–543.

214. **Richet, H., B. Hubert, G. Nitemberg, A. Andremont, A. Buu-Hoi, P. Ourbak, C. Galicier, M. Veron, A. Boisivon, A. M. Bouvier, J. C. Ricome, M. A. Wolff, Y. Pean, L. Berardi-Grassias, J. L. Bourdain, B. Hautefort, J. P. Laaban, and D. Tillant.** 1990. Prospective multicenter study of vascular-catheter-related complications and risk factors for positive central-catheter cultures in intensive care unit patients. *J. Clin. Microbiol.* **28**:2520–2525.

215. **Riebel, W., N. Frantz, D. Adelstein, and P. J. Spagnuolo.** 1986. *Corynebacterium* JK: a cause of nosocomial device-related infection. *Rev. Infect. Dis.* **8**:42–49.

216. **Roberts, L. A., P. J. Collignon, V. B. Cramp, S. Alexander, A. E. McFarlane, E.**

Graham, A. Fuller, V. Sinickas, and A. Hellyar. 1990. An Australia-wide epidemic of *Pseudomonas pickettii* bacteraemia due to contaminated "sterile" water for injection. *Med. J. Aust.* **152**:652–655.

217. Root, J. L., O. R. McInture, N. J. Jacobs, and C. P. Daghlian. 1988. Inhibitory effect of disodium EDTA upon growth of *Staphylococcus epidermidis* in vitro: relation to infection prophylaxis of Hickman catheters. *Antimicrob. Agents Chemother.* **32**:1627–1631.

218. Rose, H. D. 1978. Venous catheter-associated candidemia. *Am. J. Med. Sci.* **275**: 265–269.

219. Rotrosen, D., R. A. Calderone, and J. E. Edwards, Jr. 1986. Adherence of *Candida* species to host tissues and plastic surfaces. *Rev. Infect. Dis.* **8**:73–85.

220. Rotrosen, D., T. R. Gibson, and J. E. Edwards, Jr. 1983. Adherence of *Candida* species to intravenous catheters. *J. Infect. Dis.* **147**:594.

221. Rushforth, J. A., C. M. Hoy, P. Kite, and J. W. L. Puntis. 1993. Rapid diagnosis of central venous catheter sepsis. *Lancet* **342**:402–403.

222. Russell, P. B., J. Kline, M. C. Yoder, and R. A. Polin. 1987. Staphylococcal adherence to polyvinyl chloride and heparin-bonded polyurethane catheters is species dependent and enhanced by fibronectin. *J. Clin. Microbiol.* **25**:1083–1087.

223. Sanders, R. A., and G. F. Sheldon. 1976. Septic complications of total parenteral nutrition. A five year experience. *Am. J. Surg.* **132**:214–220.

224. Sanderson, I., and M. Deitel. 1973. Intravenous hyperalimentation without sepsis. *Surg. Gynecol. Obstet.* **136**:577–585.

225. Schadow, K. H., W. A. Simpson, and G. D. Christensen. 1988. Characteristics of adherence to plastic tissue culture plates of coagulase-negative staphylococci exposed to subinhibitory concentrations of antimicrobial agents. *J. Infect. Dis.* **157**:71–77.

226. Scheld, W. M., and M. A. Sande. 1990. Endocarditis and intravascular infections, p. 670–706. *In* G. L. Mandell, R. G. Douglas, and J. E. Bennett (ed.), *Principles and Practices of Infectious Diseases*, 3rd ed. Churchill Livingstone, New York.

227. Schuman, E. S., V. Winters, G. F. Gross, and J. F. Hayes. 1985. Management of Hickman catheter sepsis. *Am. J. Surg.* **149**:627–628.

228. Schwartz-Fulton, J., R. Colley, B. Valanis, and J. E. Fischer. 1981. Hyperalimentation dressings and skin flora. *Natl. Intravenous Ther. Assoc.* **4**:354–356.

229. Sheehan, G., K. Leicht, M. O'Brien, G. Taylor, and R. Rennie. 1993. Chlorhexidine versus povidone-iodine as cutaneous antisepsis for prevention of vascular-catheter infection, abstr. 1616. *Proc. Abstr. 33rd Intersci. Conf. Antimicrob. Agents Chemother.* American Society for Microbiology, Washington, D.C.

230. Sherertz, R. J., R. J. Falk, K. A. Huffman, C. A. Thomann, and W. D. Mattern. 1983. Infections associated with subclavian Uldall catheters. *Arch. Intern. Med.* **143**: 52–56.

231. Sherertz, R. J., K. S. Gledhill, K. D. Hampton, M. A. Pfaller, L. B. Givner, J. S. Abramson, and R. G. Dillard. 1992. Outbreak of *Candida* bloodstream infections associated with retrograde medication in a neonatal intensive care unit. *J. Pediatr.* **120**:455–461.

232. Sherertz, R. J., I. I. Raad, A. Belani, L. C. Koo, K. H. Rand, D. L. Pickett, S. A. Straub, and L. L. Fauerbach. 1990. Three-year experience with sonicated vascular catheter cultures in a clinical microbiology laboratory. *J. Clin. Microbiol.* **28**:76–82.

233. Sheth, N. K., T. R. Franson, and P. G. Sohnle. 1985. Influence of bacterial adherence to intravascular catheters on in-vitro antibiotic susceptibility. *Lancet* **ii**:1266–1268.

234. Sheth, N. K., H. D. Rose, T. R. Franson, F. L. A. Buckmire, and P. G. Sohnle. 1983. *In vitro* quantitative adherence of bacteria to intravascular catheters. *J. Surg. Res.* **34**:213–218.

235. Shinozaki, T., R. S. Deane, J. E. Mazuzan, Jr., A. J. Hamel, and D. Hazelton. 1983. Bacterial contamination of arterial lines. *JAMA* **249**:223–225.
236. Shivnan, J. C., D. McGuire, S. Freeman, E. Sharkazy, G. Bosserman, E. Larson, and P. A. Grouleff. 1991. Comparison of transparent adherent and dry sterile gauze dressings for long-term central catheters in patients undergoing bone marrow transplant. *Oncol. Nurses Forum* **18**:1349–1356.
237. Siboni, K., H. Olsen, E. Ravn, P. Sogaard, A. Hjorth, K. N. Nielsen, K. Askgaard, B. Secher, J. Borghans, L. Khing-Ting, H. Joosten, W. Fredericksen, K. Hensen, N. Mortensen, and O. Sebbensen. 1979. *Pseudomonas cepacia* in 16 non-fatal cases of postoperative bacteremia derived from intrinsic contamination of the anaesthetic Fentanyl. *Scand. J. Infect. Dis.* **11**:39–45.
238. Simmons, B. 1985. Alternative to i.v. filter usage. Letter. *Infect. Control* **6**:342–344.
239. Sitges-Serra, A., J. Linares, and J. Garau. 1985. Catheter sepsis: the clue is the hub. *Surgery* **97**:355–357.
240. Sitges-Serra, A., P. Puig, J. Linares, J. L. Pérez, N. Farreró, E. Jaurrieta, and J. Garau. 1984. Hub colonization as the initial step in an outbreak of catheter-related sepsis due to coagulase negative staphylococci during parenteral nutrition. *J. Parenter. Enteral Nutr.* **8**:668–672.
241. Sitzmann, J. V., T. R. Townsend, M. C. Siler, and J. G. Bartlett. 1985. Septic and technical complications of central venous catheterization. A prospective study of 200 consecutive patients. *Ann. Surg.* **202**:766–770.
242. Smith, R. L., S. M. Meixler, and M. S. Simberkoff. 1991. Excess mortality in critically ill patients with nosocomial bloodstream infections. *Chest* **100**:164–167.
243. Snydman, D. R., S. A. Murray, S. J. Kornfeld, J. A. Majka, and C. A. Ellis. 1982. Total parenteral nutrition-related infections. Prospective epidemiologic study using semiquantitative methods. *Am. J. Med.* **73**:695–699.
244. Snydman, D. R., B. R. Pober, S. A. Murray, J. F. Gorbea, J. A. Majka, and L. K. Perry. 1982. Predictive value of surveillance skin cultures in total-parenteral nutrition-related infection. *Lancet* **ii**:1385–1388.
245. Snydman, D. R., M. D. Reidy, L. K. Perry, and W. J. Martin. 1987. Safety of changing intravenous (IV) administration sets containing burettes at longer than 48 hour intervals. *Infect. Control* **8**:113–116.
246. Snydman, D. R., B. S. Sullivan, M. Gill, J. A. Gould, D. R. Parkinson, and M. B. Arkins. 1990. Nosocomial sepsis associated with interleukin-2. *Ann. Intern. Med.* **112**:102–107.
247. Snyder, R. H., F. J. Archer, T. Endy, T. W. Allen, B. Condon, J. Kaiser, D. Whatmore, G. Harrington, and C. J. McDermott. 1988. Catheter infection. A comparison of two catheter maintenance techniques. *Ann. Surg.* **208**:651–653.
248. Soifer, N. E., B. R. Edlin, R. A. Weinstein, and MRH IV Study Group. 1989. A randomized IV team trial, abstr. 1076. *Program Abstr. 29th Intersci. Conf. Antimicrob. Agents Chemother.* American Society for Microbiology, Washington, D.C.
249. Solomon, S. L., H. Alexander, J. W. Eley, R. L. Anderson, H. C. Goodpasture, S. Smart, R. A. Furman, and W. J. Martone. 1986. Nosocomial fungemia in neonates associated with intravascular pressure-monitoring devices. *Pediatr. Infect. Dis. J.* **5**:680–685.
250. Solomon, S. L., R. F. Khabbaz, R. H. Parker, R. L. Anderson, M. A. Geraghty, R. M. Furman, and W. J. Martone. 1984. An outbreak of *Candida parapsilosis* bloodstream infections in patients receiving parenteral nutrition. *J. Infect. Dis.* **149**:98–102.
251. Steere, A. C., M. K. Rifaat, E. B. Seligmann, Jr., H. D. Hochstein, G. Friedland, P. Dasse, K. O. Wustrack, K. J. Axnick, and L. F. Barker. 1978. Pyrogenic reactions associated with the infusion of normal serum albumin (human). *Transfusion* **18**:102.

252. **Steere, A. C., J. H. Tenney, D. C. Mackel, M. J. Snyder, S. Polakavetz, M. E. Dunne, and R. E. Dixon.** 1977. *Pseudomonas* species bacteremia caused by contaminated normal human serum albumin. *J. Infect. Dis.* **135:**729.

253. **Stillman, R. M., F. Soliman, L. Garcia, and P. N. Sawyer.** 1977. Etiology of catheter-associated sepsis. Correlation with thrombogenicity. *Arch. Surg.* **112:**1497–1499.

254. **Stotter, A. T., H. Ward, A. H. Waterfield, and A. J. W. Sim.** 1987. Junctional care: the key to prevention of catheter sepsis in intravenous feeding. *J. Parenter. Enteral Nutr.* **11:**159–162.

255. **Strand, C. L., R. R. Wajsbort, and K. Sturmann.** 1993. Effect of iodophor vs iodine tincture skin preparation on blood culture contamination rate. *JAMA* **269:**1004–1006.

256. **Strinden, W. D., R. B. Helgerson, and D. G. Maki.** 1985. Candida septic thrombosis of the great veins associated with central catheters. Clinical features and management. *Ann. Surg.* **202:**653–658.

257. **Telenti, A., J. M. Steckelberg, L. Stockman, R. S. Edson, and G. D. Roberts.** 1991. Quantitative blood cultures in candidemia. *Mayo Clin. Proc.* **66:**1120–1123.

258. **Terpenning, M. A., B. P. Buggy, and C. A. Kauffman.** 1988. Hospital-acquired infective endocarditis. *Arch. Intern. Med.* **148:**1601–1603.

259. **Thomas, F., J. P. Burke, J. Parker, J. F. Orme, J. R. M. Gardner, T. P. Clemmer, G. A. Hill, and P. MacFarlane.** 1988. The risk of infection related to radial vs. femoral sites for arterial catheterization. *Crit. Care Med.* **11:**807–812.

260. **Timmerman, C. P., A. Fleer, J. M. Besnier, L. Degraaff, F. Cremers, and J. Verhoef.** 1991. Characterization of a proteinaceous adhesion of *Staphylococcus epidermidis* which mediates attachment to polystyrene. *Infect. Immunol.* **59:**4187–4192.

261. **Tojo, M., N. Yamashita, D. A. Goldmann, and G. B. Pier.** 1988. Isolation and characterization of a capsular polysaccharide adhesion from *Staphylococcus epidermidis. J. Infect. Dis.* **157:**713–722.

262. **Tomford, J. W., and C. O. Hershey.** 1985. The I.V. therapy team. Impact on patient care and costs of hospitalization. *Natl. Intravenous Ther. Assoc.* **8:**387–389.

263. **Tomford, J. W., C. O. Hershey, C. E. McLaren, D. K. Porter, and D. I. Cohen.** 1984. Intravenous therapy team and peripheral venous catheter-associated complications. A prospective controlled study. *Arch. Intern. Med.* **144:**1191–1194.

264. **Torres-Rohas J. R., C. W. Stratton, C. V. Sanders, T. A. Horsman, H. B. Hawley, H. E. Dascomb, and L. J. Vial.** 1982. Candidal suppurative peripheral thrombophlebitis. *Ann. Intern. Med.* **96:**431–435.

265. **Tully, J. L., G. H. Friedland, L. M. Baldini, and D. A. Goldmann.** 1981. Complications of intravenous therapy with steel needles and Teflon catheters. A comparative study. *Am. J. Med.* **70:**702–706.

266. **Vanherweghem, J.-L., M. Dhaene, M. Goldman, J.-C. Stolear, J.-P. Sabot, Y. Waterlot, E. Serruys, and C. Thayse.** 1986. Infections associated with subclavian dialysis catheters: the key role of nurse training. *Nephron* **42:**116–119.

267. **Vanhuynegem, L., P. Parmentier, and C. Potvliege.** 1987. In situ bacteriologic diagnosis of total parenteral nutrition catheter infection. *Surgery* **103:**174–177.

268. **Vaudaux, P., D. Lew, and F. A. Waldvogel.** 1987. Host-dependent pathogenic factors in foreign body infection. A comparison between *Staphylococcus epidermidis* and *S. aureus. Zentralbl. Bakteriol. Suppl.* **16:**183–193.

269. **Vaudaux, P., D. Pittet, A. Haeberli, P. G. Lerch, J. J. Morgenthaler, R. A. Proctor, F. A. Waldvogel, and D. P. Lew.** 1993. Fibronectin is more active than fibrin or fibrinogen in promoting *Staphylococcus aureus* adherence to inserted intravascular catheters. *J. Infect. Dis.* **167:**633–641.

270. **Vaudaux, P., D. Pittet, A. Haeberli, E. Huggler, U. E. Nydegger, D. P. Lew, and**

F. A. Waldvogel. 1989. Host factors selectively increase staphylococcal adherence on inserted catheters: a role for fibronectin and fibrinogen or fibrin. *J. Infect. Dis.* **160:** 865–875.

271. Vaudaux, P. E., F. A. Waldvogel, J. J. Morgenthaler, and U. E. Nydegger. 1984. Adsorption of fibronectin onto polymethylmethacrylate and promotion of *Staphylococcus aureus* adherence. *Infect. Immun.* **45:**768–774.

272. Venditti, M., F. De Bernardis, A. Micozzi, E. Pontieri, P. Chirletti, A. Cassone, and P. Martins. 1992. Fluconazole treatment of catheter-related right-sided endocarditis caused by *Candida albicans* and associated with endophthalmitis and folliculitis. *Clin. Infect. Dis.* **14:**422–426.

273. Verghese, A., W. C. Widrich, and R. D. Arbeit. 1985. Central venous septic thrombophlebitis—the role of medical therapy. *Medicine* **64:**394–400.

274. Wang, E. E. L., C. G. Prober, L. Ford-Jones, and R. Gold. 1984. The management of central intravenous catheter infections. *Pediatr. Infect. Dis. J.* **3:**110–113.

275. Washington, J. A., II, and D. M. Ilstrup. 1986. Blood cultures: issues and controversies. *Rev. Infect. Dis.* **8:**792–802.

276. Watanakunakorn, C., and I. M. Baird. 1977. *Staphylococcus aureus* bacteremia and endocarditis associated with a removeable infected intravenous device. *Am. J. Med.* **63:**253–255.

277. Weightman, N. C., E. M. Simpson, D. C. E. Speller, M. G. Mott, and A. Oakhill. 1988. Bacteraemia related to indwelling central venous catheters: prevention, diagnosis and treatment. *Eur. J. Clin. Microbiol. Infect. Dis.* **7:**125–129.

278. Weinstein, M. P., L. B. Reller, H. R. Murphy, et al. 1983. The clinical significance of positive blood cultures: a comprehensive analysis of 500 episodes of bacteremia and fungemia in adults. I. Laboratory and epidemiological observations. *Rev. Infect. Dis.* **5:**35–53.

279. Wey, S. B., M. Mori, M. A. Pfaller, R. F. Woolson, and R. P. Wenzel. 1989. Risk factors for hospital-acquired candidemia. A matched case-control study. *Arch. Intern. Med.* **149:**2349–2353.

280. Williams, D. N., J. Gibson, J. Vos, and A. C. Kind. 1982. Infusion thrombophlebitis and infiltration associated with intravenous cannulae: a controlled study comparing three different cannula types. *Natl. Intravenous Ther. Assoc.* **5:**379–382.

281. Wrenn, J. E., and C. E. Speicher. 1974. Platelet concentrates: sterility of 400 single units stored at room temperature. *Transfusion* **14:**171.

282. Wurzel, C. L., C. Halom, J. G. Feldman, and L. G. Rubin. 1988. Infection rates of Broviac-Hickman catheters and implantable venous devices. *Am. J. Dis. Child.* **142:** 536–540.

283. Young, G. P., M. Alexeyeff, D. M. Russell, and R. J. S. Thomas. 1988. Catheter sepsis during parenteral nutrition: the safety of long-term OpSite dressings. *J. Parenter. Enteral Nutr.* **12:**365–370.

284. Yu, V. L., A. Goetz, M. Wagener, P. B. Smith, J. D. Rihs, J. Hanchet, and J. J. Zuravleff. 1988. *Staphylococcus aureus* nasal carriage and infections in patients on hemodialysis. Efficacy of antibiotic prophylaxis. *N. Engl. J. Med.* **318:**91–95.

285. Zinner, S. H., B. C. Denny-Brown, P. Braun, J. P. Burke, P. Toala, and E. H. Kass. 1969. Risk of infection with intravenous indwelling catheters: effect of application of antibiotic ointment. *J. Infect. Dis.* **120:**616–619.

286. Zufferey, J., B. Rime, P. Francioli, and J. Bille. 1988. Simple method for rapid diagnosis of catheter-associated infection by direct acridine orange staining of catheter tips. *J. Clin. Microbiol.* **26:**175–177.

Infections Associated with Indwelling Medical Devices, 2nd ed.
Edited by Alan L. Bisno and Francis A. Waldvogel
© 1994 American Society for Microbiology, Washington, DC 20005

Chapter 9

Infections of Prosthetic Heart Valves and Vascular Grafts

Adolf W. Karchmer and Gary W. Gibbons

PROSTHETIC VALVE ENDOCARDITIS

As cardiac valve replacement became a routine surgical procedure, prosthetic valve endocarditis (PVE) became an important disease of medical progress. In some medical centers PVE constitutes more than 15% of the total of all endocarditis, and the disease is attended by considerable morbidity and mortality (120). This chapter reviews the incidence, pathogenesis, microbiology, pathology, treatment, and prevention of PVE.

Incidence and Risk Factors

Prosthetic valve endocarditis has been reported to occur in from 1 to 9.4% of patients. Mayer and Schoenbaum in their review of 14 large series reported that 3.2% of 1,849 patients with valve replacements performed in the 1960s and 2.1% of 10,136 persons operated on in the 1970s developed PVE (74). These infection rates, however, do not provide accurate assessments of the incidence of PVE. The studies that were reviewed often lacked comprehensive follow-up information on operated patients and thus may have failed to account for infections that were not treated at the reporting institution. Similarly, patients that had been lost to follow-up or that had died were rarely detailed, causing the population at risk to be overestimated. Recent studies utilizing clear and ac-

Adolf W. Karchmer • Department of Medicine, Harvard Medical School, and Infectious Disease Section, New England Deaconess Hospital, Boston, Massachusetts 02215. **Gary W. Gibbons** • Department of Surgery, Harvard Medical School, and Division of Vascular Surgery, New England Deaconess Hospital, Boston, Massachusetts 02215.

Table 1. Actuarial estimate of the cumulative incidence of PVE

Study (years)[a]	Reference	No. of patients in initial group	Estimated risk by months after surgery (% with PVE)		
			12 mo	48 mo	60 mo
Rutledge et al. (1956–81)	96	1,598	1.4		3.2
Ivert et al. (1975–79)	50	1,465	3.0	4.1	
Calderwood et al. (1975–82)	18	2,608	3.1	5.4	5.7
Arvay and Lengyel (1981–85)	7	912			4.9

[a] Years during which surgery was performed.

ceptable definitions of PVE, detailed comprehensive follow-up of operated patients, and actuarial methods of data analysis provide a more reliable view of the incidence of PVE (Table 1). Ivert et al. identified 53 patients with PVE among 1,465 survivors of valve replacement surgery performed from January 1975 to July 1979 and estimated the cumulative risks of PVE to be 3.0% at 12 months and 4.1% at 48 months (50). Calderwood et al. found 116 patients with PVE in 2,608 patients that survived valve replacement surgery done from January 1975 through December 1982 (18). Actuarial estimates of cumulative risks in this study were 3.1% at 12 months and 5.7% at 60 months. Among 1,598 patients who underwent valve replacement from 1956 through 1981, Rutledge et al. estimated actuarially that the cumulative risks of PVE were 1.4% at 12 months and 3.2% at 66 months (96). Arvay and Lengyel, in a study of 912 patients who had valves replaced from 1981 through 1985, found 27 patients with PVE and determined actuarially a 4.9% risk of endocarditis at 5 years (7). Furthermore, each of these studies defined a higher risk period during the initial 6 to 12 months after surgery and a lower risk period thereafter. They also illustrated that prosthetic valves remain vulnerable to infection as long as they are in place.

The effect of specific factors, such as the site of valve implantation or the type of valve implanted (mechanical versus bioprosthetic valve), on the risk for developing PVE has also been examined. Initial assessments came from less detailed studies using unsophisticated analyses. Some of these studies have shown the incidence of endocarditis to be higher in patients with aortic prostheses than in those with mitral valve replacements (73, 74, 96, 117). Others have shown the incidence of PVE to be similar for prostheses at these sites (96, 103), and one study found a higher rate of endocarditis among mitral valve recipients (113). In studies based on thorough case findings and using sophisticated multivariate analyses (Cox regression model), Ivert et al. (50) and Calderwood et al. (18) found no difference in risk of PVE between patients with mitral or aortic prostheses. The risk of infection for mechanical and bioprosthetic valves at the end of the follow-up period was not significantly different in two studies (93, 96). Ivert and colleagues noted a threefold increased risk of PVE among mechanical valve recipients, compared with patients with bioprostheses, during the early months after surgery, with equivalent risks thereafter (50). Interestingly, Calderwood et al. confirmed a significantly higher risk of PVE for mechanical valves in the initial 3 months after surgery but noted that porcine valves had a higher risk of infection 12 months or more after surgery (18). In this study, the cumulative risk at the end of 5 years was similar for the two valve types. Arvay and Lengyel noted similar risks for PVE during the initial year after valve replacement for mechanical and bioprosthetic valve recipients; however, patients with bioprosthetic valves were of a greater risk a year or longer after valve surgery. Actuarial estimates indicated that at 5 years after valve replacement, 98.4% of mechanical valve recipients were free of endocarditis, whereas only 90.7% of bioprostheses were free of PVE. Of 19 cases of PVE involving bioprostheses, 14 occurred more than a year after valve replacement (7). Calderwood et al. (18) found an enhanced risk for PVE among recipients of multiple prostheses, compared with recipients of single valves, and Ivert et al. (50) noted an increased risk of PVE with a longer cardiopulmonary bypass time. These observations suggest that PVE may be associated with more prolonged or complex surgery; however, the inability of Ivert et al. (50) or Calderwood et al. (18) to associate incremental risks for PVE with concomitant coronary artery bypass grafting and of the latter study to find an increased risk with duration of cardiopulmonary bypass or aortic cross-clamping undermines this hypothesis.

Pathogenesis

The biochemical and biophysical pathogenesis of prosthetic device infection, as well as the impact of foreign materials on host defenses and the role of impaired host defenses in the pathogenesis and maintenance of foreign body infection, have been considered elsewhere in this volume (see chapters 1 through 3). The clinical events that play a role in the pathogenesis of PVE vary and are related to the time of onset of infection. Suspecting that the pathogenesis of these infections would relate to nosocomial events, particularly those occurring during or shortly after surgery, Block et al. coined the term early PVE for patients with onset of infection within 60 days of surgery (12). Indeed, several investigators have recovered bacterial species that are commonly associated with early PVE from the operative field and the cardiopulmonary bypass equipment (2, 11, 61). Additionally, postoperative infections due to bacteria that are subsequently noted to cause endocarditis have been found in 31 to 92% of patients with early PVE (29, 49, 119). Porcine bioprostheses contaminated by *Mycobacterium chelonae* during production have given rise to sporadic cases of PVE (63, 95). Furthermore, epidemiologic investigations supplemented by restriction endonuclease analysis patterns of infecting organisms have demonstrated perioperative infection of valve prosthesis by *Legionella pneumophila* and *Legionella dumoffii* (110).

Rather than defining as nosocomial only those cases of coagulase-negative staphylococcal PVE occurring within 2 months of cardiac surgery, the time interval for these cases might be extended to 12 months. The appropriateness of this categorization is suggested by the high percentage of methicillin-resistant coagulase-negative staphylococci among the organisms causing PVE throughout the initial 12 months after surgery and the association of these staphylococci with either a nosocomial acquisition or a nosocomially enhanced component of normal flora (18, 56, 59). In epidemiologic and microbiologic studies, Archer et al. identified cases of coagulase-negative staphylococcal PVE occurring at an average of 5.3 months and as long as 13 months after cardiac surgery, which had resulted from intraoperative contamination (5). In three additional reports wherein epidemiologic evidence indicated that coagulase-negative staphylococcal PVE developed as a result of intraoperative contamination, the diagnosis in 3 of 10 cases of PVE occurred long after the time of infection (84 days to 5.5 months) (14, 76, 115). These epidemiologic studies corroborate the concept of a prolonged latent period prior to the clinical onset of nosocomial PVE in some patients (5).

The bacteriology of PVE with onset 12 months or more following valve surgery suggests that these infections have been acquired outside of the hospital. Indeed, incidental infections (e.g., urinary tract infection and furunculosis) and trauma to mucosal surfaces (e.g., genitourinary tract and dental manipulation) could be identified as predisposing events for 50% of patients with late-onset PVE (defined as onset 60 days or more after surgery) (29, 49). Similarly, the passage of months and often years after surgery before fastidious gram-negative coccobacilli (*Haemophilus* species, *Actinobacillus actinomycetemcomitans*, *Cardiobacterium hominis*, *Eikenella corrodens*, and *Kingella* species), organisms that enter the blood from the oral cavity and respiratory tract, are encountered as causes of PVE suggests that late-onset PVE is primarily acquired through incidental nonnosocomial infection and bacteremia (75).

Fang et al. evaluated the frequency of PVE among patients experiencing nosocomial bacteremia. Among the 115 patients in whom the bacteremia was not the diagnostic event for PVE, 18 (16%) were shown subsequently to have developed PVE (33). These figures may be an over-estimate, because in some of these 18 patients, the bacteremia might still have been the sentinel event of undected PVE. The rate of PVE after staphylococcal bacteremia was 24%, compared with 10% after gram-neg-ative bacillus bacteremia. The duration of antibiotic therapy for the bac-teremia did not appear to alter the rate of subsequent PVE. Of 21 patients treated for 2 weeks or less, 1 developed PVE, compared with 11 of 79 patients treated for more than 14 days.

Microbiology

Complex biochemical, biophysical, and biological interactions occur between organisms, prostheses, and patients, which allow organisms to colonize devices and avoid eradication by host defenses or antimicrobial agents. These interactions have a profound influence on the microbiol-ogy of PVE. Additionally, the clinical events surrounding valve implanta-tion, the cutaneous and mucosal flora of patients, and the incidental bacteremic infections that befall patients with prosthetic valves impact importantly on the spectrum of organisms that cause PVE.

Although a wide spectrum of organisms has caused isolated cases of PVE, the microbiology of this infection during given periods after cardiac surgery is relatively predictable (Table 2). Among cases of PVE occurring prior to 1975, *Staphylococcus epidermidis, Staphylococcus aureus,* enteric and nonfermentative gram-negative bacilli, diphtheroids, and yeasts were predominant causes of PVE presenting within 2 months of surgery. PVE occurring more than 2 months after surgery was often caused by staphylococci; however, streptococci and enterococci, which were infrequent causes of PVE during the initial 2 months postopera-tively, were prominent causes during this later period. Among cases diagnosed since 1975, coagulase-negative staphylococci have been the dominant cause of PVE beginning within 2 months after surgery; only occasional cases were caused by *S. aureus,* gram-negative bacilli, diphthe-roids, and yeasts. The infrequent role of these latter organisms in early-onset PVE compared with the pre-1975 period, while not carefully stud-ied, is probably the result of multiple factors, including improved surgi-cal techniques, postoperative care that reduced nosocomial infections, and improved perioperative antibiotic prophylaxis. Among cases of PVE seen from 1975 through 1982, coagulase-negative staphylococci re-mained the strikingly dominant cause of endocarditis occurring from 2 to 12 months after surgery (18). The organisms causing PVE that occurs more than 12 months after valve implantation differ from those causing

Table 2. Microbiology of PVE

Organism	No. of cases				
	Before 1975[a]		1975–1982[b]		
	<2 mo[c]	>2 mo	<2 mo	>2–12 mo	>12 mo
Coagulase-negative staphylococci	41	36	22	19	10
S. aureus	30	22	2	3	5
Gram-negative bacilli	30	19	2	1	1
Streptococci (nonenterococcal)	9	41	0	1	12
Enterococci	6	14	0	2	4
Pneumococci	2	0	0	0	0
Diphtheroids	12	6	4	0	1
Fungi	18	9	2	2	1
Fastidious gram-negative coccobacilli	NA[d]	NA	0	1	7
Other	0	0	3	2	1
Culture negative	3	7	3	3	2
Total	151	154	38	34	44

[a] From reference 58.
[b] From reference 18. Includes fastidious gram-negative coccobacilli.
[c] Time of onset after surgery.
[d] NA, not available.

PVE during the first year and are similar to those associated with native valve endocarditis (exclusive of nosocomial and drug abuse-associated infective endocarditis). During this late postoperative period the predominant causes of infection are streptococci, coagulase-negative staphylococci, enterococci, *S. aureus*, and fastidious gram-negative coccobacilli, particularly *A. actinomycetemocomitans, C. hominis,* and *Haemophilus* species (18, 75).

Reports of PVE have often referred to coagulase-negative staphylococci as *S. epidermidis* without, in fact, careful speciation and have frequently failed to report the antibiotic susceptibility of these staphylococci (29, 50, 93, 103, 113, 122). Karchmer, Archer, and Dismukes studied the 70 unique coagulase-negative staphylococci that had caused PVE at their respective hospitals from 1975 through 1980 (56). They found resistance to methicillin, as well as to the other semisynthetic penicillinase-resistant penicillins and cephalosporins, in 34 (87%) of 39 coagulase-negative staphylococci causing PVE within 2 months of surgery and in 19 (87%) of 22 staphylococci causing PVE between 2 and 12 months postoperatively. In contrast, only 2 (22%) of the 9 coagulase-negative staphylococci isolated from patients with PVE beginning more than 12 months after surgery were methicillin resistant. Similarly, Calderwood et al. noted that 84% of coagulase-negative staphylococci that caused PVE within 12 months of surgery were resistant to methicillin, contrasted with 30% of coagulase-negative staphylococci causing infection later (18). Karchmer et al. determined that 53 of 55 unique isolates that had caused PVE were *S. epidermidis* (sensu stricto) and one each was *Staphylococcus cohnii* and *Staphylococcus haemolyticus* (56).

A broad range of bacteria have caused sporadic cases of PVE. *Corynebacterium* species, often consistent by biochemical testing with the J-K group, cause PVE occurring within the initial 6 months after surgery and are notable because of their relative resistance to many antibiotics other than vancomycin and their fastidious growth requirements (81). In addition to the variety of gram-negative bacilli that have caused PVE, gram-positive bacteria not commonly considered to cause endocarditis have been reported as the etiologic agents for sporadic cases of PVE; among these are *Nocardia asteroides* (117), *Bacillus cereus* (85), and *Listeria monocytogenes* (16, 46). *L. pneumophila* and *L. dumoffii,* organisms not previously recognized as causes of endocarditis, have been reported to cause nosocomial PVE (110).

Fungi not only account for significant numbers of cases but also are associated with high case fatality rates. *Candida* species, followed by *Aspergillus* species, are the two most common fungi causing PVE (74, 118). Invasive fungi, including *Histoplasma capsulatum* (41), *Cryptococcus neoformans* (45), and *Mucor* species (60), have caused occasional cases of PVE, as have the so-called saprophytic fungi, such as *Penicillium chrysogenum* (114), *Paecilomyces varioti* (55), and *Trichosporon cutaneum* (109). Fungal vegetations formed on prosthetic valves are bulky and may partially occlude the orifice or embolize and occlude medium-sized arteries.

Patients with PVE caused by *Legionella* species (110), mycobacteria (95), and fungi other than *Candida* spp. (74) commonly present with negative blood cultures when routine techniques are used. Similarly, in patients with PVE due to *Coxiella burnetii* (the etiologic agent for Q fever), blood cultures are negative (35). This disgnosis is suggested by finding high titers of complement-fixing antibody to the phase I antigen of *C. burnetii* and confirmed by isolation of the organism from the prosthesis itself (35).

Pathology

Infection involving prosthetic cardiac valves is rarely confined to the surface of the prosthesis. In fact, infection frequently invades the valve annulus into which the prosthetic valve has been sewn and is often associated with significant prosthesis dysfunction. The invasive perivalvular infection noted in PVE differs notably from the leaflet-confined

Table 3. Pathology of infection involving mechanical prosthetic valves

Series	Total no. of patients	No. (%) with following pathology:			
		Annulus invasion	Myocardial abscess	Valve obstruction	Pericarditis
Autopsy					
Arnett and Roberts (6)	22	22	11	6	2
Anderson et al. (1)	22	11	4	6	2
Rose (92)	30	30	9	2	2
Total	74	63 (85)	24 (32)	14 (19)	4 (5)
Autopsy/surgery					
Dismukes et al. (29)	38	8	3	2	2
Richardson et al. (89)	47	28	9	1	0
Total	85	36 (42)	12 (14)	3 (4)	2 (2)

infection of native valve endocarditis. A clear understanding of the pathology of PVE is essential to the development of effective treatment.

Infection engrafted on mechanical valves commonly extends into the annulus and adjacent myocardium (Table 3). Examination of infected mechanical valves from patients with fatal PVE revealed invasion of the annulus and myocardial abscess in 85% and 32%, respectively (1, 6, 92). Partial dehiscence of the prosthetic valve with resulting paravalvular regurgitant flow was a common consequence of annulus infection because the sutures that had anchored the valve pulled through necrotic annulus tissue. In 19% of valves examined at autopsy, extensive vegetations encroached on the valve orifice, causing functional obstruction, a finding more frequently associated with infection of mitral valve rather than aortic valve prostheses (1, 6, 92). Infection, particularly involving prostheses at the aortic site, occasionally burrows deeply into myocardial tissue, forming abscesses that drain into the pericardial space and cause pericarditis or that, as a result of inflammation or tissue destruction, interrupt the conduction system and cause first, second, or complete heart block (1, 6, 58, 67).

The data derived from autopsy experience are clearly biased by inclusion of the most severe pathology; nevertheless, the image of invasive infections causing frequent valve dysfunction is accurate. A less distorted view is provided by series that include all patients as the population at risk and use pathology derived from valves examined at surgery or autopsy (Table 3). In the 85 patients reported by Dismukes et al. and Richardson et al., infection of the annulus and myocardial abscess were documented in 42 and 14%, respectively (29, 89). Among 58 patients

with PVE, Ismail et al. reported infection of the valve annulus with dehiscence in 38 (82%) of 41 infected mechanical valves examined at surgery
or necropsy (49). In these 41 patients, valve ring abscess and extension
of infection into adjacent cardiac structures were more common with
infection of aortic than of mitral prostheses, whereas valve thrombosis
occurred more commonly with mitral than with aortic PVE. Baumgartner
et al. reported abscess formation in 65% of patients undergoing operation
for mechanical valve endocarditis (10).

Early studies of infected porcine bioprosthetic valves (glutaraldehyde-preserved porcine leaflets mounted in a cloth-covered rigid supporting strut) suggested that endocarditis was confined to the porcine
leaflets. Ferrans et al. described the pathology associated with infected
bioprosthetic valves from 4 patients and reviewed the data published
for 43 other patients. These investigators identified ring abscess in only
3 (6%) cases and valve dehiscence in one (2%) patient and noted that
infection could involve the cusps with invasion of the leaflet substance
and breakdown of heterograft collagen (37). They also reported that vegetations resulted in stenosis of 13% of infected bioprostheses. Among
10 infected bioprostheses, Bortolotti et al. noted ring abscess and dehiscence in one, regurgitation due to cusp tears or perforations of four
valves, and stenosis of two mitral prostheses due to thrombotic vegetations (13). Infected cusps were notable for collagen disruption and infiltration by microorganisms and inflammatory cells.

Subsequently, it has become clear that bioprosthetic valve infection
is not confined to the cusp but often invades paravalvular tissue. Paravalvular abscess formation was noted in 2 of 11 infected bioprostheses described by Magilligan et al. (69), 3 of 20 valves reported by Nunez et al.
(82), and 14 of 39 infected bioprostheses removed at surgery by Baumgartner et al. (10). Fernicola and Roberts found that infection involved the
sewing ring-annulus in 20 of 37 infected bioprosthetic valves removed
from patients at surgery or autopsy (36). In 26 patients reoperated for
porcine bioprosthetic valve endocarditis, Sett et al. noted valve dehiscence in 11 and annular abscess formation in 7 cases (100). Cortina et
al. found that the frequency of invasive infection extending into adjacent
myocardium was similar for explanted mechanical valves and bioprostheses (24). Among 85 patients treated for porcine bioprosthetic valve endocarditis at the Massachusetts General Hospital, 38 (45%) were found
to have infection invading the annulus or myocardium (A. W. Karchmer
and S. B. Calderwood, unpublished observations) (Table 4). Invasive
pathology was found more frequently when the onset of PVE occurred
within 12 months of cardiac surgery (59%) than with later-onset infection

Table 4. Pathology of porcine bioprosthetic valve endocarditis at Massachusetts General Hospital, 1975–1983[a]

Time of onset after surgery (mo)	Total no. of patients	No. (%) with:		
		Invasive infection	Leaflet infection	Site not examined
≤12	49	29 (59)[b]	2	18
>12	36	9 (25)[b]	9	18

[a] A. W. Karchmer and S. B. Calderwood, unpublished.
[b] $P < 0.05$.

(25%) ($P < 0.05$). Of interest in this regard, in a multivariate analysis of 96 patients with PVE involving a single valve, complicated infection, defined by clinical features that correlate with invasive infection, was significantly associated with onset of PVE within 12 months of operation and the aortic position but not with the type of prosthesis (17).

Magilligan has provided an important clinical perspective to the histopathology and evolution of infected porcine cusps that had been described by Ferrans et al. (37), Bortolotti et al. (13), and Nunez et al. (82). Magilligan noted that 9 of 27 patients treated medically for PVE required valve replacement for dysfunction developing 2 to 98 months after PVE (68). Additionally, one patient who died 3 months after successful medical treatment of *Streptococcus faecalis* infection of bioprosthetic aortic and mitral valves was found to have severe stenosis of these valves, caused by fusion of healed vegetations along commissures. Thus, structural changes in the collagen of cusps caused by infection may shorten the period of effective bioprosthesis function despite eradication of infection. Additionally, clinically significant bioprosthetic valve dysfunction during active PVE may result from prosthesis dehiscence due to annulus infection or from fenestrations of cusps. Fernicola and Roberts detected tears or perforations of cusps in 16 of 37 infected bioprosthetic valves (36).

Clinical and Laboratory Features

The clinical features of PVE, while rarely diagnostic in themselves, are important because they prompt consideration of the diagnosis and provide critical information for decisions regarding therapy. The features of PVE are, with the exception of more frequent signs of valve dysfunction and myocardial invasion, similar to those of native valve endocarditis. The symptoms, signs, and laboratory features noted in patients with PVE beginning within 2 months of cardiac surgery, particularly among patients develoing endocarditis before discharge from the hospital after surgery, are often altered by the impact of surgery and postoperative complications.

Dismukes and Karchmer described the clinical characteristics of 79 patients with PVE treated at the Massachusetts General Hospital from 1964 to 1975 (Table 5) (28). Leport et al., in a study of 50 cases of PVE with onset more than 2 months after surgery, found new murmurs in 48%, congestive heart failure in 56%, splenomegaly in 24%, and cerebrovascular complications in 26% (64). In 48 patients with PVE (16 early and 32 late onset), Masur and Johnson reported congestive heart failure in 19 (40%) and central nervous system complications in 15 (31%) (73). Wilson et al. noted a septic shock presentation in 5 patients; this was seen only among 16 patients with early-onset PVE (122). On the other hand, Karchmer et al. noted an acute fulminant presentation with hypotension in 4 of 43 patients with late PVE; these infections were caused by *S. aureus* or *Streptococcus pyogenes* (57).

The laboratory studies of greatest use in the diagnosis and management of PVE are those that provide insight into the etiology of the infection, the function of prosthesis, and the presence of invasive infections. Blood cultures, the primary method by which the cause of PVE is established, are positive in 85 to 95% of patients (28, 64, 73, 74, 93). Because of the continuous nature of bacteremia in endocarditis, when one blood culture is positive, it can be anticipated that multiple cultures will be

Table 5. Clinical features of PVE at the Massachusetts General Hosptial, 1964–1975[a]

Feature	No. (%) with feature by time of onset after cardiac surgery	
	≤2 mo (*n* = 36)	>2 mo (*n* = 43)
Fever	35 (97)	43 (100)
Regurgitant murmur	17 (47)	27 (63)
Splenomegaly	13 (36)	18 (42)
Petechiae (skin/conjunctiva)	20 (56)	23 (53)
Peripheral signs[b]	5 (14)	12 (28)
Congestive heart failure	13 (36)	19 (44)
Central nervous system emboli	4 (11)	13 (28)
Hematocrit of <35%	32 (89)	31 (72)
Leukocytosis (>12,000 leukocytes/mm³)	28 (78)	22 (51)
Hematuria (>5 erythrocytes/high-power field)	NE[c]	28 (65)

[a] From reference 28.
[b] Janeway lesions, Osler nodes, or Roth spots.
[c] NE, not evaluable because of indwelling catheter.

positive, irrespective of body temperature. In fact, the documented persistence of bacteremia over an extended time is a clue to the diagnosis of PVE. Negative blood cultures in patients with PVE are seen most commonly when antibiotics have been administered in the recent past. Occasionally, PVE due to fastidious organisms such as the gram-negative coccobacilli or pyridoxal-requiring streptococci may present with negative cultures. Although in PVE due to C. *burnetii* (Q fever) and *Legionella* species the routine blood cultures are negative, the diagnosis can be established serologically or with special cultures of valve tissue (or blood in *Legionella* PVE) (35, 110). Fungi causing PVE (except *Candida* species and perhaps other yeast forms when new special blood culture techniques are used) are rarely isolated in blood cultures but can be recovered in embolized vegetations that have been removed from arteries or from the infected valve (74, 114).

Cardiac chamber size, ventricular function, and blood flow can be assessed by two-dimensional and Doppler echocardiography and thus indirectly indicate prosthesis function. In addition, vegetations, paravalvular regurgitation, annulus abscess, and prosthesis dehiscence can be detected by echocardiography. Detection of vegetations on infected prosthetic valves by the use of transthoracic echocardiography is difficult, with a sensitivity as low as 30%. In contrast, using a transesophageal approach to evaluate 22 infected valves, Mugge et al. identified definite vegetations on 17 valves and probable vegetation on an additional 2 valves (80). Several smaller studies have confirmed the increased sensitivity of the transesophageal echocardiogram, compared with the transthoracic study, in the detection of lesions indicative of PVE (101, 107). Alternatively, a negative transesophageal study may be false; among 21 patients with bacteremia in the presence of a prosthesis, the negative predictive value of the transesophageal study was 86% (104). The transesophageal approach provides excellent views of a mitral prosthesis and the posterior portion of an aortic prosthesis. The anterior aortic root area is better visualized from a transthoracic approach. Consequently, to obtain an optimal echocardiographic evaluation, the site of suspected infection must be considered. Additionally, in patients at high risk of PVE, repeat studies may detect diagnostic abnormalities not noted on the initial echocardiogram (104). Finally, the transesophageal echocardiogram is strikingly more sensitive for the detection of myocardial abscess in patients with PVE than is the transthoracic study, 87 and 28%, respectively. Enhanced sensitivity is noted for abscesses in association with infection of mitral or aortic prostheses and occurs without significant loss of specificity (26).

Other studies may help to define the pathology associated with PVE.

Cardiac catheterization and angiography may disclose prosthetic valve dysfunction or paravalvular abscess cavities (82). Although not a sensitive test, the electrocardiogram, by demonstrating new or progressive conduction system disturbances, can provide indirect evidence of a septal abscess (67, 120). These electrocardiographic changes are more likely to be encountered with aortic valve infections than with mitral valve endocarditis. Baumgartner et al. found abscesses at cardiac surgery in 11 of 16 patients with PVE complicated by atrioventricular conduction disturbances (10). Patients with new conduction system abnormalities require evaluation for a myocardial abscess.

It is important to recognize that no laboratory abnormality is absolutely diagnostic of PVE. Bacteremia may be unrelated to endocarditis. Sande et al. suggested that gram-negative bacteremia during the initial 85 days after surgery was unlikely to be associated with PVE, particularly if potential peripheral sources of septicemia were apparent (98). Similarly, Fang et al. found that of 171 valve recipients with nosocomial bacteremia, only 74 (43%) had or subsequently developed PVE; in 97 patients (57%), bacteremia was unassociated with ongoing or subsequent PVE (33). Valve dysfunction may be due to a technical or mechanical problem rather than PVE, and a systemic embolus may result from bland thrombus formation rather than from an infected vegetation. Hence, data from tests must not be taken out of context but rather must be integrated with clinical observations to help confirm or refute the diagnosis of PVE (28).

Treatment

The guiding principles for treating native valve endocarditis provide the basis for the treatment of PVE. However, to achieve optimal results from therapy, these principles must be used in concert with an understanding of the microbiology of PVE, the antimicrobial susceptibility of causative organisms, and the unique aspects of the pathology of PVE, including valve site and prosthesis-specific considerations. After appropriate consideration of adverse drug effects, bactericidal antibiotics or combinations of antibiotics are selected and administered parenterally in appropriate doses. Antibiotic treatment for 6 weeks is commonly used. Recovery of the causative organism and determination of its antimicrobial susceptibility is essential if the selected therapy is to be optimal. Consequently, it is important that the etiology of PVE not be obscured by premature treatment. Indolent endocarditis, in the absence of hemodynamic instability that mandates early surgical intervention, does not require immediate antimicrobial therapy. Antibiotics should be withheld briefly pending the isolation of an organism from blood cultures. If oral antibiotics that might render initial blood cultures sterile have been given, this delay (3 to 5 days) is particularly important because it allows blood cultures to be repeated without the interference of additional therapy. Presentations of PVE that are acute or complicated by hemodynamic instability due to prosthetic valve dysfunction require that blood cultures be obtained and antibiotics be administered promptly.

Antimicrobial therapy

While the details of antimicrobial therapy for the various organisms causing PVE are beyond the scope of this discussion, comments regarding treatment of several organisms are warranted (Table 6). For PVE caused by penicillin-susceptible (MIC ≤ 0.1 μg/ml) nonenterococcal streptococci, treatment with penicillin plus an aminoglycoside is recommended. However, if aminoglycoside therapy is relatively contraindicated by potential adverse effects, successful therapy has been provided with penicillin, cephalothin, or vancomycin (12, 29, 79; A. Karchmer, unpublished data). It may be desirable when treating PVE caused by streptococci that are relatively resistant to penicillin (MIC > 0.1 μg/ml) to administer an aminoglycoside with the penicillin for more than 2 weeks, i.e., 4 to 6 weeks.

The majority of coagulase-negative staphylococci causing PVE are resistant to methicillin as well as other semisynthetic penicillinase-resistant penicillins and cephalosporins. This resistance pattern should be assumed until susceptibility to methicillin has been conclusively established using techniques such as those described by Archer (3) or Karchmer et al. (56). Data from both experimental endocarditis models and retrospective clinical studies of PVE due to methicillin-resistant coagulase-negative staphylococci demonstrated that regimens in which vancomycin was used were superior to those in which beta-lactam antibiotics were used and that vancomycin in combination with rifampin and an aminoglycoside was more efficacious than vancomycin alone (4, 56, 62, 116). In a retrospective study, vancomycin used alone or in combination with rifampin and/or an aminoglycoside yielded an 81% (21 of 26 patients) cure rate, compared with a cure rate of 50% (10 of 20 patients) for a beta-lactam antibiotic alone or in combination with rifampin and/or an aminoglycoside (56). A prospective randomized treatment trial for PVE due to methicillin-resistant coagulase-negative staphylococci, compared vancomycin plus rifampin for 6 weeks with this combination plus gentamicin administered during the initial 2 weeks (56a). Overall, 78% of the patients enrolled in the study were cured, and no difference was noted in the cure rates between the two regimens. However, in 37% of the patients receiving the vancomycin and rifampin regimen, the coagulase-negative staphylococci became resistant to rifampin during therapy. Continued combination therapy with effective agents in these patients required administration of vancomycin and gentamicin. Rifampin resistance did not develop when patients were treated with vancomycin and rifampin plus gentamicin during the initial 2 weeks. Accordingly, to prevent the development of rifampin resistance in infecting coagulase-negative staphylococci and thus to spare patients the potential nephrotoxicity of prolonged therapy (4 to 6 weeks) with an aminoglycoside-containing regimen, the three-drug regimen that limits gentamicin to only 2 weeks is recommended (Table 6).

The coagulase-negative staphylococci causing PVE have usually been highly susceptible to gentamicin and rifampin; however, strains resistant to gentamicin have been encountered recently. Because resistance to rifampin may emerge rapidly after initiation of therapy with vancomycin and rifampin, it may be prudent to delay beginning rifampin until susceptibility of the causative strain to gentamicin has been determined. In the event of resistance to gentamicin, this delay will avoid an inadvertent period of vancomycin and rifampin therapy (vancomycin, rifampin, and gentamicin versus a gentamicin-resistant strain) with the inherent potential for emergence of resistance to rifampin. If the infecting coagulase-negative staphylococcus is resistant to gentamicin, an alternative aminoglycoside to which the strain remains highly susceptible should be sought. If available, the alternative aminoglycoside should be administered in combination with vancomycin, and thereafter, treatment with rifampin can be initiated. If there are no aminoglycosides to which the strain is susceptible, a quinolone can be used in combination with vancomycin and rifampin. In the rabbit model of S. epidermidis endocarditis, treatment with ciprofloxacin plus rifampin was as efficacious as the regimen of vancomycin, gentamicin, and rifampin (94). Additionally, in a subcutaneous tissue cage model of S. aureus foreign body infection, fleroxacin used in combination treatment with rifampin or with vancomycin plus rifampin prevented the emergence of the rifampin-resistant staphylococci that were noted when treatment with rifampin alone or vancomycin plus rifampin was administered (20, 66). If the strain is resistant to all aminoglycosides and quinolones, treatment should be attempted with vancomycin plus rifampin.

Although the susceptibility of diphtheroids to beta-lactam antibiotics is variable, when strains are susceptible to gentamicin (MIC $\leq$ 4 μg/ml), a synergistic bactericidal effect can be anticipated from the combination of penicillin and gentamicin. This synergy, however, is not achievable when strains are resistant to gentamicin (81). Vancomycin is bactericidal against these organisms and provides an alternative for therapy

Table 6. Antimicrobial therapy for PVE[a]

Organism	Regimen of choice[b]	Duration (wk)	Alternative regimen[b,c]	Duration (wk)
Streptococci Penicillin susceptible (MIC, ≤0.1 μg/ml) nonenterococcal	1. Aqueous crystalline penicillin G, 20 MU/day i.v. in divided q4h doses	6	1. Cephalothin, 2.0 g i.v. q4h	6
	plus		or	
	Gentamicin, 1 mg/kg body wt (not to exceed 80 mg) i.v. or i.m. q8h	2	2. Cefazolin, 2.0 g i.v. q8h	6
Staphylococci S. aureus (methicillin susceptible)	1. Nafcillin or oxacillin, 2 g i.v. q4h	6	1. Cephalothin, 2 g i.v. q4h	6
	plus		plus	
	Gentamicin, 1 mg/kg body wt (not to exceed 80 mg) i.v. or i.m. q8h	2	Gentamicin, 1 mg/kg body wt (not to exceed 80 mg) i.v. or i.m. q8h	2
			or	
			2. Vancomycin,[d] 30 mg/kg body wt i.v. divided in q12h or q6h doses	6
S. aureus (methicillin resistant)	1. Vancomycin,[d] 30 mg/kg body wt i.v. divided in q12h or q6h doses	6	None	
Coagulase negative (methicillin resistant)	1. Vancomycin,[d] 30 mg/kg body wt i.v. divided in q12h or q6h doses	6	See text	
	plus			

Organism	Regimen	wk
	Gentamicin, 1 mg/kg (not to exceed 80 mg) i.v. or i.m. q8h	2
	plus	
	Rifampin, 300 mg p.o. q8h	6
Diphtheroids		
Gentamicin susceptible (MIC, ≤4 μg/ml)	1. Aqueous crystalline penicillin G, 20 MU/day in q4h divided doses	6
	plus	
	Gentamicin, 1 mg/kg body wt (not to exceed 80 mg) i.v. or i.m. q8h	6
	1. Vancomycin,[d] 30 mg/kg body wt i.v. divided in q12h or q6h doses	6
Gentamicin resistant (MIC, >4 μg/ml)	1. Vancomycin,[d] 30 mg/kg body wt i.v. divided in q12h or q6h doses	6
Fastidious gram-negative coccobacilli[e]	1. Ampicillin, 2 g i.v. q4h or	6
	2. Ampicillin, 2 g i.v. q4h plus either	6
	Streptomycin, 7.5 mg/kg body wt (not to exceed 500 mg) i.m. q12h	6
	or	
	Gentamicin, 1 mg/kg body wt (not to exceed 80 mg) i.m. or i.v. q8h	6
	1. Cefotaxime,[f] 2 g i.v. q4h (benefit of adding aminoglycoside not established)	6

[a] Doses assume average weight and normal renal function. Where necessary, doses must be modified for marked obesity or decreased renal function.

[b] Abbreviations: i.v., intravenously; i.m., intramuscularly; p.o., orally; q4h, every 4 h.

[c] For patients who are allergic to penicillin; avoid cephalosporins if immediate-type hypersensitivity to penicillin is suspected.

[d] Vancomycin dose not to exceed 2 g/day unless serum concentrations monitored.

[e] Includes *Haemophilus* species, *A. actinomycetemcomitans*, *C. hominis*, *Eikenella corrodens*, and *Kingella* species.

[f] Ceftizoxime, ceftriaxone, or ceftazidime in comparable dose could be used.

when a synergistic combination is not available. On the basis of these in vitro observations and the reported clinical experiences, regimens for treating patients with diphtheroid PVE hve been formulated (Table 6).

Meyer and Gerding, in a brief review, noted that all 21 of the reported cases with PVE caused by fastidious gram-negative coccobacilli had been cured and that only 4 required surgical intervention (75). Antibiotic therapy with ampicillin or penicillin, combined with an aminoglycoside in nine patients, was used commonly; however, in four patients a cephalosporin was used for part of the treatment. Hindes et al. reported 17 cases of PVE due to these organisms; using antibiotic regimens similar to those noted by Meyer and Gerding, 11 of 13 were cured medically, and 2 of 3 were cured with antibiotics and surgery. One patient died prior to initiation of treatment (46a).

Optimal therapy for PVE caused by enterococci requires a synergistic combination of antibiotics with a net bactericidal effect. This is usually achieved by combining gentamicin (or occasionally streptomycin) with penicillin, ampicillin, or vancomycin. Although a detailed consideration of antimicrobial therapy for enterococcal PVE is beyond the scope of this chapter, excellent recent reviews, which include consideration of treatment in the light of increasing antimicrobial resistance among enterococci, are available (30–32). Of interest, the outcome of therapy for enterococcal PVE has been relatively favorable, often without valve replacement (88).

If antimicrobial therapy is initiated before culture results are available or for putative culture-negative PVE, a combination of vancomycin, gentamicin, and ampicillin (or a "third-generation" cephalosporin) should be used. Because fastidious gram-negative coccobacilli are important causes of late PVE, the beta-lactam component of the regimen is particularly important when the onset of PVE in these patients is 6 or more months after surgery. Special blood culture techniques and serologic tests for fungi, *Legionella* species, *C. burnetii*, and *Mycoplasma* species should be considered when routine blood cultures are negative.

Surgical treatment

In spite of therapy with increasingly potent antimicrobial regimens during the 1970s, the outcome of patients with PVE did not improve over that noted previously. Combining studies reported through 1969, Mayer and Schoenbaum noted mortality rates of 74% and 48% for early PVE (onset less than 60 days after valve placement) and late PVE, respectively. For studies reported from 1970 through 1979, the mortality rates were 69% and 45% for early and late PVE, respectively (74). Increased mortality rates due to PVE were noted in patients with specific clinical features (10, 49, 57, 73). For example, mortality rates of 84% and 29% were found among PVE patients with moderate to severe congestive heart failure and those with mild or no heart failure, respectively (57). Additionally, a mortality rate of 67% was noted in patients with murmurs indicative of prosthesis dysfunction, while the mortality rate among patients without these murmurs was 31%. The mortality rate of PVE caused by streptococci was 39%, while that of PVE caused by other organisms was 64% (57). PVE patients with fever persisting for 10 or more days in spite of appropriate antibiotic therapy experienced a fatality rate of 63%, while only 30% of those who became afebrile more promptly died (57). Careful review of surgical and necropsy pathology from PVE patients revealed that these clinical features, as well as new onset and persistent electrocardiographic conduction disturbances and relapse of PVE after appropriate antibiotic treatment, reflected invasive infection or valvular dysfunction that was unlikely to respond to even the most potent antimicrobial therapy (57). The pathology suggested the need for surgical debridement of infection and repair of hemodynamically impaired prosthetic valves if the outcome of patients with these features was to be improved. In fact, several groups found that the motality rate for PVE was often lower in surgically treated patients than in those treated with antibiotics alone, although the differences were not statistically significant (29, 73, 103, 122). Subsequently, Saffle et al. pooled data from three major centers and demonstrated a significantly lower mortality rate among patients treated with antibiotics plus surgery (23%) than among those treated with antibiotics alone (60%) (97). These results were obtained in spite of the prevailing opinion that surgical treatment should be reserved as a final effort for desperately ill patients failing antibiotic treatment.

Calderwood et al. used a stepwise logistic regression with backward deletion to identify independent factors associated with the outcome of PVE (17). They found the best predictor of death during initial treatment of PVE to be the presence of complicated PVE, wherein complicated endocarditis was defined by clinical features indicative of invasive infection or valve dysfunction (congestive heart failure, murmur of prosthesis dysfunction, new electrocardiographic conduction disturbance, or fever persisting for 10 or more days during appropriate antibiotic therapy). In turn, complicated PVE was significantly associated with a prosthesis in the aortic position or the onset of symptoms within 12 months after surgery but not with the type of prosthetic valve. The outcome of 74 patients with complicated PVE was evaluated. Among the 41 patients treated with medical-surgical therapy, 12 (29%) died during the initial hospitalization; in contrast, among 33 patients treated medically, 12

(36%) died. Furthermore, among the 29 who survived initial medical-surgical therapy, there were 4 late PVE-related deaths, 2 relapses of PVE, and 2 operations for late sequelae of PVE. Among the 21 who survived initial medical treatment, there were 3 additional PVE-related deaths, 2 relapses, and 9 operations for late sequelae. Overall, 21 (51%) of 41 patients with complicated PVE receiving initial medical-surgical therapy survived and did not experience subsequent PVE-related complications, compared with only 7 (33%) of 33 patients with complicated PVE who received medical therapy ($P = 0.008$). The clinical constellation called complicated PVE defines a patient population that has a higher mortality rate than patients with uncomplicated PVE and a group of patients that is best treated with medical-surgical therapy. Many patients with complicated PVE require operations during initial therapy. Some have infection that can be eradicated by medical therapy; however, these patients remain at high risk for relapse and progressive prosthesis dysfunction, and thus they require careful follow-up.

The potential for salvaging patients with complicated PVE or unresponsive infection through prompt aggressive cardiac surgical intervention is increasingly accepted. Elaborate reconstruction of infection-damaged cadiac tissues may be required and is feasible. By reconstruction of the aortic annulus and root, using a Dacron tube graft and saphenous vein bypass grafts to the coronary arteries, or by placing a mitral prosthesis in the distal left atrium, patients can be salvaged in spite of extensive destructive endocarditis (52, 91). Additionally, antibiotic-impregnated cryopreserved aortic root homografts have been used successfully to reconstruct the aortic outflow tract of patients with aortic PVE complicated by annular abscess formation (42).

Indications for surgical intervention have evolved (Table 7) (10, 57, 64, 83, 120). Some of these indications are not absolute but rather serve to prompt careful considerations of surgical therapy. Moderate to severe congestive heart failure (New York Heart Association class III or IV) associated with prosthesis dysfunction is a commonly accepted indication for surgery. Few patients with this degree of PVE-induced heart failure are alive 6 months after medical treatment, while surgical-medical treatment has resulted in survival rates of 44 (89) to 64% (A. W. Karchmer, unpublished data). Patients with relapse of PVE after appropriate antibiotic therapy have been found to have invasive paravalvular infection; they are more likely to survive PVE if treated surgically (17, 57). While not a uniformly accepted indication for surgical treatment of PVE, several investigators favor a surgical therapy for PVE caused by *S. aureus* or coagulase-negative staphylococci (56, 57, 83, 89, 120). Rather than an indication for surgery, the potential for additional systemic em-

Table 7. Indications for cardiac surgery in patients with PVE

---

1. Moderate to severe heart failure due to prosthesis dysfunction (incompetence or obstruction)
2. Invasive and destructive paravalvular infection
   A. Partial valve dehiscence
   B. New or progressive conduction system disturbances
   C. Fever persisting 10 or more days during appropriate antibiotic therapy
   D. Purulent pericarditis
   E. Sinus of Valsalva aneurysm or intracardiac fistula
3. Uncontrolled bacteremic infection during therapy
4. Infection caused by selected organisms
   A. Fungi
   B. *Staphylococcus aureus*[a]
   C. Coagulase-negative staphylococci[a]
5. Relapse after appropriate antimicrobial therapy
6. Persistent temperature during therapy for culture-negative PVE in absence of other causes of fever
7. Recurrent arterial emboli[a]

---

[a] Relative indication (see text).

boli is often viewed as a factor that in combination with other considerations might help to justify surgery. In fact, a recent review notes that recurrent emboli are rare in patients with PVE who are receiving appropriate antimicrobial therapy (27). Patients with culture-negative endocarditis who continue to experience fever during empiric antibiotic therapy are candidates for surgical intervention. Surgery will allow a definitive microbiologic diagnosis and development of specific effective antimicrobial therapy. Additionally, some of these patients will be found to have fungal endocarditis or unrecognized invasive infection that warrants surgery.

Some investigators have recommended that patients with renal dysfunction or early PVE (within 2 months of surgery) and some with aortic PVE be treated surgically (10, 24). Nunez et al. have recommended surgery for patients with bioprosthetic valve endocarditis who have two-dimensional echocardiographic evidence of vegetations, because of the strong association of this finding with significantly increased transvalvular pressure gradients (82). In reality, these are additional situations in which there is likely to be invasive infection or prosthesis dysfunction.

The timing of cardiac surgical therapy for patients with PVE must be individualized. The hemodynamic status of the patient is the most important consideration in determining the time of cardiac surgery. As in patients with native valve endocarditis, the likelihood of patients with PVE surviving valve replacement surgery is inversely related to the severity of the patient's heart failure at the time of surgery. Thus, while in theory it may be desirable to control infection with antibiotic therapy prior to surgery, this must not be attempted at the expense of progressive paravalvular tissue destruction and further deterioration in the patient's hemodynamics. Baumgartner et al. have demonstrated that longer periods of antibiotic therapy prior to surgery do not correlate with inability to recover bacteria from intraoperative cultures or with a more favorable outcome (10). In an analysis of outcome among patients with PVE who were treated surgically, they found that renal dysfunction prior to surgery was one of the most important predictors of both increased operative mortality and overall long-term unsatisfactory outcome (10). Renal failure indicated advanced decompensated heart failure and low cardiac output. Cortina et al. also found that renal dysfunction was an important independent predictor of increased operative mortality (24). Both studies recommended earlier surgical intervention, before decompensated heart failure and renal dysfunction supervene. Similarly, survival rates among patients with endocarditis that is invasive and unresponsive to antibiotic therapy will be higher with earlier surgery than with continued therapy with antibiotics and delay of surgery (10, 15, 67).

In selected patients with PVE, the results of therapy with antibiotics alone are comparable to the results of medical-surgical therapy; for these patients, medical therapy is recommended. They include patients with late-onset PVE (12 months or more after surgery) who are infected with less virulent organisms (viridans group streptococci, enterococci, and fastidious gram-negative coccobacilli) and who do not develop complicated endocarditis (lack indications for surgery) (57, 75, 88, 97). Several studies have suggested that successful therapy of bioprosthetic valve endocarditis is commonly achieved with antibiotics alone (68, 93). However, the finding that bioprosthetic valve infection is frequently complicated by annulus invasion and valve dehiscence or by a cusp destruction indicates an important role for medical-surgical therapy in many patients with bioprosthetic valve endocarditis (10, 17, 24, 36, 82, 100). Many patients with PVE, regardless of the type of prosthesis, are likely to benefit from surgical therapy. Among 56 patients with infection involving a porcine bioprosthesis, 27 (48%) required surgical replacement of the infected prosthesis. Furthermore, 74% of surgically treated patients survived, compared with 62% of those treated with antibiotics alone (100). Of the 116 patients with PVE studied by Calderwood et al., 45 (39%) received medical-surgical therapy, and among the patients who were treated medically, at least 33 were candidates for surgical treatment by virtue of having complicated PVE (17). This suggests, as do data from other studies, that as many as 65% of patients with PVE may be candidates for medical-surgical therapy during their initial hospitalization (17, 97).

Anticoagulant therapy. Careful anticoagulation therapy has been advocated for patients with PVE involving prostheses that would usually warrant maintenance anticoagulation (57, 99, 120, 121). The initial data, while limited, suggested that the risk of central nervous system complications was higher among patients not receiving adequate anticoagulation therapy than among those who were anticoagulated (99, 120). Although a recent examination of this issue failed to confirm this benefit of anticoagulation therapy, increased risk of hemorrhagic stroke was not associated with anticoagulation therapy (27). Anticoagulation should be reversed temporarily if a patient experiences a hemorrhagic central nervous system event. Anticoagulation is not recommended for patients with PVE involving devices that do not under usual circumstances require anticoagulant therapy.

Prevention

The morbidity and mortality of PVE remain high in spite of improved therapy. Thus, prevention of this entity must be assigned a high priority. Patients with PVE continue to experience mortality rates of 30 to 35%, and 40 to 60% require cardiac surgry as an essential element of therapy. The increased hazard of developing PVE during the initial 6 to 12 months after cardiac surgery (18, 50) and the association of operative field and bypass equipment contamination, as well as postoperative infections, with early PVE (2, 11, 29, 61, 119) suggest that prevention efforts be focused on the perioperative period. This need is further supported by the increased mortality associated with the early onset of PVE (10, 17, 24, 49).

In addition to scrupulous attention to surgical technique, efforts to prevent serious postoperative infections after cardiac surgery (e.g., mediastinitis or PVE) have focused on prophylactic antibiotics. Placebo-controlled trials demonstrated a significant reduction in wound infections when prophylactic antibiotics were administered to patients undergoing cardiac surgery (8, 39). Although similar studies have never demonstrated a significant reduction in PVE, prophylactic antibiotics are assumed to have this effect and are accepted as routine during cardiac valve replacement surgery (47). Selection of specific regimens for use in this surgery must consider individual hospital flora (for example, the prevalence of methicillin-resistant *S. aureus*), the common causes of PVE during the 6 to 12 months after surgery, the spectrum of antibiotic activity and the potential toxicities of candidate antibiotics, and the demonstrated efficacy of these agents in properly designed and executed trials. Additionally, specific regimens must be designed so that antibiotic concentrations exceeding the MICs of the expected pathogens are present in tissues before and throughout the surgical procedure. The failure of prophylaxis may relate to inadequate serum concentrations at the end of prolonged surgery (43, 86); thus the pharmacokinetics and dosing of individual agents must be carefully considered. Longer courses (5 days) of prophylaxis have been shown to be no more effective than single-dose or short-course (48 h) prophylaxis; furthermore, the former may result in colonization of the patient with more resistant organisms (22, 43).

Although regimens vary among medical centers, cefazolin (1 g intravenously) preoperatively and every 6 h thereafter for 48 h is preferred by many, including the authors, unless nosocomial infections caused by methicillin-resistant *S. aureus* are prevalent (53, 86). For patients unable to tolerate a beta-lactam antibiotic, vancomycin (15 mg/kg intravenously) immediately preoperatively, and 10 mg/kg after initiation of bypass and every 8 h postoperatively for 48 h is recommended (34). Vancomycin is also recommended when the prophylactic regimen must include methicillin-resistant *S. aureus*. Recent studies of antibiotic prophylaxis wherein doses have been adjusted to provide adequate serum concentrations have questioned whether cephalosporins with similar in vitro activity patterns provide comparable protection. Cefamandole was more effective than cefazolin in preventing wound infections, particularly those caused by *S. aureus*, in cardiac surgery patients (54). In a second study, cefazolin tended to be less effective than cefuroxime and cefamandole in preventing wound infections after cardiac surgery (102). A third randomized double-blind trial found similar operative site infection rates among cardiac surgery patients who received perioperative prophylaxis with cefamandole, cefazolin, or cefuroxime (112). The routine use of vancomycin for prophylaxis in valve replacement surgery has been recommended because of the hazard of early PVE caused by methicillin-resistant coagulase-negative staphylococci. While vancomycin prophylaxis may be justified in institutions where methicillin-resistant *S. aureus* is a frequent nosocomial pathogen, its superiority to cefazolin or cefamandole in preventing PVE caused by coagulase-negative staphylococci has not been established. In one randomized double-blind trial, patients undergoing cardiac or major vascular surgery who received vancomycin experienced fewer surgical wound infections than did those who received cefazolin or cefamandole (70). However, in this study there was no significant difference in surgical wound infection rates between recipients of the various prophylactic antibiotic regimens when one considered patients undergoing cardiac surgery.

Patients must also be protected against later-onset prosthetic valve endocarditis. Existing problems likely to give rise to transient bacteremia in the future (e.g., existing dental or gingival disease) should be addressed prior to performing an elective valve replacement. Furthermore, regardless of the time elapsed since cardiac surgery, prosthetic valve recipients should always receive prophylactic antibiotics when undergoing procedures that are associated with bacteremia. The most vigorous prophylaxis regimens recommended in the guidelines of the American Heart Association (chapter 14) should be followed whenever possible (25). Minor bacterial infections (e.g., furuncles, sinusitis) should be considered a significant threat to the prosthetic valve and treated with antibiotics.

INFECTIONS OF VASCULAR GRAFTS

Since the 1950s, technological advances in artificial conduits have made vascular reconstructive surgery to any accessible artery in the body possible. While almost every textile material has been tried as a substitute for the arterial homograft, Dacron and polytetrafluoroethylene (Gore-Tex) are the two synthetic graft materials that have withstood the test of time. From the outset, their use has been complicated by the occurrence of graft-related infections. While autologous venous and arterial grafts can become infected, the incidence of infections involving autologous grafts is low. Consequently, this discussion focuses on infections associated with synthetic grafts. The complications of graft infections are potentially devastating and include sepsis, anastomotic disruption with bleeding or pseudoaneurysm formation, graft thrombosis, limb loss, and high perioperative and late mortality.

Incidence

While the ideal prosthetic arterial graft would endothelialize and become incorporated with human tissue, none has done so entirely; consequently, the graft remains a foreign body. The placement of synthetic grafts has increased steadily, as they are used not only as arterial and venous conduits but also as points of access for dialysis and drug delivery. The combination of improved prosthetic design allowing better incorporation, optimal surgical technique, and antimicrobial prophylaxis has reduced the frequency of graft infection to the range of 1 to 5% (23, 40, 48, 51, 65, 106). This rate has remained stable during the past decade. Greco has estimated that in the United States approximately 10,000 patients have a prosthetic arterial graft infection yearly (45). The frequency of graft infection varies markedly, however, depending upon the anatomic site of the prosthesis. The highest rates have been observed in grafts that traverse the inguinal area (44).

Pathogenesis

The great majority of arterial prosthetic infections are thought to arise from contamination at the time of implantation. The high incidence of graft infections in the groin may be due to (i) the superficial location of the graft, which favors cutaneous contamination; (ii) the increased incidence of wound infections that occur at this site and that may secondarily contaminate the prosthesis; (iii) disruption of local lymphatics, increasing vulnerability to local infection; and (iv) the presence of devitalized tissue and local purulent lesions distal to the site of vascular occlusion in an ischemic lower extremity.

The pathogenesis of infections associated with intra-abdominal grafts is likely more complex. It is possible that intestinal erosion secondary to prosthesis-induced trauma may be the inciting event or, conversely, that a primary graft infection initiates suture line leak, pseudoaneurysm formation, and enteric erosion (108).

Data from an experimental animal model indicate that vascular prostheses may be contaminated during episodes of bacteremia (71), particularly in the first 4 months postoperatively when the pseudointimal lining is incomplete. In practice, however, hematogenous seeding of an arterial graft is quite infrequent.

Microbial Etiology

Staphylococcal species are the microorganisms most frequently isolated from vascular prosthetic infections, but gram-negative bacilli are encountered also. Recently, Bandyk noted that the less virulent S. epidermidis rivaled S. aureus as the most prevalent pathogen (9). Goldstone and Moore (44) found that S. aureus was the major organism recovered from groin infections occurring within 3.5 months of surgery, while coagulase-negative staphylococci predominated among groin infections presenting beyond that interval. Liekweg and Greenfield (65) reviewed data on 164 well-documented cases of vascular prosthetic infection reported through 1974. S. aureus was isolated in fully one-half of these infections. Other organisms isolated, either alone or in combination, were as follows (in percentages): Escherichia coli, 13.4; Streptococcus spp., 8.5; Pseudomonas spp., 6.1; Klebsiella spp., 5.4; Proteus spp., 4.8; and coagulase-negative staphylococci, 3.6. There were also rare isolates of micrococci, enterococci, salmonellae, and anaerobes. S. aureus was isolated from 73% of infections involving aortofemoral grafts and 55% involving femoropopliteal grafts. In contrast, *S. aureus* was isolated from less than one-third of aortoiliac graft infections.

Clinical Manifestations

The clinical manifestations of graft infection are varied. Signs and symptoms depend on three main factors: the time interval between implantation and appearance of graft sepsis, graft location, and the type of bacteria involved.

Graft infections may occur within the early postoperative period, but many cases, especially those involving *S. epidermidis,* may not become evident for months or years. The mean interval between surgery and the recognition of infection in 128 cases reviewed by Liekweg and Greenfield (65) was 27 weeks; nevertheless, 80% of groin infections became apparent within 5 weeks. Only a few of the late-onset cases appear to be due to hematogenous spread from other bodily sites.

Approximately one-half of all graft infections present as localized wound infections, often with a draining sinus or graft exposure or both (44, 65). This presentation commonly occurs in close proximity to the original site of surgery. Anastomotic false aneurysm, hemorrhage, and graft thrombosis may also herald a localized graft-wound infection; this sequence usually occurs as a delayed presentation. Presentations centered around a surgical wound infection are characteristic of infections involving femoropopliteal, ileofemoral, or aortofemoral grafts and most commonly occur in the groin incision. Infections may involve only a segment of the prosthesis or may spread extensively along its length, depending on the virulence of the pathogen, the magnitude of the host defense response, and whether the graft had become integrated with surrounding tissue prior to infection.

Infection involving an intra-abdominal aortic prosthesis may be cryptic. During the early postoperative period, infection may be associated with a prolonged ileus or unexplained sepsis and multiorgan failure. Less than 20% of aortic graft infections will be recognized within 1 month of surgery; the mean interval from surgery to the diagnosis of aortic graft infection is almost 25 months. Aortic graft infection may present with nonspecific symptoms including malaise, anorexia, weight loss, back or abdominal pain, and low-grade fever. The infection may also manifest itself as an aortoenteric fistula with gastrointestinal bleeding occurring as hematemesis or melena (105). Bleeding may be acute and extensive with symptoms compressed into a period of hours or may be indolent and recur over days to weeks. Although bleeding is suggestive of a fistula, in less than one-half of the patients is the diagnosis established with certainty prior to exploratory laparotomy.

More overt signs and symptoms of infection such as fever, leukocytosis, absence of graft incorporation with perigraft inflammation and localized exudate, pseudoaneurysm, graft thrombosis, or a draining pulsatile mass in the groin may be present in only one-half of the patients with graft infection. Blood cultures are positive in less than 50% of cases. It is important, therefore, for clinicians to realize that infections of vascular prosthetic grafts, in general, may be quite subtle in presentation.

The detection and localization of infections involving an intra-abdominal or intrathoracic segment of a prosthetic graft may present particular difficulties. Positive blood cultures only document the presence of an intravascular infection and establish the responsible pathogen. The findings on physical examination are limited when infection of a totally intra-abdominal or thoracoabdominal graft is suspected. Evaluation must include a careful review of the previous operating room reports and hospital course to identify predisposing factors. Vascular imaging techniques with which to assess the vascular anastomosis, the degree of graft incorporation, or a localized inflammatory process include ultrasonography, computed tomography, magnetic resonance imaging, arteriography, contrast sinography, and radionuclide scans using gallium or labeled white blood cells. Needle aspiration of perigraft collections under ultrasound or computed tomographic guidance can provide additional information regarding an abnormality visualized on vascular imaging. In evaluating a patient with suspected aortoenteric fistula, fiberoptic gastrointestinal endoscopy visualizing the entire upper gastrointestinal tract, including the third and fourth portions of the duodenum, is essential. Because the sensitivity of vascular imaging and radionuclide studies is modest, a negative study does not exclude vascular graft infection. When clinical data are compelling, operative management should not be delayed. In fact, in some patients, a definitive diagnosis of graft infection can only be established by surgical exploration (9).

Management

Antibiotic therapy

The current management of prosthetic graft infections includes removal of the involved infected prosthetic graft, appropriate antibiotic therapy, and revascularization. Purulent secretions in association with an exposed graft should be examined by Gram stain and cultured. Graft infections frequently are caused by staphylococci. For infections caused by beta-lactam-susceptible staphylococci, appropriate antibiotic therapy consists of high-dose intravenous nafcillin or oxacillin; if the infection is due to methicillin-resistant staphylococci, vancomycin is required. Penicillin-allergic patients infected with methicillin-susceptible staphylococci can usually safely be treated with cephalosporins, provided their hypersensitivity is not of the immediate type. Patients who have experienced prior anaphylactic-type reactions to penicillin should be treated with vancomycin. The role of rifampin in combination with a beta-lactam antibiotic or vancomycin in the treatment of staphylococcal graft infection has not been evaluated.

If the bacteriologic diagnosis is in doubt, initial therapy should also encompass the possibility of infection with gram-negative bacilli. A variety of expanded-spectrum penicillins, cephalosporins, and aminoglycosides are available for this purpose. Should the infection be intra-abdominal, raising the possibility of an enteroprosthetic fistula, the regimen should include agents effective against anaerobic intestinal flora. Examples of such agents are cefoxitin, beta-lactam–β-lactamase inhibitor combinations, imipenem, clindamycin, and metronidazole. Patients are treated with intravenous antibiotics for prolonged periods of time (although data are scant, the authors prefer 6 weeks of parenteral therapy), and some patients are placed on lifelong regimens of suppressive oral antibiotics. The latter often is exercised when it seems likely that the newly implanted graft may have been contaminated at the anastamotic site or when the arterial stump that was closed proximal to an infected site may have been contaminated (72).

Surgical management

The current surgical management of prosthetic graft infection is based on the premise that the infected prosthetic graft must be removed. Traditionally, the therapy of choice includes excision of the infected graft and revascularization by an extra-anatomic bypass or an in situ autologous arterial or venous conduit (19, 90). Many procedures are recommended, but no method is without problems. Extra-anatomic graft patency is not ideal, and subsequent limb loss associated with a failed extra-anatomic bypass is as high as 34% (11, 87). Mortality in the course of reconstructive efforts has been reported to be as high as 25%, with late mortality as high as 82% at 5 years (84). For this reason, new strategies are under consideration in selected patients. In situ reconstruction of primary vascular infections along with surgical debridement and prolonged antibiotic administration has yielded some successes. Most authorities agree that certain criteria must be met if in situ reconstruction is to be attempted. The resection must be as complete as possible, removing all infected artery, aneurysm, and neighboring tissue, and any new anastomosis must use uninfected healthy tissue (19, 38). A vascularized tissue flap should cover the prosthesis and all suture lines (78). Adequate antibiotic therapy should be instituted promptly, with a prolonged duration of treatment. These procedures have been advocated for patients with an incorporated proximal graft who have a low-grade graft infection with negative blood and perigraft cultures and no evidence of anastomotic breakdown. Some authors have concluded that an infected vascular prosthesis can be replaced in situ by an antibiotic-bonded graft (21, 111). Polytetrafluoroethylene has been chosen by some as the prosthetic material of choice in treating infected grafts (77). Most vascular surgeons still believe that in situ graft replacement has limited or no application in the setting of frank pus surrounding a vascular graft anastomosis.

Prevention

Infection following arterial reconstruction presents a major challenge to modern vascular surgery. Regardless of the therapeutic measures employed, graft infections continue to demonstrate high rates of perioperative and late morbidity and mortality. Consequently, prevention of infection, wherever possible, is highly desirable. Potential sites of bacteremic seeding (urinary tract infection, dental abscess, etc.), as well as local infections of ischemic extremities, should be eradicated before placement of a bypass graft. During the operative procedure, strict attention should be given to asepsis and to fastidious surgical technique (108). Although data are limited, prophylactic antibiotics are believed to be responsible, at least in part, for the decline in infection rates associated with the insertion of vascular prostheses. The use of such prophylaxis is now conventional. Readers are referred to chapter 14 for an analysis of published controlled trials, as well as a suggested prophylactic regimen.

Data are inadequate to allow a determination of the necessity for antimicrobial prophylaxis in patients with arterial prostheses undergoing dental and surgical procedures. The rationale for such prophylaxis would be to prevent the development of an infective arteritis. It would thus be analogous to the prophylaxis recommended to prevent infective endocarditis in patients with prosthetic heart valves. The incidence, however, of graft infections induced by bacteremia is quite low. Nevertheless, considering the intravascular location of the prosthesis and the grave implications of such an infection, prophylaxis seems to be reasonable, particularly for the first 4 months postoperatively, when experimental data indicate that the graft is most susceptible to bacteremic seeding (71). Should prophylaxis be elected, the regimens suggested by the American Heart Association (27) for prevention of infective endocarditis are applicable. For dental prophylaxis, the nonparenteral regimen recommended by the American Heart Association for endocarditis prophylaxis (as opposed to the parenteral regimen recommended for patients with prosthetic cardiac valves) would be appropriate.

REFERENCES

1. **Anderson, D. J., B. H. Bulkley, and G. M. Hutchins.** 1977. A clinicopathologic study of prosthetic valve endocarditis in 22 patients: morphologic basis for diagnosis and therapy. *Am. Heart J.* **94:**325–332.
2. **Ankeney, J. L., and R. J. Parker.** 1969. Staphylococcal endocarditis following open heart surgery related to positive intraoperative blood cultures, p. 719–728. *In* L. A. Brewer III, D. A. Cooley, J. C. Davila, K. A. Merendino, and H. D. Sirak (ed.), *Prosthetic Heart Valves.* Charles C Thomas, Publisher, Springfield, Ill.
3. **Archer, G. L.** 1978. Antimicrobial susceptibility and selection of resistance among *Staphylococcus epidermidis* isolates recovered from patients with infections of indwelling foreign devices. *Antimicrob. Agents Chemother.* **14:**353–359.
4. **Archer, G. L., J. L. Johnston, G. J. Vazquez, and H. B. Haywood III.** 1983. Efficacy of antibiotic combinations including rifampin against methicillin-resistant Staphylococcus epidermidis: in vitro and in vivo studies. *Rev. Infect. Dis.* **5:**S538–S542.
5. **Archer, G. L., N. Vishniavsky, and H. G. Stiver.** 1982. Plasmid pattern analysis of *Staphylococcus epidermidis* isolates from patients with prosthetic valve endocarditis. *Infect. Immun.* **35:**627–632.
6. **Arnett, E. N., and W. C. Roberts.** 1976. Prosthetic valve endocarditis. *Am. J. Cardiol.* **38:**281–291.
7. **Arvay, A., and M. Lengyel.** 1988. Incidence and rsk factors of prosthetic valve endocarditis. *Am. J. Cardiothorac. Surg.* **2:**340–346.
8. **Austin, T. W., J. C. Coles, R. Burnett, and M. Goldback.** 1980. Aortocoronary bypass procedures and sternotomy infections: a study of antistaphylococcal prophylaxis. *Can. J. Surg.* **23:**483.
9. **Bandyk, D. F.** 1991. Diagnosis of aortic graft infection, p. 430–435. *In* C. B. Ernst and J. C. Stanley (ed.), *Current Therapy in Vascular Surgery,* 2nd ed. B. C. Decker, Inc., Philadelphia.
10. **Baumgartner, W. A., D. C. Miller, B. A. Reitz, P. E. Oyer, S. W. Jamieson, E. B. Stinson, and N. E. Shumway.** 1983. Surgical treatment of prosthetic valve endocarditis. *Ann. Thorac. Surg.* **35:**87–102.
11. **Blakemore, W. S., G. J. McGarrity, R. J. Thurer, H. W. Wallace, H. MacVaugh III, and L. L. Coriell.** 1971. Infection by air-borne bacteria with cardiopulmonary bypass. *Surgery* **70:**830–837.
12. **Block, P. C., R. W. DeSanctis, A. N. Weinberg, and W. G. Austen.** 1970. Prosthetic valve endocarditis. *J. Thorac. Cardiovasc. Surg.* **60:**540–548.
13. **Bortolotti, U., G. Thiene, A. Milano, G. Panizzon, M. Valente, and V. Gallucci.** 1981. Pathological study of infective endocarditis on Hancock porcine bioprostheses. *J. Thorac. Cardiovasc. Surg.* **81:**934–942.
14. **Boyce, J. M., G. Potter-Bynoe, S. M. Opal, L. Dziobek, and A. A. Medeiros.** 1990. A common-source outbreak of *Staphylococcus epidermidis* infections among patients undergoing cardiac surgery. *J. Infect. Dis.* **161:**493–499.
15. **Boyd, A. D., F. C. Spencer, O. W. Isom, J. N. Cunningham, G. E. Reed, A. J. Acinapura, and D. A. Tice.** 1977. Infective endocarditis: an analysis of 54 surgically treated patients. *J. Thorac. Cardiovasc. Surg.* **73:**23–30.
16. **Breyer, R. H., E. N. Arnett, T. L. Spray, and W. C. Roberts.** 1978. Prosthetic valve endocarditis due to Listeria monocytogenes. *Am. J. Clin. Pathol.* **69:**186–187.

17. **Calderwood, S. B., L. A. Swinski, A. W. Karchmer, C. M. Waternaux, and M. J. Buckley.** 1986. Prosthetic valve endocarditis: analysis of factors affecting outcome of therapy. *J. Thorac. Cardiovasc. Surg.* **92:**776–783.

18. **Calderwood, S. B., L. A. Swinski, C. M. Waternaux, A. W. Karchmer, and M. J. Buckley.** 1985. Risk facors for the development of prosthetic valve endocarditis. *Circulation* **72:**31–37.

19. **Calligaro, K. D., F. J. Veith, S. K. Gupta, et al.** 1990. A modified method for management of prosthetic graft infections involving an anastomosis to the common femoral artery. *J. Vasc. Surg.* **11:**485–492.

20. **Chuard, C., M. Herrmann, P. Vaudaux, F. A. Waldvogel, and D. P. Lew.** 1991. Successful therapy of experimental chronic foreign-body infection due to methicillin-resistant *Staphylococcus aureus* by antimicrobial combinations. *Antimicrob. Agents Chemother.* **35:**2611–2616.

21. **Coburn, M. D., W. S. Moore, M. Chvapil, H. A. Gelabert, and W. J. Quinones-Baldrich.** 1992. Use of an antibiotic-bonded graft for in situ reconstruction after prosthetic graft infections. *J. Vasc. Surg.* **16:**651–660

22. **Conte, J. E., Jr., S. N. Cohen, B. B. Roe, and R. M. Elashoff.** 1972. Antibiotic prophylaxis and cardiac surgery: a prospective double-blind comparison of single-dose versus multiple-dose regimens. *Ann. Intern. Med.* **76:**943–949.

23. **Cormier, J. M., A. S. Ward, P. Lagneau, and D. Janneau.** 1980. Infection complicating aortoiliac surgery. *J. Cardiovasc. Surg.* **21:**303–314.

24. **Cortina, J. M., J. Martinell, V. Artiz, J. Fraile, S. Serrano, and G. Rabago.** 1987. Surgical treatment of active prosthetic valve endocarditis. Results in 66 patients. *Thorac. Cardiovasc. Surg.* **35:**209–214.

25. **Dajani, A. S., A. L. Bisno, K. J. Chung, D. T. Durack, M. Freed, M. A. Gerber, A. W. Karchmer, D. Millard, S. Rahimtoola, S. T. Shulman, and C. Watanakunakorn.** 1990. Prevention of bacterial endocarditis: recommendations by the American Heart Association. *JAMA* **264:**2919–2922.

26. **Daniel, W. G., A. Mugge, R. P. Martin, O. Lindert, D. Hausmann, B. Nonnast-Daniel, J. Laas, and P. R. Lichtlen.** 1991. Improvements in the diagnosis of abscesses associated with endocarditis by transesophageal echocardiography. *N. Engl. J. Med.* **324:**795–800.

27. **Davenport, J., and R. G. Hart.** 1990. Prosthetic valve endocarditis 1976–1987: antibiotics, anticoagulation and stroke. *Stroke* **21:**993–999.

28. **Dismukes, W. E., and A. W. Karchmer.** 1976. The diagnosis of infected prosthetic heart valves: bacteremia versus endocarditis, p. 61–80. *In* R. J. Duma (ed.), *Infections of Prosthetic Heart Valves and Vascular Grafts.* University Park Press, Baltimore.

29. **Dismukes, W. E., A. W. Karchmer, M. J. Buckley, W. G. Austen, and M. N. Swartz.** 1973. Prosthetic valve endocarditis: analysis of 38 cases. *Circulation* **48:**365–377.

30. **Eliopoulos, G. M.** 1992. Enterococcal endocarditis, p. 209–223. *In* D. Kaye (ed.), *Infective Endocarditis,* 2nd ed. Raven Press, Ltd., New York.

31. **Eliopoulos, G. M.** 1993. Increasing problems in the therapy of enterococcal infections. *Eur. J. Clin. Microbiol. Infect. Dis.* **12:**409–412.

32. **Eliopoulos, G. M., and C. T. Eliopoulos.** 1990. Therapy of enterococcal infections. *Eur. J. Clin. Microbiol. Infect. Dis.* **9:**118–126.

33. **Fang, G., T. F. Keys, L. O. Gentry, A. A. Harris, N. Rivera, K. Getz, P. C. Fuchs, M. Gustafson, E. S. Wong, A. Goetz, M. M. Wagener, and V. L. Yu.** 1993. Prosthetic valve endocarditis resulting from nosocomial bacteremia: a prospective, multicenter study. *Ann. Intern. Med.* **119:**560–567.

34. **Farber, B. F., A. W. Karchmer, M. J. Buckley, and R. C. Moellering, Jr.** 1983. Vanco-

mycin prophylaxis in cardiac operations: determination of an optimal dosage regimen. *J. Thorac. Cardiovasc. Surg.* **85**:933–935.

35. **Fernandez-Guerrero, M. L., J. M. Muelas, J. M. Aguado, G. Renedo, J. Fraile, F. Soriano, and E. DeVillalobos.** 1988. Q fever endocarditis on porcine bioprosthetic valves: clinicopathologic features and microbiologic findings in three patients treated with doxycycline, cotrimoxazole, and valve replacement. *Ann. Intern. Med.* **108:** 209–213.

36. **Fernicola, D. J., and W. C. Roberts.** 1993. Frequency of ring abscess and cuspal infection in active infective endocarditis involving bioprosthetic valves. *Am. J. Cardiol.* **72**:314–323.

37. **Ferrans, V. J., S. W. Boyce, M. E. Billingham, T. L. Spray, and W. C. Roberts.** 1979. Infection of glutaraldehyde-preserved porcine valve heterografts. *Am. J. Cardiol.* **43:** 1123–1136.

38. **Fichelle, J. M., G. Tabet, P. Cormier, J. C. Farkas, C. Laurian, F. Gigo, J. Marzelle, J. Acar, and J. M. Cormier.** 1993. Infected infrarenal aortic aneurysms: when is in situ reconstruction safe? *J. Vasc. Surg.* **17**:635–645.

39. **Fong, J. W., C. B. Baker, and D. C. McKee.** 1979. The value of prophylactic antibiotics in aorta-coronary bypass operations: a double blind randomized trial. *J. Thorac. Cardiovasc. Surg.* **78**:908–913.

40. **Fry, W. J., and S. M. Lindenauer.** 1967. Infection complicating the use of plastic arterial implants. *Arch. Surg.* **94**:600–609.

41. **Gaynes, R. P., P. Gardner, and W. Causey.** 1981. Prosthetic valve endocarditis caused by Histoplasma capsulatum. *Arch. Intern. Med.* **141**:1533–1537.

42. **Glazier, J. J., J. Verwilghen, R. M. Donaldson, and D. N. Ross.** 1991. Treatment of complicated prosthetic aortic valve endocarditis with annular abscess formation by homograft aortic root replacement. *J. Am. Coll. Cardiol.* **17**:1177–1182.

43. **Goldmann, D. A., C. C. Hopkins, A. W. Karchmer, R. M. Abel, M. T. McEnany, C. Akins, M. J. Buckley, and R. C. Moellering, Jr.** 1977. Cephalothin prophylaxis in cardiac valve surgery: a prospective, double-blind comparison of two-day and six-day regimens. *J. Thorac. Cardiovasc. Surg.* **73**:470–479.

44. **Goldstone, J., and W. S. Moore.** 1974. Infection in vascular prostheses: clinical manifestations and surgical management. *Am. J. Surg.* **128**:225–232.

45. **Greco, R. S.** 1991. Utilizing vascular prostheses for drug delivery. *J. Vasc. Surg.* **5:** 753–755.

46. **Higgins, T. L., J. A. Mallek, and P. H. Slugg.** 1983. Listeria monocytogenes endocarditis on a prosthetic heart valve. *South. Med. J.* **76**:675–676.

46a.**Hindes, R. G., A. W. Karchmer, and S. B. Calderwood.** 1987. Prosthetic valve endocarditis caused by fastidious gram-negative rods. *Program Abstr. 27th Intersci. Conf. Antimicrob. Agents Chemother.*, abstr. no. 121.

47. **Hirschmann, J. B., and T. S. Inui.** 1980. Antimicrobial prophylaxis. A critique of recent trials. *Rev. Infect. Dis.* **2**:1–23.

48. **Hoffert, P. W., S. Gensler, and H. Haimovici.** 1965. Infection complicating arterial grafts: personal experience with 12 cases and a review of the literature. *Arch. Surg.* **90**:427–435.

49. **Ismail, M. B., N. Hannachi, F. Abid, Z. Kaabar, and J. F. Rouge.** 1987. Prosthetic valve endocarditis: a survey. *Br. Heart J.* **58**:72–77.

50. **Ivert, T. S. A., W. E. Dismukes, C. G. Cobbs, E. H. Blackstone, J. W. Kirklin, and L. A. L. Bergdahl.** 1984. Prosthetic valve endocarditis. *Circulation* **69**:223–232.

51. **Jamieson, G. G., J. A. DeWeese, and C. G. Rob.** 1975. Infected arterial grafts. *Ann. Surg.* **181**:850–852.

52. Jault, F., I. Gandjbakhch, J. C. Chastre, J. P. Levasseur, V. Bors, C. Gilbert, A. Pavie, and C. Carbol. 1993. Prosthetic valve endocarditis with ring abscesses: surgical management and long-term results. *J. Thorac. Cardiovasc. Surg.* **105:**1106–1113.

53. Kaiser, A. B. 1986. Antimicrobial prophylaxis in surgery. *N. Engl. J. Med.* **315:** 1129–1138.

54. Kaiser, A. B., M. R. Petracek, J. W. Lea IV, D. S. Kernodle, A. C. Roach, W. C. Alford, Jr., G. R. Burrus, D. M. Glassford, Jr., C. S. Thomas, Jr., and W. S. Stoney. 1987. Efficacy of cefazolin, cefamandole, and gentamicin as prophylactic agents in cardiac surgery: results of a prospective, randomized, double-blind trial in 1030 patients. *Ann. Surg.* **206:**791–797.

55. Kalish, S. B., R. Goldschmidt, C. Li, R. Knop, F. V. Cook, G. Wilner, and T. A. Victor. 1982. Infective endocarditis caused by Paecilomyces varioti. *Am. J. Clin. Pathol.* **78:**249–252.

56. Karchmer, A. W., G. L. Archer, and W. E. Dismukes. 1983. Staphylococcus epidermidis causing prosthetic valve endocarditis: microbiologic and clinical observations as guides to therapy. *Ann. Intern. Med.* **98:**447–455.

56a. Karchmer, A. W., G. L. Archer, and National Collaborative Endocarditis Study Group. 1984. Methicillin-resistant *Staphylococcus epidermidis* prosthetic valve endocarditis: a therapeutic trial. *Program Abstr. 24th Intersci. Conf. Antimicrob. Agents Chemother.*, abstr. no. 476.

57. Karchmer, A. W., W. E. Dismukes, M. J. Buckley, W. G. Austen. 1978. Late prosthetic valve endocarditis: clinical features influencing therapy. *Am. J. Med.* **64:**199–206.

58. Karchmer, A. W., and M. N. Swartz. 1977. Infective endocarditis in patients with prosthetic heart valves, p. 58–61. *In* E. L. Kaplan and A. V. Taranta (ed.), *Infective Endocarditis.* American Heart Association symposium monograph no. 52. American Heart Association, Dallas.

59. Kernodle, D. S., N. L. Barg, and A. B. Kaiser. 1988. Low-level colonization of hospitalized patients with methicillin-resistant coagulase-negative staphylococci and emergence of the organisms during surgical antimicrobial prophylaxis. *Antimicrob. Agents Chemother.* **32:**202–208.

60. Khicha, G. J., R. B. Berroya, F. B. Escano, Jr., and C. S. Lee. 1972. Mucormycosis in a mitral prosthesis. *J. Thorac. Cardiovasc. Surg.* **63:**903–905.

61. Kluge, R. M., F. M. Calia, J. S. McLaughlin, and R. B. Hornick. 1974. Source of contamination in open heart surgery. *JAMA* **230:**1415–1418.

62. Kobasa, W. D., K. L. Kaye, T. Shapiro, and D. Kaye. 1983. Therapy for experimental endocarditis due to Staphylococcus epidermidis. *Rev. Infect. Dis.* **5:**S533–S537.

63. Laskowski, L. F., J. J. Marr, J. F. Spernoga, N. J. Frank, H. B. Barner, G. Kaiser, and D. H. Tyras. 1977. Fastidious mycobacteria grown from porcine prosthetic-heart-valve cultures. *N. Engl. J. Med.* **297:**101–102.

64. Leport, C., J. L. Vilde, F. Bricaire, A. Cohen, B. Pangon, C. Gaudebout, and P. E. Valere. 1987. Fifty cases of late prosthetic valve endocarditis: improvement in prognosis over a 15 year period. *Br. Heart J.* **58:**66–71.

65. Liekweg, W. G., Jr., and L. J. Greenfield. 1977. Vascular prosthetic infections: collected experience and results of treatment. *Surgery* **81:**335–342.

66. Lucet, J. C., M. Herrmann, P. Rohner, R. Auckenthaler, F. A. Waldvogel, and D. P. Lew. 1990. Treatment of experimental foreign body infection caused by methicillin-resistant *Staphylococcus aureus. Antimicrob. Agents Chemother.* **34:**2312–2317.

67. Madison, J., K. Wang, F. L. Gobel, and J. E. Edwards. 1975. Prosthetic aortic valvular endocarditis. *Circulation* **51:**940–949.

68. Magilligan, D. J., Jr. 1986. Bioprosthetic valve endocarditis, p. 253–263. *In* D. J.

Magilligan, Jr., and E. L. Quinn (ed.), *Endocarditis: Medical and Surgical Management.* Marcel Dekker, New York.

69. **Magilligan, D. J., E. L. Quinn, and J. C. Davila.** 1977. Bacteremia, endocarditis, and the Hancock valve. *Ann. Thorac. Surg.* **24:**508–518.

70. **Maki, D. G., M. J. Bohn, S. M. Stolz, G. M. Kroncke, C. W. Acher, and P. D. Myerowitz.** 1992. Comparative study of cefazolin, cefamandole, and vancomycin for surgical prophylaxis in cardiac and vascular operations: a double-blind randomized trial. *J. Thorac. Cardiovasc. Surg.* **104:**1423–1434.

71. **Malone, J. M., W. S. Moore, G. Campagna, and B. Bean.** 1975. Bacteremic infectability of vascular grafts: the influence of pseudointimal integrity and duration of graft function. *Surgery* **78:**211–216.

72. **Malone, J. M., S. G. Lalka, K. E. McIntyre, V. M. Bernhard, and T. S. Pabst.** 1988. The necessity for long-term antibiotic therapy with positive arterial wall cultures. *J. Vasc. Surg.* **8:**262–267.

73. **Masur, H., and W. D. Johnson.** 1980. Prosthetic valve endocarditis. *J. Thorac. Cardiovasc. Surg.* **80:**31–37.

74. **Mayer, K. H., and S. C. Schoenbaum.** 1982. Evaluation and management of prosthetic valve endocarditis. *Prog. Cardiovasc. Dis.* **25:**43–54.

75. **Meyer, D. J., and D. N. Gerding.** 1988. Favorable prognosis of patients with prosthetic valve endocarditis caused by gram-negative bacilli of the HACEK group. *Am. J. Med.* **85:**104–107.

76. **Michelson, P. A., J. J. Plorde, K. P. Gordon, C. Hargiss, J. McLure, F. D. Schoenknecht, F. Condie, F. C. Tenover, and L. S. Tompkins.** 1985. Instability of antibiotic resistance in a strain of *Staphylococcus epidermidis* isolated from an outbreak of prosthetic valve endocarditis. *J. Infect. Dis.* **152:**50–58.

77. **Miller, J. H.** 1993. Partial replacement of an infected arterial graft by a new prosthetic polytetrafluoroethylene segment: a new therapeutic option. *J. Vasc. Surg.* **17:**546–558.

78. **Mixter, R. C., W. D. Turnipseed, D. J. Smith, Jr., et al.** 1989. Potential muscle flaps: a new technique for covering infected vascular grafts. *J. Vasc. Surg.* **9:**472–478.

79. **Moore-Gillon, J., S. J. Eykyn, and I. Phillips.** 1983. Prosthetic valve endocarditis. *Br. Med. J.* **287:**739–741.

80. **Mugge, A., W. G. Daniel, G. Frank, and P. R. Lichtlen.** 1989. Echocardiography in infective endocarditis: reassessment of prognostic implications of vegetation size determined by the transthoracic and the transesophageal approach. *J. Am. Coll. Cardiol.* **14:**631–638.

81. **Murray, B. E., A. W. Karchmer, and R. C. Moellering, Jr.** 1980. Diphtheroid prosthetic valve endocarditis: a study of clinical features and infecting organisms. *Am. J. Med.* **69:**838–848.

82. **Nunez, L., R. de la Llana, M. G. Aguado, A. Iglesias, J. L. Larrea, and D. Celemin.** 1983. Bioprosthetic valve endocarditis: indicators for surgical intervention. *Ann. Thorac. Surg.* **35:**262–270.

83. **Oakley, C. M.** 1987. Treatment of prosthetic valve endocarditis. *J. Antimicrob. Chemother.* **20:**181–186.

84. **O'Hara, P. J., N. R. Hertzer, E. G. Beven, and L. P. Krajewski.** 1986. Surgical management of infected abdominal aortic grafts: review of a 25 year experience. *J. Vasc. Surg.* **3:**725–731.

85. **Oster, H. A., and T. Q. Kong.** 1982. Bacillus cereus endocarditis involving a prosthetic valve. *South Med. J.* **75:**508–509.

86. **Platt, R., A. Munoz, J. Stella, S. VanDevanter, and J. K. Koster, Jr.** 1984. Antibiotic prophylaxis for cardiovascular surgery: efficacy with coronary artery bypass. *Ann. Intern. Med.* **101:**770–774.

87. **Quinones-Baldrich, W. J., J. J. Hermaneley, and W. S. Moore.** 1991. Long-term results following surgical management of aortic graft infection. *Arch. Surg.* **126:** 507–511.
88. **Rice, L. B., S. B. Calderwood, G. M. Eliopoulos, B. F. Farber, and A. W. Karchmer.** 1991. Enterococcal endocarditis: a comparison of prosthetic and native valve disease. *Rev. Infect. Dis.* **13:**1–7.
89. **Richardson, J. V., R. B. Karp, J. W. Kirklin, and W. E. Dismukes.** 1978. Treatment of infective endocarditis: a 10-year comparative analysis. *Circulation* **58:**589–597.
90. **Reilly, L. M., and J. Goldstone.** 1986. The infected aortic graft, p. 231–252. *In* J. J. Bergin and J. S. T. Yao (ed.), *Reoperative Arterial Surgery.* Grune & Stratton, New York.
91. **Rocchiccioli, C., J. Chastre, Y. Lecompte, I. Gandjbakhch, and C. Gibert.** 1986. Prosthetic valve endocarditis. *J. Thorac. Cardiovasc. Surg.* **92:**784–789.
92. **Rose, A. G.** 1986. Prosthetic valve endocarditis: a clinicopathological study of 31 cases. *S. Afr. Med. J.* **69:**441–445.
93. **Rossiter, S. J., E. B. Stinson, P. E. Oyer, D. C. Miller, J. N. Schapira, R. P. Martin, and N. E. Shumway.** 1978. Prosthetic valve endocarditis: comparison of heterograft tissue valves and mechanical valves. *J. Thorac. Cardiovasc. Surg.* **76:**795–803.
94. **Rouse, M. S., R. M. Wilcox, N. K. Henry, J. M. Steckelberg, and W. R. Wilson.** 1990. Ciprofloxacin therapy of experimental endocarditis caused by methicillin-resistant *Staphylococcus epidermidis. Antimicrob. Agents Chemother.* **34:**273–276.
95. **Rumisek, J. D., R. A. Albus, and J. S. Clarke.** 1985. Late Mycobacterium chelonei bioprosthetic valve endocarditis: activation of implanted contaminant? *Ann. Thorac. Surg.* **39:**277–279.
96. **Rutledge, R., J. Kim, and R. E. Applebaum.** 1985. Actuarial analysis of the risk of prosthetic valve endocarditis in 1,598 patients with mechanical and bioprosthetic valves. *Arch. Surg.* **120:**469–472.
97. **Saffle, J. R., P. Gardner, S. C. Schoenbaum, and W. Wild.** 1977. Prosthetic valve endocarditis: a case for prompt valve replacement. *J. Thorac. Cardiovasc. Surg.* **73:** 416–420.
98. **Sande, M. A., W. D. Johnson, E. W. Hook, and D. Kaye.** 1972. Sustained bacteremia in patients with prosthetic cardiac valves. *N. Engl. J. Med.* **286:**1067–1070.
99. **Santinga, J. T., M. Kirsh, and R. Fekety.** 1984. Factors affecting survival in prosthetic valve endocarditis: review of the effectiveness of prophylaxis. *Chest* **84:**471–475.
100. **Sett, S. S., M. P. J. Hudon, W. R. E. Jamieson, and A. W. Chow.** 1993. Prosthetic valve endocarditis: experience with porcine bioprostheses. *J. Thorac. Cardiovasc. Surg.* **105:**428–434.
101. **Shively, B. K., F. T. Gurule, C. A. Roland, J. H. Leggett, and N. B. Schiller.** 1991. Diagnostic value of transesophageal compared with transthoracic echocardiography in infective endocarditis. *J. Am. Coll. Cardiol.* **18:**391–397.
102. **Slama, T. G., S. J. Sklar, J. Misinski, and S. W. Fess.** 1986. Randomized comparison of cefamandole, cefazolin, and cefuroxime prophylaxis in open-heart surgery. *Antimicrob. Agents Chemother.* **29:**744–747.
103. **Slaughter, L., J. E. Morris, and A. Starr.** 1973. Prosthetic valvular endocarditis: a 12 year review. *Circulation* **47:**1319–1325.
104. **Sochowski, R. A., and K. L. Chan.** 1993. Implication of negative results on a monoplane transesophageal echocardiographic study in patients with suspected infective endocarditis. *J. Am. Coll. Cardiol.* **21:**216–221.
105. **Szilagyi, D. E.** 1979. Management of complications after arterial reconstruction. *Surg. Clin. North Am.* **59:**659–668.

106. **Szilagyi, D. E., R. F. Smith, J. P. Elliott, and M. P. Vrandecic.** 1972. Infection in arterial reconstruction with synthetic grafts. *Ann. Surg.* **176:**321–332.
107. **Taams, M. A., E. J. Gussenhoven, E. Bos, P. deJacgere, J. R. T. C. Roelandt, G. R. Sutherland, and N. Bom.** 1990. Enhanced morphological diagnosis in infective endocarditis by transesophageal echocardiography. *Br. Heart J.* **63:**109–113.
108. **Talkington, C. M., and J. E. Thompson.** 1982. Prevention and management of infected prostheses. *Surg. Clin. North Am.* **62:**515–530.
109. **Thomas, D., A. Mogahed, and J. P. Leclerc.** 1984. Prosthetic valve endocarditis caused by Trichosporon cutaneum. *Int. J. Cardiol.* **5:**83.
110. **Tompkins, L. S., B. J. Roessler, S. C. Redd, L. E. Markowitz, and M. L. Cohen.** 1988. Legionella prosthetic-valve endocarditis. *N. Engl. J. Med.* **318:**530–535.
111. **Torsello, G., W. Sandmann, A. Gehrt, and R. M. Jungblut.** 1993. In situ replacement of infected vascular prostheses with rifampin-soaked vascular grafts: early results. *J. Vasc. Surg.* **17:**768–773.
112. **Townsend, T. R., B. A. Reitz, W. B. Bilker, and J. G. Bartlett.** 1993. Clinical trial of cefamandole, cefazolin, and cefuroxime for antibiotic prophylaxis in cardiac operations. *J. Thorac. Cardiovasc. Surg.* **106:**664–670.
113. **Turina, M.** 1982. Prosthetic valve endocarditis. *Thorac. Cardiovasc. Surg.* **30:**350–353.
114. **Upshaw, C. B., Jr.** 1974. Penicillium endocarditis of aortic valve prosthesis. *J. Thorac. Cardiovasc. Surg.* **68:**428–431.
115. **van den Broek, P. J., A. S. Lampe, G. A. M. Berbee, J. Thompson, and R. P. Mouton.** 1985. Epidemic of prosthetic valve endocarditis caused by *Staphylococcus epidermidis. Br. Med. J.* **291:**949–950.
116. **Vazquez, G. J., and G. L. Archer.** 1980. Antibiotic therapy of experimental *Staphylococcus epidermidis* endocarditis. *Antimicrob. Agents Chemother.* **17:**280–285.
117. **Vlachakis, N. D., P. C. Gazes, and P. Hariston.** 1973. Nocardial endocarditis following mitral valve replacement. *Chest* **63:**276–278.
118. **Watanakunakorn, C.** 1979. Prosthetic valve infective endocarditis. *Prog. Cardiovasc. Dis.* **22:**181–192.
119. **Wilson, W. R.** 1977. Prosthetic valve endocarditis: incidence, anatomic location, cause, morbidity and mortality, p. 61–78. *In* R. J. Duma (ed.), *Infections of Prosthetic Heart Valves and Vascular Grafts: Prevention Diagnosis and Treatment.* University Park Press, Baltimore.
120. **Wilson, W. R., G. K. Danielson, E. R. Giuliani, and J. E. Geraci.** 1982. Prosthetic valve endocarditis. *Mayo Clin. Proc.* **57:**155–161.
121. **Wilson, W. R., J. E. Geraci, G. K. Danielson, R. L. Thompson, J. A. Spittell, Jr., J. A. Washington II, and E. R. Giuliani.** 1978. Anticoagulant therapy and central nervous system complications in patients with prosthetic valve endocarditis. *Circulation* **57:**1004–1007.
122. **Wilson, W. R., P. M. Jaumin, G. K. Danielson, E. R. Giuliani, J. A. Washington, and J. E. Geraci.** 1975. Prosthetic valve endocarditis. *Ann. Intern. Med.* **82:**751–756.

Infections Associated with Indwelling Medical Devices, 2nd ed.
Edited by Alan L. Bisno and Francis A. Waldvogel
© 1994 American Society for Microbiology, Washington, DC 20005

Chapter 10

Pacemaker Infections

F. Waldvogel

GENERAL ASPECTS OF PACEMAKER (PM) INFECTIONS

The field of cardiac pacing has expanded rapidly in recent years because of engineering improvements as well as progress in microprocess technology. Although the present PMs have a battery life span of 4 to 12 years, depending on current drain, both the broadening indications for PM implantation and the growth of the geriatric population increase the population subjected to PM surgery and hence at risk of PM infection—a rare but dreaded complication (1).

The PM is made of two essential components, i.e., the pulse generator (a power source with associated technical circuits, to deliver the electrical stimulus) and the insulated electrical conductor (a mixture of alloys with a sheath made of polyurethane var silicone) linked to its pacing electrode (either an endocardial or an epicardial lead) (1). PM infection has been defined as (i) local inflammation and abscess in the pulse generator pocket, (ii) erosion of the skin in the pacing system with subsequent concomitant infection, and (iii) fever with positive blood cultures in a patient with a PM and with no obvious other focus of infection (5). This definition is incomplete and obviously will miss some indolent cases of PM infections and those presenting with pericardial disease, and conversely, it may falsely diagnose PM infections in bacteremic patients (4). Basically, however, it is worth subdividing PM infections into those involving the pulse-generator pocket only (often contaminated during PM implantation or change), those involving the conducting system only (often due to bacteremic spread), and those involving all components of the implanted material (mostly cases due to surgical contamination).

F. Waldvogel • Department of Medicine, University Hospital, 1211 Gevena 14, Switzerland.

For the reasons inherent to the definitions mentioned above, it is difficult to obtain concordant figures regarding PM infections. Between 1968 and 1981, a prevalence of 0.13 to 12% has been reported (reviewed by Bluhm [2]). In another review of 18 PM analyses published between 1973 and 1979, the mean infection rate of 939 procedures was 2.9% (14). More recent data report a prevalence of 1 to 7% (19), with an increased risk at reintervention (25). A recent study aimed at evaluating specifically the complications after single- versus dual-chamber PM implantation in a series of 337 consecutive cases gave similar rates of infection for both procedures, i.e., 0.77% and 1 to 3%, respectively (13). Thus, one can conclude that PM infection has become a rather rare complication of PM implantation. Although no data are available, it can be surmised that the risk of infection decreases with time, since pocket infections are usually postsurgical and the conducting system will become progressively coated by a neoendothelium and fibrous tissue (see below).

The pathological changes induced by cardiac pacemakers have been recently reviewed in detail (6). Since both the generator and the conducting leads behave like foreign material, they are submitted to the biological conditions associated with foreign body infections described in chapter 1. Regarding the leads, it has been demonstrated that neoendothelialization begins at implantation and that fibrosis becomes evident at 6 to 8 weeks (17, 21). *Staphylococcus* colonization of both the plastic electrode sheaths and the pulse generator has been studied both in clinical infection (12, 18) and experimentally (11); in both conditions, adherence of the organism to the artificial surface and heavy production of slime have been demonstrated. Thus, one can assume that PM component infections will follow the same pathophysiology as other foreign body infections, until the prosthetic surface becomes covered by neoendothelium and/or fibrous tissue. It is worth mentioning that the intravenous PM leads are subjected to additional problems conducive to bacterial contamination because of their close contact with the thrombogenic proteins of the coagulation cascade.

CLINICAL PRESENTATION

The clinical presentation of PM infection will depend on many variables including the site of infection (pulse-generator pocket and/or conducting or electrode systems), the type of electrode implantation (intraventricular or epicardial), the mode of infection (local contamination or secondary to bacteremic spread), the organism involved, the complications following the primary infectious event (e.g., mediastinitis, endocarditis). No comprehensive review is available regarding all of these various modes of presentations. Schematically, the clinical problem can be summarized as follows.

In the case of pulse-generator pocket infection, the mode of presentation corresponds to a localized prosthetic infection: localized edema and pain, possibly complicated by local ulceration and fistula formation, are the hallmarks of infection. Low-grade fever, chills, or even a septic state can be part of the clinical picture. Under some conditions, infection can be indolent and is suspected because of a positive blood culture without any other focus of infection.

In electrode infections with an epicardial implantation, the above described symptoms and signs may be accompanied by pericarditis and complicated by mediastinitis. Pleural effusions and bronchocutaneous fistula have also been described (for review, see reference 6).

With transvenously inserted PMs, the lead may theoretically become infected without concomitant contamination of the generator pocket. This seems to be rare, although osteomyelitis of the clavicle and of the first rib, associated with trauma at the time of catheterization, has been described (22). Cases of localized transvenous lead infections are probably rarely reported as PM infections, since they present clinically as primary nosocomial bacteremias. Secondary infection of the intravenous PM leads is described below.

An interesting problem is the evaluation of the frequency of endocarditis secondary to transvenous-ventricular PM lead infections. A recent French study identified 58 such cases over a 16-year period, of which only 27 cases could be formally confirmed by echocardiography, surgery, or autopsy as bona fide endocarditis (10). Fortunately, this complication remains a rarity—0.15% of the implantations and changes of PM pulse generators (10). Most of these patients presented with chills, fever, positive blood cultures, and pulmonary emboli. Tricuspid valve insufficiency could be demonstrated in 30 to 50% of the cases (10).

The clinical challenge of sustained gram-negative bacteremia with an endocardial PM has been shown to be unrelated to the pacing system and is rapidly cured with antibiotics alone without removal of the pacing leads. In the case of staphylococcal bacteremia, whether related or not to the pacing system, it had to be assumed that the pacing leads were infected; the rate of recovery from the wires was 82% and 75% under either condition, similar to that of the pulse generator (80%). These numbers are corroborated by the study by Choo et al. (5), which showed an 88% recovery rate under similar conditions. The most common portal of entry in staphylococcal bacteremia is probably the subcutaneous site of implantation of the PM. Extension along the wire into the vascular system is the best explanation for the probably subsequent, sustained bacteremia. Hematogenous colonization of the PM conducting system during the course of a bacteremia from a distant focus has often been evoked as a pathogenic mechanism but rarely been documented (7, 8). It is probably an exceptional mechanism, since the intravenous pacing system is rapidly covered by a neoendothelium and fibrous tissue, which precludes the foreign surface from being coated by microorganisms (chapter 1).

Besides standard bacteriological techniques, few laboratory tests make a decisive contribution to the diagnosis of PM infections. Recently, anecdotal reports of recognition of PM lead infections by transesophageal echocardiography (24, 27) and by percutaneous intravascular and intracardiac ultrasound examination (9) have been published. These techniques, as well as various neutrophil-labelling techniques, will probably remain exceptional procedures for exceptional clinical situations, without possible statistical validation.

MICROBIOLOGY

In the light of our present understanding of prosthesis-associated infections, it can be predicted that most infections will be due to gram-positive organisms. This is indeed the case. In his analysis of 11 series of PM infections, Bluhm (2) showed that *Staphylococcus aureus* and *S. epidermidis* encompassed 75%of the causative organisms in 180 infections. Other gram-negative organisms were members of the family *Enterobacteriaceae*. As for other prosthetic infections, an ever-growing list of unusual microorganisms responsible for individual infections have been described, including *Candida albicans, Aspergillus* species, and *Petrellidium boydii* (for review, see reference 26). Interestingly enough, and despite the fact that we are typically dealing with a hospital-based procedure, no report has been published yet regarding nosocomial epidemics or particular resistance problems in this setting.

TREATMENT

Once PM infection is identified and the responsible organism isolated, the next step is to make an appropriate choice of antibiotics. This choice will also be determined by the susceptibility studies performed. Under most circumstances, a β-lactamase-resistant penicillin should be administered in "septicemia" dosage by the intravenous route. This is as far as the consensus goes; neither the duration of antibiotic treatment nor the necessity for the removal of the power generator and conduction leads has been subjected to controlled studies, thus leaving space for personal interpretations and decisions.

Basically, PM infection has to be considered as a serious illness with high morbidity and mortality. It would be—in my opinion—unwise to give antibiotic therapy of less than 4 weeks duration in most cases. After cessation of therapy, the patient should be carefully monitored over several months regarding recurrence of infection.

If the infectious process has been clearly demonstrated to reside in the pulse-generator pocket only, the generator should be removed and another one implanted at a distant site. The timing of this intervention has never been defined, but it would be prudent to plan the operation early in the therapeutic program. The situation is more complicated if the conducting system and/or leads are infected. Under such circumstances, it is generally illusory to cure the infection without removing the whole pacing system, including the PM leads. Such interventions have to be weighed against each patient's life expectancy and the risk of the operative procedure. Indications for lead extraction must therefore pointedly be subdivided into mandatory (life-threatening situation), necessary (significant morbidity), and discretionary (optional) (3), taking into account that failure to remove infected leads can result in a mortality as high as 66% (20). Another study showed that lead retention after infection of the pacing system resulted in a 51% complication rate, the majority of which were major (e.g., septicemia, superior vena cava syndrome) (16). In their study on sustained bacteremia with permanent endocardial pacemakers, Camus et al. (4) showed that in staphylococcal infection, cure was only achieved when the whole pacemaker system was removed. Whereas replacement of a new pulse generator at another site does not cause any major difficulties, removal of the PM leads by external traction is associated with many risks to the patient, including chest pain, bradycardia, ventricular arrhythmias, invagination and avulsion of the right ventricle, lesions to the tricuspid valves, and tamponade (for review, see reference 15). The various techniques for lead extraction have been described in detail in several recent reviews (3, 15, 20, 26). Under some circumstances, cardiopulmonary bypass has been used to remove the infected material (23). Whether the leads should be removed under any circumstances is not settled. In pocket infections, the original lead may be left in place and the connector end may be moved to the new generator site. In most circumstances, however, it will be difficult to exclude lead contamination, and removal of the whole pacemaker system may be indicated.

In conclusion, PM infection will require a careful evaluation of the site of infection (generator, leads, or both) and identification of the responsible organism. Isolation of a gram-positive organism from the PM surroundings or from the bloodstream strongly suggests PM infection. Parenteral administration of "septicemic" doses of the appropriate antibiotic should be given for 4 weeks. Removal of PM components warrants careful discussion and evaluation. Under most circumstances, removal is indicated, with remote implantation of the PM generator and placement of epicardial leads, provided that transvenous electrodes were used initially.

PREVENTION OF PM INFECTIONS

In his very thorough work on PM infections, Bluhm (2) used several prophylactic regimens to show their efficacy in generator implantations or replacements. In a single-blinded study, 2 g of cloxacillin intravenously, 1 to 2 h preoperatively, followed by 4 g/day intravenously for 2 days and 4 g/day orally for another 8 days was highly effective. This study can now be criticized in the light of our present knowledge regarding too high an infection rate in the control group (14%) and an abnormally long treatment period. Finally, during a subsequent validation period with the same apparently efficacious prophylaxis regimen, an infection rate as high as 4% was found. At present, no well-controlled study has allowed firmer conclusions regarding prevention of infection during PM replacement or implantation. In the light of the above data and of the information accrued regarding indwelling prosthetic material, it would seem prudent to administer preventive antistaphylococcal agents to achieve appropriate tissue levels during the operative procedure and shortly thereafter. There is no indication to apply a similar preventive approach to prevent PM infection during medical or surgical manipulations at a distant, potentially infected site conducive to bacteremia. Finally, there is no need to remove uninfected, abandoned intracardiac leads, because the likelihood of subsequent infection is remote.

CONCLUSION AND REMAINING PROBLEMS

PM infections remain a dreaded, but fortunately relatively rare, complication of PM insertion and replacement. Adequate preventive methods (choice of antibiotics, duration, etc.) still require better documentation. Identification of staphylococcal carrier states may help to define patients at higher risk. Once the catastrophic event, i.e., infection, has occurred, parenteral antibiotic treatment for a prolonged period is mandatory. The risks inherent to the removal and reimplantation procedures have to be evaluated individually in the light of the patient's comorbidities, life expectancy, and indications for permanent pacing. A better understanding of the unresponsiveness to antibiotics demonstrated by bacteria associated with the indwelling foreign material and improved treatment modalities may, one day, obviate the traumatic intervention of PM change.

REFERENCES

1. **Barold, S. S., and D. P. Zipeas,** 1992. Cardiac pacemakers and antiarrhythmic devices, p. 726–755. In E. Braunwald (ed.), *Heart Disease,* 4th ed. The W. B. Saunders Co., Philadelphia.
2. **Bluhm, G.** 1985. Pacemaker infections. *Acta Med. Scand. Suppl.* **699:**1–62.
3. **Byrd, C. L., S. J. Schwartz, and N. Hedin.** 1992. Lead extraction. *Cardiol. Clin.* **10:** 735–746.
4. **Camus, C. H., C. Leport, F. Raffi, C. H. Michelet, F. Cartier, and J. L. Vilde.** 1993. Sustained bacteremia in 26 patients with a permanent endocardial pacemaker: assessment of wire removal. *Clin. Infect. Dis.* **17:**46–55.
5. **Choo, M. H., D. R. Holmes, B. J. Gersh, et al.** 1981. Permanent pacemaker infections: characterization and management. *Am. J. Cardiol.* **48:**559–564.
6. **Cox, J. N.** 1994. Pathology of cardiac pacemakers and central catheters. *Curr. Top. Pathol.* **86:**200–257.
7. **Glock, Y., J. Sabatier, M. Salvador-Mazenq, and P. Puel.** 1986. Les endocardites sur electrodes endocavitaires de stimulateurs cardiaques: a propos de 7 cas. *Arch. Mal. Coeur Vaiss.* **4:**483–488.
8. **Harthorne, J. W.** 1985. Complications of permanent cardiac pacemakers: in reply. *N. Engl. J. Med.* **313:**1086–1087. (Letter.)
9. **Kerber, S., C. Fechtrup, U. Karbenn, and G. Breithart.** 1993. Nachweis einer Schrittmacherelektroden-infektion mittels intravasckularem Ultraschall. *Z. Kardiol.* **82:**172–174.
10. **Kugener, H., J. L. Rey, C. Tribouilloy, J. S. Hermide, G. Jarry, P. Anivee, and Y. Maingourd.** 1993. Endocarditis infectieuses sur sondes de stimulation endocavitaire permanents: interet de l'echocardiographic et revue de la litterature. *Ann. Cardiol. Angeiol.* **42:**331–338.
11. **Marrie, T. J., and J. W. Costerton.** 1984. Morphology of bacterial attachment to cardiac pacemaker leads and powerpacks. *J. Clin. Microbiol.* **19:**911.
12. **Marrie, T. J., J. Nelligan, and J. W. Costerton.** 1982. A scanning and transmission electron microscopic study of an infected endocardial pacemaker lead. *Circulation* **66:** 1339–1341.
13. **Mueller, X., H. Sadeghi, and L. Kappenberger.** 1990. Complications after single versus dual chamber pacemaker implantation. *PACE* **13:**711–714.
14. **Muers, M. F., A. G. Arnold, and P. Sleight.** 1981. Prophylactic antibiotics for cardiac pacemaker implantation. A prospective trial. *Br. Heart J.* **46:**539–544.
15. **Myers, M. R., V. Parsonnet, and A. D. Bernstein.** 1991. Extraction of implanted transvenous pacing leads: a review of a persistent clinical problem. *Am Heart J.* **3:** 881–887.
16. **Parry, G., J. Goudevenos, S. Jameson, P. C. Adams, and R. G. Gold.** 1991. Complications associated wih retained pacemaker leads. *PACE* **14:**1251–1256.
17. **Parsonnet, V., L. Gilbert, and I. R. Zucker.** 1973. The natural history of pacemaker wires. *J Thorac. Cardiovasc. Surg.* **65:**315–322.

18. Peters, G., F. Saborowski, R. Locci, and G. Pulverer. 1984. Investigations on staphylococcal infection of transvenous endocardial pacemaker electrodes. *Am. Heart J.* **108:** 359–365.
19. Phibbs, B., and H. J. L. Marriott. 1985. Complications of permanent transvenous pacing. *N. Engl. J. Med.* **312:**1428–1432.
20. Rettig, G., P. Doeneche, S. Sen, et al. 1979. Complications with retained transvenous pacemaker electrodes. *Am. Heart J.* **98:**587–594.
21. Robboy, S. J., J. W. Harthorne, R. C. Leinbach, C. A. Sanders, and W. G. Austen. 1969. Autopsy findings with permanent perivenous pacemakers. *Ciculation* **39:**495–501.
22. Rosenfeld, L. E. 1985. Osteomyelitis of the first rib presenting as a cold abscess nine months after subclavian venous catheterization. *PACE* **8:**897–899.
23. Rubio-Alvarez, J., D. Duran-Munoz, J. Sierra-Quiroga, and J. B. Garcia-Bengochera. 1988. Right heart endocarditis and endocardial pacemakers (correspondence). *Ann. Thorac. Surg.* **48:**147.
24. Van Camp, G., and J. L. Vandendossche. 1991. Recognition of pacemaker lead infection by transesophageal echocardiography. *Br. Heart J.* **65:**229–230.
25. Wade S., and C. G. Cobbs. 1988. Infections in cardiac pacemakers. *Curr. Clin. Infect. Dis.* **9:**44–61.
26. Wilson, H. A., T. R. Downes, J. S. Julian, W. L. White, and E. F. Haponik. 1993. Candida endocarditis: a treatable form of pacemaker infection. *Chest* **103:**283–284.
27. Zehender, M., C. Buchner, A. Geibel, W. Kasper, T. Meinertz, and H. Just. 1989. Diagnosis of hidden pacemaker lead sepsis by transesophageal echocardiography and a new technique for lead extraction. *Am. Heart J.* **118:**1050–1053.

Infections Associated with Indwelling Medical Devices, 2nd ed.
Edited by Alan L. Bisno and Francis A. Waldvogel
© 1994 American Society for Microbiology, Washington, DC 20005

Chapter 11

Prosthetic Joint Infections

James M. Steckelberg and Douglas R. Osmon

Prosthetic joint implantation is among the most remarkable advances in surgery and medicine to occur during the last three decades. Although the results of this procedure are usually highly satisfactory (42, 50, 137), infection was recognized early as a serious cause of postoperative morbidity and prosthesis failure (32, 35, 166) (Fig. 1). Infection of the prosthesis occurs in only a small proportion of patients (5, 59, 95), but this dreaded complication results in major morbidity due to pain, immobility, failure and loss of the prosthesis, reoperation, and in some cases loss of limb or life. Successful treatment of these infections is difficult, usually requiring both multiple operative interventions and prolonged antimicrobial therapy to achieve microbial sterilization as well as a satisfactory functional result. Other implanted orthopedic foreign bodies, including a variety of fixation devices for the stabilization of fractures, are also subject to infection. While the pathogenesis and general principles of treatment are similar in many ways to those of prosthetic joints, a full discussion of these infections is beyond the scope of this chapter.

EPIDEMIOLOGY

Mechanisms of Infection

Two major mechanisms by which microorganisms cause prosthetic joint infection have been postulated. Microorganisms may colonize the prosthesis at the time of implantation, either through direct inoculation

James M. Steckelberg and Douglas R. Osmon • Division of Infectious Diseases, Orthopedic Infectious Diseases Focus Group, Mayo Clinic and Mayo Foundation, Rochester, Minnesota 55905.

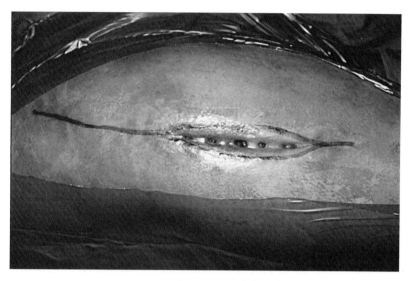

Figure 1. Infected total hip arthroplasty with four draining sinus tracts.

during tissue or implant manipulation or as a result of airborne contamination of the wound (84). Alternatively, microorganisms may reach a previously sterile implant either through hematogenous seeding during a bacteremia or through direct contiguous spread from an adjacent focus of infection (89). Knowledge of the proportion of cases due to these different mechanisms is especially important in anticipating rational approaches to the prevention of infection.

Unfortunately, because of the sometimes long latency period between the onset of infection and the onset of symptoms and/or diagnosis, many infections are difficult to classify etiologically except by arbitrary definitions or assumptions (10, 144). It is clear, for example, that prosthetic joint infection, like osteomyelitis, may remain asymptomatic for many years before the late occurrence of symptoms and that conversely, hematogenous infection may occur early, in the immediate postoperative period. The time after implantation at which diagnosis of infection is first made is therefore inadequate by itself to categorize the mechanism of infection. Consequently the relative importance of operating room-acquired infection compared with hematogenous seeding has remained controversial (108).

Despite this controversy, several lines of evidence suggest that the majority of prosthetic joint infections are acquired in the operating room. First, clinical trials document that diverse types of perioperative prophylaxis, including systemic and local antimicrobial prophylaxis as well as ultraclean operating room environments, all designed to reduce intraoperative contamination of the prosthesis, significantly decrease the incidence of prosthetic joint infection (64, 83, 93). Secondly, systemic antimicrobial prophylaxis has been shown to also reduce the incidence of late prosthetic joint infection (31), further supporting the concept that even though a prosthetic joint infection is not diagnosed until years after prosthesis insertion, the infection may be due to intraoperative contamination. Finally, several investigators in both retrospective and prospective studies have reported a low proportion of cases acquired through hematogenous seeding when large series of patients have been critically reviewed. For example, among 490 total hip arthroplasty infections in Sweden, a hematogenous source was found for only 33 (7%) (5); in Britain, Ainscow and Denham (6) prospectively followed 1,112 total joint arthroplasties for a mean of 6 years and observed just 22 deep infections, only 3 of which were attributable to hematogenous seeding.

Incidence

Progress in understanding the epidemiology of orthopedic prosthesis infections has been hampered by methodological problems in the published literature, including the reliance on case series rather than well-designed epidemiological cohort studies, the frequent lack of an explicit case definition, incomplete case ascertainment and selection biases, and especially failure to account for differences in duration or completeness of follow-up, resulting in confusion between incidence (a rate) and risk (a proportion) (82). Estimates of cumulative risk (a percentage) should be interpreted or compared with caution, since it is quite difficult to estimate the true incidence rate or annual risk when the denominator for the rate (person-years) is unspecified. Studies that have longer follow-up will ultimately report higher cumulative risk, even when the true incidence in the study cohort is low; failure to account for differences in completeness and duration of follow-up between treatment groups will inevitably lead to erroneous conclusions (82).

The overall rate (hazard) of prosthetic joint infection is highest in the first 6 months postoperatively and declines continuously thereafter. In our experience, the combined incidence rates of total hip and knee arthroplasty infection during the first postoperative year, during the second postoperative year, and after 2 years are approximately 6.5, 3.2, and 1.4 infections per 1,000 joint-years, respectively (unpublished observations). The higher early incidence and subsequent declining rate of infection over time after implantation likely reflects a combination of the effects of the predominance of operating room-acquired infection (as discussed above), variable delays in symptom onset and diagnosis of infection after implantation, and the increasing resistance of prostheses to hematogenous seeding over time (149). The rate of total knee arthroplasty infection is approximately twofold higher than the rate of hip arthroplasty infection at any time period after implantation (unpublished observations). There are insufficient data currently to accurately compare the true incidence rates of infection of arthroplasties in other anatomic locations, but risks (as opposed to incidence rates), with variable follow-up periods, of 7 to 9% for elbows, 1% for shoulders, 2.4% for wrists, and 2.4% for ankles have been reported (134).

Risk Factors

Host factors

A number of host characteristics have been implicated either anecdotally or in controlled studies as factors increasing the risk for prosthetic joint infection (see chapter 1). The primary factors predisposing to infection appear not to be systemic humoral or cellular immune defects but rather local abnormalities of host defenses, primarily related to the presence of the foreign body itself and the opportunities for and degree of exposure of the prosthesis to microorganisms. Systemic immunodeficiency states have been associated with unusual orthopedic infections (22), but opportunistic pathogens are notably uncommon causes of prosthetic joint infection.

Among potential host factors predisposing to prosthesis infection, prior joint surgery, perioperative wound complications, and rheumatoid arthritis are consistently observed and well established. Poss and colleagues (124), in a review of 4,240 large joint arthroplasties with a mean follow-up of 2.5 to 3.5 years, found that the risk of deep infection was eightfold higher among patients undergoing a revision total hip arthroplasty than among patients with primary arthroplasty. Similarly, Ahnfelt et al. found that the relative risk of deep infection increased with the number of prior hip operations and was approximately sixfold higher among hips with five prior surgeries than among those with no prior operations (5). Patients who have undergone prior knee procedures and who subsequently undergo a total knee arthroplasty are at two- to fourfold increased risk of subsequent deep infection (133, 165). The reasons for the increased risk of infection after revision surgery remain unknown.

Postoperative wound healing complications, including "superficial" infection, hematomas, delayed healing, necrosis of the wound edge, and dehiscence, occur commonly among patients who ultimately manifest deep infection and are an important risk factor for subsequent deep infection (11, 120, 124, 133, 171). In one study, 25 of 26 patients who developed perioperative deep infections had a history of postoperative wound healing problems (124). In a carefully analyzed prospective study with short-term (1 year) follow-up, Wymenga et al. found that although multiple indicators of poor wound healing were associated with an increased risk of joint infection in univariate analyses, only superficial wound infection per se, defined as erythema more than 1 cm from the incision, and an unhealed wound at discharge were independently associated with an increased risk of deep infection in multivariate analyses (171). The relative risk of joint infection among patients with wound healing problems was increased from 13- to 20-fold after total knee arthroplasty and from 22- to 52-fold after total hip arthroplasty.

A number of studies have demonstrated higher risk of prosthesis infection among patients with rheumatoid arthritis, with a relative risk increased approximately two- to fourfold, compared with that of patients with osteoarthritis (41, 47, 68, 124, 138, 171). This increased risk is less evident in studies with shorter follow-up (124, 171). Whether the increased risk of prosthetic joint infection among rheumatoid arthritis patients relates to the greater frequency of early wound infection (163), the greater prevalence of multiple joint surgeries, higher rates of skin and wound colonization with staphylococcal species, greater prevalence of skin ulcerations and skin infection, use of T-cell-suppressive agents, or the immunological abnormalities of rheumatoid arthritis itself cannot yet be answered with certainty.

Other host characteristics identified as risk factors for prosthesis infection in some studies but not in others include diabetes mellitus, the use of steroids, obesity, extreme age, joint dislocation, poor nutrition, distant infection, psoriasis, hemophilia, sickle cell hemoglobinopathy, joint implantation for malignancy, and prior septic arthritis (1, 47, 48, 51, 61, 66, 71, 81, 97, 104, 124, 147, 152, 171). The data supporting an increased risk associated with these factors are less consistent than the findings associated with prior surgery, wound complications, or rheumatoid arthritis.

Implant factors

As previously mentioned, prostheses at different anatomic sites are associated with different risks of deep infection. However, confirmation of these findings in studies utilizing formal epidemiological tools that control for potential confounders including severity of comorbid illnesses (53) is lacking. Furthermore, even at the same anatomic site, different types of prostheses seem to carry different risks of infection. For example, Poss and colleagues found that metal-to-metal hinged knee prostheses had a 20-fold increased risk of infection, compared with that of metal-to-plastic knee prostheses (124). It has been speculated that this increased risk of infection may be due to the deleterious effects of the metal debris released by these implants on local immune defense mechanisms (see below).

PATHOGENESIS

Like that of other infections of implanted materials, the pathogenesis of prosthetic joint infection involves a complex interplay among host factors, microbial factors, and the biology of foreign implanted materials. The distribution of microorganisms causing prosthetic joint infections differs from the distribution of commensal and pathogenic microorganisms that would be expected to contact these biomaterials by random exposure, through either direct inoculation or hematogenous seeding. A common characteristic of microorganisms that are pathogenic for orthopedic appliances is, however, their ability to adhere to these foreign materials (59) (see chapters 1 to 3).

Implant Factors

A number of recent reviews provide an excellent overview of the chemical and physical properties of various biomaterials, including metal alloys, affecting the potential for microbial adhesion and infection (9, 38, 39, 59). As is the case with biomaterials implanted at other sites, the presence of a joint prosthesis significantly lowers the number of bacteria required to establish infection. Southwood et al. demonstrated in a rabbit model of prosthetic hip replacement that only a few *Staphylococcus aureus* inoculated at the time of joint replacement were required for the development of infection, but bacteremic seeding 3 weeks after implantation was significantly more difficult (149).

The complex host responses to the presence of metal alloy and polymers commonly used in orthopedic implants have been extensively studied. An inflammatory reaction typically occurs in response to the metallic particulate and ionic debris released from arthroplasty components (13, 141, 142). The response to cement appears to be more marked than the response to metallic debris (13). The T cell immunological response to prosthesis-associated infection differs from the host response observed in sterile prosthesis-associated inflammation, reactive synovitis, or rheumatoid synovitis (141). While an increased risk of bland loosening may occur because of an exuberant host sterile inflammatory reaction, this reaction has also been hypothesized to decrease local immunocompetence and thus predispose to infection. Possible mechanisms include macrophage and neutrophil exhaustion due to oxidative preemption by reaction to sterile debris, resulting in diminished killing capacity in the presence of implanted biomaterials (56, 57, 59, 60, 73, 100, 142, 172). Unpolymerized polymethylmethacrylate cement has also been shown in vitro to inhibit phagocyte, lymphocyte, and complement function (115, 117–119, 121). In vivo polymerization has been shown, in an experimental dog model, to reduce the number of bacteria required to establish bone infection, compared with that of prepolymerized polymethylmethacrylate or metal foreign bodies (21, 117).

In addition to the promotion of bacterial adherence and inhibition of local immune mechanisms, prosthetic arthroplasty biomaterials may also impair the activity of antimicrobial agents against microorganisms in the vicinity of the foreign body (57, 103, 107). While physical penetration through extracellular glycocalyx barriers may partially explain this phenomenon, other mechanisms have also been postulated, including phenotypic changes in adherent microorganisms (59, 142).

MICROBIOLOGY

Several investigators have published data on the microbiology of prosthetic joint infection (67, 125, 140). However, because of a lack of a uniform definition of infection, different methods of intraoperative culture ascertainment, variable reporting of microbiological data, small sample size, and a variety of selection biases among different investigations, these data are difficult to interpret.

We have recently studied 1,033 cases of total hip and total knee prosthetic arthroplasty infections seen at the Mayo Clinic between 1969 and 1991, which were classified as definite infection according to a strict case definition. A case was defined as a definite prosthetic joint infection if at least one of the following criteria were satisfied: (i) two or more cultures from sterile joint aspirates or intraoperative cultures were positive for the same organism, (ii) purulence was observed at the time of surgical inspection, (iii) acute inflammation consistent with infection was present on histopathologic examination of intracapsular tissue, or (iv) a sinus tract that communicates with the joint space was present. The pathogens identified in these cases are shown in Table 1.

The majority of infections (61%) are caused by aerobic gram-positive cocci, most commonly S. aureus, coagulase-negative staphylococci, beta-hemolytic streptococci, viridans group streptococci, and enterococci. Aerobic gram-negative bacilli including members of the family Enterobac-

Table 1. Microbiology of 1,033 prosthetic joint infections[a] seen at Mayo Clinic from 1969 to 1991

Microorganism(s)	No. (%) of PJI[b]
Coagulase-negative staphylococci	254 (25)
S. aureus	240 (23)
Polymicrobial	147 (14)
Gram-negative bacilli	114 (11)
Streptococci[c]	79 (8)
Unknown[d]	83 (8)
Anaerobes	62 (6)
Enterococci	29 (3)
Other microorganisms	25 (2)
Total	1,033 (100)

[a] All cases met case definition of definite infection. See text for discussion.
[b] PJI, prosthetic joint infections.
[c] Includes beta-hemolytic streptococci and viridans group streptococci.
[d] Includes cases in which there was no growth on routine bacterial cultures, routine bacterial cultures were not obtained, or microbiological information was not available.

teriaceae (*Escherichia coli, Proteus mirabilis,* and others) and *Pseudomonas aeruginosa* cause infection less frequently. Anaerobes such as peptostreptococci account for 6% of infections in our series, consistent with other investigators' experience (67, 125). *Bacteroides* spp. are an unusual cause of anaerobic infection. Polymicrobial infections account for 14% of cases.

Rare microbial causes of prosthetic joint infection that have been reported and should be considered in the correct clinical and epidemiological setting include *Haemophilus parainfluenzae* (126), *Pasteurella multocida* (110), *Candida* spp. (157), *Brucella melitensis* (2), *Mycobacterium tuberculosis* (168), *Mycobacterium fortuitum* (17), *Echinococcus* spp. (159), *Gemella haemolysans* (43), *Yersinia enterocolitica* (109), *Listeria monocytogenes* (7), *Aspergillus* spp. (8), and *Mycoplasma hominis* (148).

Although some authors have suggested that the microbiology of prosthetic joint infection may vary with time after implantation (67, 125), the proportion of cases due to any one particular microorganism in 130 primary total hip arthroplasty infections seen at our institution between 1969 and 1987 was not significantly different between early and late infections (Table 2) (29). This information suggests that the mechanism of infection of early and late postoperative infections may be similar. If, on the other hand, hematogenous infections were the major source of late infections, one would expect to see an increased proportion of site-specific pathogens in later postoperative infections. These data are also useful in guiding empirical antimicrobial therapy while waiting for the results of cultures and antimicrobial susceptibility testing (see below).

Table 2. Microbiology of early and late primary THA infections at the Mayo Clinic from 1969 to 1987

Microorganism(s)	No. (%) of infections		
	Early[a]	Late[b]	Total
Coagulase-negative staphylococci	12 (18)	10 (15)	22 (17)
S. aureus	18 (28)	17 (26)	35 (27)
Other	35 (54)	38 (58)	73 (56)
Total	65 (100)	65 (100)	130 (100)

[a] 0–24 mo.
[b] >24 mo.

DIAGNOSIS

The clinical presentation of prosthetic joint infection is highly variable, ranging from the syndrome of acute septic arthritis with joint pain and erythema, swelling, fever, and systemic symptoms to a syndrome of indolent loosening and chronic pain, which is difficult to distinguish from bland loosening on the basis of symptoms and clinical examination alone. A fulminant presentation is more common with virulent organism such as *S. aureus* or pyogenic beta-hemolytic streptococci, while a chronic indolent course is more typical of infection with less-virulent micoorganisms such as coagulase-negative staphylococci. Laboratory, radiographic, and scintigraphic evaluations are most helpful in the latter situation in order to distinguish infection from bland loosening preoperatively and thus provide an appropriate basis for anticipating operative decisions such as staged reimplantation. What follows is a discussion of the utility of various diagnostic tests used to diagnose prosthetic joint infection.

Laboratory Studies

The leukocyte count and the erythrocyte sedimentation rate are the two most commonly used laboratory tests in the diagnosis of prosthetic joint infection. Unfortunately neither of these tests has a positive or negative predictive value sufficiently high to allow the physician to rely on the results of these tests alone to predict the presence or absence of infection (36).

Radiologic Studies

The principal imaging modalities useful for the detection of infection of a prosthetic joint include plain radiographs or tomograms, arthro-

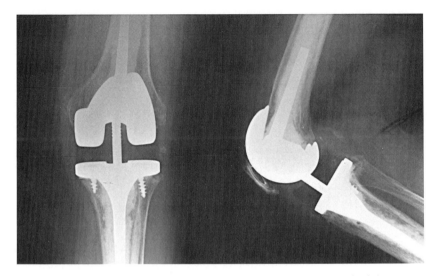

Figure 2. Plain radiograph of an infected TKA illustrating lucency at the bone-cement interface of both the femoral and tibial components.

grams, and radioisotopic imaging, particularly indium and technetium (^{99m}Tc) scanning. Abnormalities associated with infection on plain radiography are not specific for infection but may include loosening of the prosthesis, lucency at the bone-cement interface, periostitis, or other evidence of osteomyelitis (Fig. 2) (36, 87). Arthrograms (or sinograms in the presence of a sinus tract) may demonstrate communication between the joint space and the bone-cement interface, thus confirming the presence of a loose prosthesis (87). Nuclear scintigraphy may detect periprosthetic inflammation and suggest infection on the basis of characteristic combinations and timing of abnormalities. Technetium bone scanning, while sensitive for infection, lacks specificity and is frequently abnormal in inflammation because of arthritis, fractures, previous surgery, and heterotopic bone formation as well as infection. Johnson et al. reported an accuracy of 65% for the detection of prosthesis infection by indium leukocyte scanning alone (74). The accuracy of scintigraphy was increased to 93% when sequential technetium and indium scanning were correlated (Fig. 3). The advantages and disadvantages of available scintigraphic imaging techniques have recently been reviewed (116, 129, 161).

Microbiological Studies

Optimal antimicrobial therapy depends on identification of the etiologic micoorganism(s) and susceptibility testing. Adequate deep culture

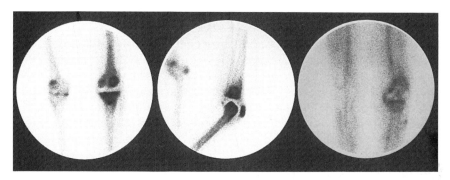

Figure 3. Technetium-99 bone scan and indium-labelled leukocyte scan demonstrating uptake around both components of the infected TKA shown in Fig. 2.

specimen collection and handling, preferably without recent antimicrobial pretreatment, is therefore essential. Multiple positive cultures, either from aspiration or from intraoperatively obtained tissue, are diagnostic and in our experience provide the single most useful diagnostic and therapeutic information. Cultures of drainage from sinus tracts do not reliably identify the etiologic microorganism(s) (88).

Recently the usefulness of a single positive culture from a sterile joint aspiration for the diagnosis of prosthetic joint infection was reviewed (36). A positive culture in this setting has an average sensitivity of 68%, specificity of 85%, and accuracy of 79%. Surveillance cultures (that is, cultures obtained intraoperatively when there is no clinical suspicion of infection) have very low predictive value in the setting of primary arthroplasties (111). The predictive value of a single positive surveillance culture at the time of revision arthroplasty for a failed prosthesis is unknown; such a result requires careful correlation with the clinical context.

Because of the critical importance of making a microbiological diagnosis, in most nonacute cases antimicrobial therapy should be withheld until all aspirate and/or intraoperative specimens for culture have been obtained from the joint. If antimicrobial therapy has already been started, it should be stopped when possible for 10 to 14 days prior to any diagnostic procedure, to avoid false-negative culture results. As much fluid for culture as possible should be obtained at the time of diagnostic joint aspiration. If sterile saline is used for aspiration, a nonbacteriostatic formulation should be used. Furthermore, when prosthesis debridement or removal is performed, the surgeon should obtain multiple tissue samples. Intraoperative cultures should include tissue from the bone-cement interface, if possible, as well as samples of any purulence that may be present (132).

All microbiological specimens should be sent promptly to the microbiology laboratory and processed as recently reviewed (62).

We suggest routinely obtaining specimens to culture for aerobic and anaerobic bacteria unless the causative organism is already known at the time of specimen collection. When the history, physical examination, or intraoperative findings suggest the possibility of unusual infection, special culturing techniques for organisms such as fungi, mycobacteria, or other organisms may be required. Failure to obtain specimens for these cultures at the time of initial debridement may result in unnecessary procedures to obtain further culture material or, ultimately, treatment failure.

The pathologist, although primarily looking for the presence or absence of acute inflammation suggestive of infection, may also find evidence of a specific type of inflammation (e.g., granulomas) that may provide a clue to the etiology of the infection. In this circumstance, it is useful to perform additional tissue stains for fungi or mycobacteria.

Once the microorganism responsible for the infection has been identified, antimicrobial susceptibility tests should be performed (101, 102). An MIC obtained by broth or agar dilution is the best guide to therapy (136). When only disk-diffusion (Kirby-Bauer disk) sensitivities are available, antimicrobial agents with intermediate or resistant results should not be used. Some investigators also advocate determining a serum bactericidal titer (SBT) (162, 167). However, these tests are difficult to reproduce within and among laboratories, and we do not advocate their use.

MANAGEMENT

There are no adequately designed, randomized, controlled, prospective trials with sufficient follow-up comparing therapeutic alternatives for the treatment of infected joint arthroplasties. Nonetheless, a number of medical and surgical approaches have been described. Surgical management and medical decisions about the duration and intensity of antimicrobial management are closely related. The optimal, but not always attainable, goal of treatment is a pain-free, functional joint with satisfactory mobility. Eradication of infection is often the most direct method of achieving this goal, but in selected cases, chronic antimicrobial suppression may be an appropriate alternative. Basic treatment options that have been proposed include, in addition to chronic suppressive antimicrobial therapy, surgical debridement with retention of the prosthesis, resection arthroplasty, arthrodesis, amputation, and one- or two-stage reimplantation. Antimicrobial agents may be delivered locally via antibiotic-impregnated polymethylmethacrylate as well as systemically.

Treatment Options

Suppressive antimicrobial therapy

Antimicrobial therapy without concomitant surgical intervention is not considered standard therapy for prosthetic joint infection. In one study of 25 patients, no patient had a satisfactory functional outcome after a mean of 1.3 years of follow-up (72); another study found that only 3 of 13 prostheses were retained after a mean of 37.6 months among patients treated with chronic antimicrobial suppression (156). Success, defined as suppression of symptoms and maintenance of a functioning joint, is greater with carefully selected patients (54), especially when suppression can be combined with initial debridement. Chronic antimicrobial suppression might be contemplated when (i) removal of the prosthesis is not feasible, (ii) the microorganism is of low virulence and highly susceptible to orally administered antimicrobial agents, (iii) there are no signs of systemic infection, (iv) the patient is compliant and tolerant of the antimicrobial agent, and (v) the prosthesis is not already loose (20, 54, 133).

Debridement with retention of the prosthesis

Attempts at salvage of a prosthesis by debridement and aggressive initial antibiotic therapy have generally been disappointing, with relapse rates as high as 77 to 88% by 2 to 4 years (145, 165). Infection with *S. aureus* or gram-negative organisms and chronicity of infection appear to be particularly poor prognostic indicators. With careful patient selection, this method may occasionally salvage a prosthesis, especially when fulminant infection occurs within 2 to 3 weeks of implantation and debridement can occur within 24 to 36 hours (18, 26, 63, 133, 145, 154).

Prosthesis removal

In order to consistently achieve a microbiological cure in prosthetic joint infection, it is necessary to remove the prosthesis and all associated cement and completely debride devitalized tissue and bone. Options after hardware removal and debridement depend on the joint site and include resection arthroplasty, arthrodesis, or exchange (one- or two-stage) arthroplasty.

Resection arthroplasty. Prior to the development of techniques that allowed successful reimplantation of an infected prosthesis, resection arthroplasty was the traditional therapeutic modality used to treat infected prostheses. The procedure involves complete removal of the infected prosthesis and any associated cement as well as infected bone or synovial tissue and the administration of 4 to 6 weeks of intravenous antibiotics.

Table 3. Success of resection arthroplasty for the treatment of THA infection

Author (year published)	Reference	No. of THA infections	No. (%) without recurrent infection	Follow-up (yr) (range [mean])
Grauer (1989)	55	33	30 (91)	2–10.5 (3.8)
Kantor (1986)	77	41	24 (59)	1–10 (3.9)
Canner (1984)	28	33	27 (82)	0.5–9 (4.1)
McElwaine (1984)	92	22	18 (82)	1.2–9 (N/A)[a]
Bourne (1984)	19	33	32 (97)	3–13 (6.2)
Bittar (1982)	14	14	11 (79)	0.17–4 (1.5)
Petty (1980)	122	21	16 (76)	1–8 (2.8)
Ahlgren (1980)	4	19	11 (58)	1–5.7 (3.3)
Mallory (1978)	90	10	10 (100)	3–5 (N/A)
Campbell (1978)	27	45	33 (71)	≥0.5 (2.2)
Clegg (1977)	34	30	24 (80)	1–6 (N/A)
Total		301	236 (78)	

[a] N/A, not available.

Resection arthroplasty results in successful eradication of infection in 58 to 100% of cases of total hip arthroplasty (THA) infection (Table 3) (4, 14, 19, 27, 28, 34, 55, 77, 90, 92, 122). Microbiological cure seems to correlate with the extent of debridement and the thoroughness of removal of the residual methylmethacrylate cement (28). After resection arthroplasty, hip function is often severely compromised. This limits the procedure's usefulness (55, 77, 122). For THA infection, this procedure is currently recommended only in situations in which exchange arthroplasty is not feasible—for example, patients who have major bone loss due to infection or prior surgery, nonambulatory patients, patients with recurrent infections, and patients with infections due to organisms for which effective antimicrobial therapy is unavailable (51).

Less information is available regarding the utility of resection arthroplasty as definitive surgical therapy for total knee arthroplasty (TKA) infection (45, 78). Falahee et al. reported that 89% of 28 TKAs were free of infection 6 months after the procedure (45). Three knees continued to have chronic drainage for up to 9 years. The mean length of antimicrobial therapy was 7.5 months. Fifteen (54%) patients walked independently following the procedure; six (21%) patients were unsatisfied with the procedure and elected to undergo arthrodesis. Resection knee arthroplasty is most often used for patients who have minimal ambulatory demands or who, because of poor bone stock or some other technical reason, are unable to undergo arthrodesis or reimplantation (128).

Arthrodesis. Until exchange arthroplasty was found to be a viable alternative, arthrodesis was the therapy of choice for TKA infection. A successful arthrodesis outcome depends on the ability to achieve adequate healthy bone apposition (79, 128). Thus, patients with large hinged knee prostheses, which sacrifice large amounts of bone, or patients who have had multiple revisions will have a decreased chance of a successful arthrodesis (23). Bone grafting can sometimes be performed in these situations (80).

The two surgical techniques most often utilized to provide a stable arthrodesis are implant removal with subsequent external fixation by use of a multiplaner external fixitor (96, 131) or prosthesis removal with subsequent internal fixation with an intramedullary nail (80). The advantages and disadvantages of these procedures have recently been reviewed (128). External fixation is recommended in cases of active TKA infection, although an intramedullary nail can be used as part of a two-stage procedure (80).

Arthrodesis is associated with prolonged periods of immobility. Time to achieve union can range from 2.5 months to 22 months (23, 40). Success rates vary considerably from study to study, likely because of differences in operative technique, patient population, and length of follow-up. In one recent study with a mean 3.8-year follow-up period, Morrey et al. reported a 70% efficacy of arthrodesis in 43 selected patients (96). There was evidence of recurrence of infection in two (6%) patients who had achieved union. Despite adequate fusion, 9% of patients experienced residual pain after the arthrodesis.

Arthrodesis is often the treatment of choice for TKA infection when patient mobility is important and reimplantation of a prosthesis is not feasible for technical reasons (128). When arthrodesis is the surgical therapy of choice, we recommend 4 to 6 weeks of parenteral antimicrobial therapy (114). In some instances, further oral antimicrobial therapy may be useful. This aggressive approach is dictated by the goal of achieving a microbiological cure and is used because persistent infection is a serious cause of arthrodesis failure (131).

Reimplantation. The best functional results in the treatment of prosthetic joint infection have been achieved with reimplantation of a new prosthesis (36, 51, 128). Unfortunately, there are no randomized prospective studies comparing the various reimplantation regimens utilized by different investigators. Thus, the clinician is left to compare the published results of various case series in order to determine the optimal approach to reimplantation for any given patient. Because case series often differ in patient population, surgical technique, duration and type of antimicrobial therapy, length and thoroughness of follow-up, and definition of an unsuccessful outcome (reinfection with a different organism, relapse of the original organism, reinfection and relapse, or a painful joint), these comparisons can sometimes be difficult.

Issues about reimplantation that remain controversial include the optimal time to reimplantation, the role of antibiotic-impregnated cement, the need for antibiotic-impregnated polymethylmethacrylate spacers in two-stage reimplantation for TKA infection, and the optimal type and duration of administration of intravenous and oral antimicrobial agents. Although several authors in recent years have reviewed the issues of time to reimplantation and the in vitro characteristics and clinical usefulness of antibiotic-impregnated polymethylmethacrylate (58, 91, 128, 155), relatively little attention has been paid to the optimal type and duration of parenteral therapy needed to eradicate prosthetic joint infection (139, 167).

THA infection. Surgical options that have been evaluated most extensively include one- and two-stage exchange arthroplasty. One-stage exchange arthroplasty involves removal of the infected prosthesis and associated cement, debridement of all devitalized tissue and bone, and immediate reimplantation of a second prosthesis. Success rates with variable lengths of follow-up have ranged from 38 to 92% (Table 4) (24, 28, 30, 33, 65, 76, 94, 98, 139, 143, 158, 170). Most investigators have used antibiotic-impregnated cement, most often with gentamicin, in combination with intravenous and oral antimicrobial therapy based on in vitro susceptibility testing. The duration of systemic antimicrobial therapy has been extremely variable, ranging from none to 9 weeks of intravenous therapy and from no oral therapy to more than 2 years of oral antibiotics (24, 28, 30, 33, 65, 76, 94, 98, 139, 143, 158, 170).

Two-stage exchange arthroplasty involves at least two separate operations. The first operation is a standard resection arthroplasty. Four to 6 weeks of intravenous antimicrobial agents, chosen on the basis of in vitro susceptibility testing, are then usually administered (91, 114, 139). Some investigators also use oral antimicrobial therapy for several weeks after the conclusion of intravenous therapy. Following a variable period of time, ranging from months to several years, a new prosthesis is reimplanted. Antibiotic-impregnated cement may or may not be utilized with the reimplanted joint. Success rates have varied from 68 to 100% with variable lengths of follow-up (Table 5) (33, 65, 91, 97, 139, 143).

In one early, small study involving 82 infected THAs reimplanted using a two-stage technique without antibiotic-impregnated cement, McDonald et al. (91) investigated factors associated with recurrence of

Table 4. Success of one-step exchange arthroplasty for THA infection

Author (year published)	Reference	No. of THA infections	No. (%) without recurrent infection	Follow-up (yr) (range [mean])[a]
Without antibiotic-impregnated cement				
Jupiter (1981)	76	17	14 (82)	2–6 (3.7)
Salvati (1982)	139	32	29 (91)	6–10 (N/A)
Miley (1982)	94	101	94 (92)	≥2.7 (N/A)
Cherney (1983)	33	5	4 (80)	3.0–7.25 (6.0)
Canner (1984)	28	5	4 (80)	0.5–9 (4.1)
Total		160	145 (90)	
With antibiotic-impregnated cement				
Carlsson (1978)	30	59	54 (91)	≥0.5 (N/A)
Murray (1981)	98	13	5 (38)	N/A (N/A)
Bucholz (1984)	24	825	645 (78)	≥2 (N/A)
Wroblewski (1986)	170	102	93 (91)	2.2–5.2 (2.2)
Sanzen (1988)	143	72	55 (76)	2–9.75 (6.0)
Hope (1989)	65	72	63 (87)	0.4–10 (3.75)
Total		1,143	915 (80)	

[a] NA, not available.

Table 5. Success of two-stage exchange arthroplasty for THA infection

Author (year published)	Reference	No. of THA infections	No. (%) without recurrent infection	Follow-up (yr) (range [mean])
Without antibiotic-impregnated cement				
Salvati (1982)	139	18	18 (100)	2–6 (4)
Cherney (1983)	33	28	19 (68)	0.17–7 (4.1)
McDonald (1989)	91	82	71 (87)	2–13 (5.5)
Total		202	115 (84)	
With antibiotic-impregnated cement				
Murray (1981)	97	22	21 (96)	1–10 (N/A)[a]
Sanzen (1988)	143	30	22 (73)	2–9.75 (6)
Hope (1989)	65	8	8 (100)	0.17–8 (1.75)
Total		60	51 (85)	

[a] N/A, not available.

infection. Variables studied included presence or absence of retained cement after resection arthroplasty, reconstruction less than 1 year after resection arthroplasty, intravenous antimicrobial therapy for less than 28 days, and infection due to aerobic gram-negative bacilli or enterococci. In univariate analysis, all factors were significant. In the multivariate analysis, only reimplantation within 1 year of resection arthroplasty was statistically significant, although the statistical power was limited.

TKA infection. Most investigators have favored delayed two-stage exchange arthroplasty with reimplantation 4 to 6 weeks after joint resection for the treatment of established TKA infection (128, 167). Reasons for this opinion have included the relatively low probability of microbiological cure with immediate and early (less than 3 weeks) reimplantation (Table 6) and the lack of a satisfactory functional outcome reported by some authors after early reimplantation (52, 130). Additionally, staged reimplantion provides the opportunity to perform multiple debridements and to identify the responsible microorganisms in order to direct antimicrobial therapy prior to reimplantation (128).

Various surgical techniques have been used by investigators when reporting their results of delayed two-stage exchange arthroplasty. The use of antibiotic-impregnated polymethylmethacrylate cement and spacers as well as the time to reimplantation has varied from series to series (Table 6). The overall success rate combining the results of numerous series is 88% (Table 6) (12, 15, 16, 18, 52, 69, 70, 96, 106, 135, 154, 160, 164, 165, 167, 169). It is tempting to suggest, on the basis of the series in Table 6, that the use of antibiotic-impregnated cement and antibiotic-impregnated spacers as adjunctive therapy provides additional protection against reinfection. However, definitive recommendations regarding these adjunctive therapies must await controlled clinical trials.

When two-stage exchange arthroplasty is the surgical therapy of choice, we agree with Rand (128) that a delay of 4 to 6 weeks between prosthesis removal and reimplantation is optimal. Parenteral antimicrobial therapy is usually administered up to and until the confirmatory bacterial cultures of specimens obtained at the time of joint reimplantation have remained negative for 5 days. In general, infection caused by more virulent organisms (*S. aureus*, aerobic gram-negative bacteria) or relatively resistant organisms (such as *P. aeruginosa*) or infection in relatively compromised hosts justifies antimicrobial treatment at the longer end of the 4 to 6 week range. We do not routinely use serum bactericidal titers to guide antimicrobial therapy for the reasons cited earlier in this chapter. Outpatient parenteral antimicrobial therapy is often feasible in our patient population.

Currently available data (Table 6) neither support nor refute the use

Table 6. Success of various surgical procedures for TKA infection

Author (year published)	Reference	No. of TKA infections	No. (%) without recurrent infection	Follow-up (yr) (range [mean])	Weeks to reimplantation (range [mean])
One-stage exchange procedures					
Freeman (1985)	49	8	8 (100)	1–3.3 (N/A)[a]	0[b]
Bengston (1986)	12	8	2 (25)	1.1–9.7 (5)	0[b]
Borden (1987)	18	3	3 (100)	2.5–4.5 (3.5)	0[b]
Teeny (1990)	154	1	1 (100)	>2 (N/A)	0[c]
Buechel (1990)	25	12	11 (92)	0.17–9.1 (6.1)	0[b]
Total		32	25 (78)		
Two-stage reimplantation Early reimplant (<3 weeks)					
Rand (1983)	130	14	8 (57)	2–4.7 (3.3)	(<2)[c]
Grogan (1986)	61	2	2 (100)	6.6–8.1 (7.3)	(<3)[c]
Total		16	10 (63)		
Without antibiotic cement					
Nelson (1982)	106	5	5 (100)	N/A (N/A)	N/A (6)
Insall (1983)	69	11	10 (91)	2.8 (1–6)	5.4–11.7 (6)
Woods (1983)	169	3	3 (100)	N/A (N/A)	12–24 (N/A)
Walker (1984)	160	11	9 (82)	2.7–7.4 (4.5)	2–114 (38.3)
Morrey (1989)	96	15	8 (53)	1–10 (8.0)	2–114 (N/A)
Jacobs (1989)	70	7	7 (100)	2–4.17 (3)	N/A (6)
Wilson (1990)	165	12	11 (92)	2–5 (2.8)	6–24 (12)
Teeny (1990)	154	9	9 (100)	2–6 (3.5)	4–>12 (N/A)
Windsor (1990)	167	29	26 (90)	2.5–6 (4)	6–11 (7.14)
Total		102	88 (86)		
With antibiotic cement					
Bliss (1985)	15	5	4 (80)	0.75–3 (1.6)	>6 (N/A)
Rosenberg (1988)	136	24	24 (100)	1–5.8 (2.5)	6–8 (6)
Wilson (1990)	165	8	5 (63)	2–5 (2.8)	6–24 (12)
Total		37	33 (89)		
Antibiotic cement plus antibiotic-impregnated spacers or beads					
Bengston (1986)	12	5	3 (60)	1.1–9.7 (5)	4–8 (N/A)
Borden (1987)	18	18	17 (100)	>1 (N/A)	N/A (3)
Wilde (1988)	164	10	9 (90)	1–4.7 (2.6)	3–12 (6)
Booth (1989)	16	25	24 (96)	0.5–5 (2)	3–204 16
Total		58	53 (91)		

[a] N/A, not available.
[b] Antibiotic-impregnated cement used.
[c] No antibiotic-impregnated cement used.

of antibiotic-impregnated cement or polymethylmethacrylate spacers. When these adjunctive therapies are used, we recommend that antimicrobial agents be chosen that are active against the microorganism causing infection and have a low risk of hypersensitivity reaction.

Amputation. Amputation or limb disarticulation should be reserved for those patients with life-threatening infection, intractable pain, or severe loss of bone stock (128). Cure of infection is accomplished surgically, but unfortunately functional outcome is usually poor (127). Parenteral antimicrobial agents are used as prophylaxis against surgical wound infection and to prevent dissemination perioperatively.

PREVENTION

Operative Contamination

Antimicrobial prophylaxis

Antimicrobial prophylaxis has been utilized traditionally in operative procedures that have a high rate of postoperative wound infection, when foreign materials must be implanted, or in operative procedures in which the wound infection rate is low but the development of a wound infection would result in a catastrophic event. Because prosthetic joint replacement falls in the latter categories, interest in perioperative prophylaxis has been intense. Six prospective clinical trials have evaluated the efficacy of perioperative antimicrobial prophylaxis in prosthetic joint surgery (30, 44, 64, 83, 123, 146). Although each of them has limitations (e.g., lack of a definition of infection, inadequate power to detect a clinically meaningful difference between study groups, or high rates of infection in control arms), the preponderance of evidence clearly favors the use of antimicrobial prophylaxis compared with no prophylaxis (51, 108).

Prophylactic antimicrobial agents should be directed against the common organisms that cause postoperative wounds infections (51). Because staphylococci and streptococci are the most common organisms to cause these infections, agents directed against these pathogens, such as penicillinase-resistant penicillins and cephalosporins (cefazolin), are most often used. However, because of an increasing frequency of infections caused by methicillin-resistant staphylococci and gram-negative aerobic bacilli, some investigators have advocated broader-spectrum prophylaxis, although no data regarding the efficacy or cost-effectiveness are available (99).

Prophylactic antimicrobial agents should be administered not more than 30 to 60 min prior to surgery. Concentrations of antimicrobial agents in tissue should be present throughout the period of time that the wound is open (51). For lengthy procedures or antimicrobial agents with short half-lives, an additional dose may need to be administered intraoperatively. There is no benefit to beginning antimicrobial therapy prior to the perioperative period or continuing therapy beyond two to three postoperative doses (105, 108, 123). This practice should be discouraged because of the possibility of added antimicrobial toxicity, selection of resistant organisms, and unnecessary expense.

Recent retrospective and prospective studies also suggest that antibiotic-impregnated cement may be effective in the prophylaxis of deep wound infection following total joint replacement (75, 86, 93). We agree with Norden that further studies with longer follow-up periods need to be conducted before an unequivocal endorsement of this practice can be given (108). If antibiotic cement is utilized prophylactically, antimicrobial agents active in vitro against staphylococci (such as vancomycin) and which are relatively nonallergenic would seem to be the preferred agents.

Ultraclean operating room environments

The utility of laminar airflow devices in preventing prosthetic joint infection remains controversial (51, 108, 128). Studies showing that the use of such devices reduces the risk of prosthetic joint infection have been published (83). However, studies have also been reported showing that the use of laminar airflow may actually increase the risk of infection, depending upon positioning of the operating personnel (138). Preliminary data from a randomized, prospective, double-blind trial at the Mayo Clinic involving more than 7,000 patients showed no significant difference in the risk of infection between patients with implants placed in conventional operating rooms and those whose implants were placed in operating rooms containing laminar airflow devices (46). Routine antimicrobial prophylaxis with cefazolin was used in both groups. Definitive recommendations regarding this costly method of prophylaxis await the results of further clinical trials.

Hematogenous seeding

Several authors have reviewed the numerous cases in the medical literature of prosthetic joint infection attributed to hematogenous seeding (3, 10, 89). In the majority of cases, it is difficult to document bacteremia preceding prosthesis infection. Fifty percent of these presumed hematogenous infections have been caused by *S. aureus*, coagulase-negative staphylococci, and beta-hemolytic streptococci, predominantly from skin sources. Urinary tract, respiratory tract, and other remote infections have also been implicated as sources of hematogenous joint infection.

It seems clear that it is prudent to aggressively diagnose and treat remote infections in patients with joint prostheses, in order to prevent hematogenous seeding (108). Effective antimicrobial selection in this situation will depend upon the site of infection, the likely in vitro susceptibility of the microorganism causing infection, and the patient's history of antibiotic intolerance.

Antimicrobial prophylaxis for patients with a prosthetic joint who undergo a dental procedure or an invasive procedure such as endoscopy or cystoscopy is controversial (51, 108) and has been recently reviewed. Certainly, there are case reports of prosthetic joint infection temporally related to these procedures and caused by flora indigenous to the appropriate body site (viridans group streptococci or *Actinomyces israelii* from the oral cavity) (85, 153). It is unknown, however, whether the incidence rate of hematogenous infection caused by these procedures is sufficiently high to outweigh the potential risk and cost of antimicrobial prophylaxis.

In a preliminary report, Osmon, Steckelberg and coworkers studied whether the incidence rate of large joint implant infection epidemiologically linked to an oral source justifies the risk and cost of antimicrobial prophylaxis. In a series of controlled epidemiological studies, the presence of teeth was a risk factor for large joint implant infection due to viridans group streptococci (odds ratio, 6.4; 95% confidence interval, 2.2 to 18.0; $P \leq 0.001$) but not for infection due to other microorganisms (112). Despite this epidemiological link, the overall incidence rate of large joint implant infection due to viridans group streptococci was only 0.06 cases per 1,000 joint-years (95% confidence interval, 0.03 to 0.1) among an incidence cohort of more than 39,000 large joint implants with approximately 275,000 joint-years of follow-up (113). This low incidence is similar to the rate of viridans group streptococcal infective endocarditis among patients with mitral valve prolapse and no murmur (151) or endocarditis in the general population (150), groups for which the American Heart Association recommends no antimicrobial prophylaxis because the risk-benefit ratio is judged to be adverse (37).

Because the rate of prosthetic joint infection due to viridans group streptococci in patients with a THA or TKA is very low, we feel that a blanket recommendation for antimicrobial prophylaxis for routine, clean dental procedures in all patients with a large joint arthroplasty does not appear warranted at present. As is the current practice with infective endocarditis, rational recommendations regarding antimicrobial prophylaxis for clean dental procedures in patients with large orthopedic implants will depend on identifying groups of patients at substantially increased risk for infection following these procedures. Patients with overt dental infection, such as dental abscesses, should receive appropriate empiric or culture-directed antibiotic treatment.

Data are also currently inadequate to formulate prophylaxis recommendations for genitourinary or gastrointestinal procedures in the absence of infection. If a physician elects to recommend antimicrobial prophylaxis for the prevention of hematogenous infection, the potential rare, but life-threatening, adverse reaction as well as the more common drug toxicities should be considered. If utilized, antimicrobial agents should be chosen on the basis of the expected flora at the site of the procedure.

SUMMARY

Although uncommon, infection of prosthetic joints causes serious morbidity and presents a major clinical and therapeutic challenge. Several mechanisms of infection have been postulated, but most infections probably occur through inoculation of the prosthesis at or near the time of implantation. The incidence rate of infection, based on the time of diagnosis, declines with time after implantation. Late cases may represent either latent infections with delayed manifestation or, in some cases, hematogenous seeding. Although the spectrum of microorganisms capable of causing prosthetic joint infection is quite broad, the majority of cases are due to gram-positive cocci, especially staphylococcal species. Medical and surgical treatment decisions for infected joint prostheses are complex and should be individualized in each case.

REFERENCES

1. **Acurio, M. T., and R. J. Friedman.** 1992. Hip arthroplasty in patients with sickle-cell hemoglobinopathy. *J. Bone Jt. Surg. Br. Vol.* **74:**367–371.
2. **Agarwal, S., M. S. Orth, M. C. Orth, S. K. Kadhi, and R. J. Rooney.** 1991. Brucellosis complicating bilateral total knee arthroplasty. *Clin. Orthop. Relat. Res.* **267:**179–181.
3. **Ahlberg, A., A. S. Carlsson, and L. Lindgren.** 1978. Hematogenous infection in total joint replacement. *Clin. Orthop. Relat. Res.* **137:**69–75.
4. **Ahlgren, S. A., G. Gudmundsson, and E. Bartholdsson.** 1990. Function after removal of a septic total hip prosthesis. *Acta Orthop. Scand.* **51:**541–545.
5. **Ahnfelt, L., P. Herberts, H. Malchau, and G. B. Andersson.** 1990. Prognosis of total hip replacement. A Swedish multicenter study of 4,664 revisions. *Acta Orthop. Scand. Suppl.* **238:**1–26.
6. **Ainscow, D. A. P., and R. A. Denham.** 1984. The risk of haematogenous infection in total joint replacements. *J. Bone Jt. Surg. Br. Vol.* **66B:**580–582.
7. **Allerberger, F., M. J. Kasten, F. R. Cockerill, M. Krismer, and M. P. Dierich.** 1992. *Listeria monocytogenes* infection in prosthetic joints. *Int. Orthop.* **16:**237–239.
8. **Austin, K. S., N. N. Testa, R. K. Luntz, J. B. Greene, and S. Smiles.** 1992. Aspergillus infection of total knee arthroplasty presenting as a popliteal cyst. Case report and review of the literature. *J. Arthroplasty* **7:**311–314.

9. **Beachey, E. H.** (ed.) 1980. *Bacterial Adherence: Receptors and Recognition,* series B. Chapman & Hall, Ltd., London.

10. **Bengtson, S., G. Blomgren, K. Knutson, A. Wigren, and L. Lidgren.** 1987. Hematogenous infection after knee arthroplasty. *Acta Orthop. Scand.* **58:**529–534.

11. **Bengston, S., K. Knutson, and L. Lidgren.** 1989. Treatment of infected knee arthroplasty. *Clin. Orthop. Relat. Res.* **245:**173–178.

12. **Bengston, S., K. Knutson, and L. Lidgren.** 1986. Revision of infected knee arthroplasty. *Acta Orthop. Scand.* **57:**489–494.

13. **Betts, F., T. Wright, E. A. Salvati, A. Boskey, and M. Bansal.** 1992. Cobalt-alloy metal debris in periarticular tissues from total hip revision arthroplasties. Metal contents and associated histologic findings. *Clin. Orthop Relat. Res.* **276:**75–82.

14. **Bittar, E. S., and W. Petty.** 1982. Girdlestone arthroplasty for infected total hip arthroplasty. *Clin. Orthop. Relat. Res.* **170:**83–87.

15. **Bliss, D. G., and G. G. Mcbride.** 1985. Infected total knee arthroplasties. *Clin. Orthop. Relat. Res.* **199:**207–214.

16. **Booth, R. E., and P. A. Lotke.** 1989. The results of spacer block technique in revision of infected total knee arthroplasty. *Clin. Orthop. Relat. Res.* **248:**57–60.

17. **Booth, J. E., J. A. Jacobson, T. A. Kurrus, and T. W. Edwards.** 1979. Infection of prosthetic arthroplasty by *Mycobacterium fortuitum.* Two case reports. *J. Bone Jt. Surg. Am. Vol.* **61:**300–302.

18. **Borden, L. S., and P. F. Gearen.** 1987. Infected total knee arthroplasty. A protocol for management. *J. Arthroplasty* **2:**27–36.

19. **Bourne, R. B., G. A. Hunter, C. H. Rorabeck, and J. J. Macnab.** 1984. A six-year follow-up of infected total hip replacements managed by Girdlestone's arthroplasty. *J. Bone Jt. Surg. Br. Vol.* **66:**340–343.

20. **Brause, B. D.** 1982. Infected total knee replacement. *Orthop. Clin. North Am.* **13:** 245–249.

21. **Brause, B. D.** 1989. Infected orthopedic prostheses, p. 111–127. *In* A. L. Bisno and F. A. Waldvogel (ed.), *Infections Associated with Indwelling Medical Devices.* American Society for Microbiology, Washington, D.C.

22. **Brennan, P. J., and M. Pia DeGirolamo.** 1991. Musculoskeletal infections in immunocompromised hosts. *Orthop. Clin. North Am.* **22:**389–399.

23. **Brodersen, M. P., R. H. Fitzgerald, Jr., L. F. A. Peterson, M. B. Coventry, and R. S. Bryan.** Arthrodesis of the knee following failed total knee arthroplasty. *J. Bone Jt. Surg. Am. Vol.* **61:**181–185.

24. **Bucholz, H. E., R. A. Elson, and K. Heinert.** 1984. Antibiotic-loaded acrylic cement: current concepts. *Clin. Orthop. Relat. Res.* **190:**96–108.

25. **Buechel, F. F.** 1990. Primary exchange revision arthroplasty using antibiotic-impregnated cement for infected total knee replacement. *Orthop. Rev.* **XIX**(Suppl.):83–87.

26. **Burger, R. R., T. Basch, and C. N. Hopson.** 1991. Implant salvage in infected total knee arthroplasty. *Clin. Orthop. Relat. Res.* **273:**105–112.

27. **Campbell, A., R. H. Fitzgerald, W. D. Fisher, and D. L. Hamblen.** 1978. Girdlestone pseudoarthrosis for failed total hip replacement. *J. Bone Jt. Surg. Br. Vol.* **60:**441–442.

28. **Canner, G. C., M. E. Steinberg, R. B. Heppenstall, and R. Balderston.** 1984. The infected hip after total hip arthroplasty. *J. Bone Jt. Surg. Am. Vol.* **66:**1393–1399.

29. **Carbone, L., J. M. Steckelberg, and W. R. Wilson.** 1991. Microbiology of primary prosthetic joint infections. *Program Abstr. 5th Eur. Congr. Clin. Microbiol. Infect. Dis.,* abstr. 5.

30. **Carlsson, A. S., G. Josefsson, and I. Lindberg.** 1978. Revision with gentamicin-impregnated cement for deep infections in total hip arthroplasties. *J. Bone Jt. Surg. Am. Vol.* **60:**1059–1064.

31. Carlsson, A. S., L. Lidgren, and L. Lindberg. 1977. Prophylactic antibiotics against early and late deep infections after total hip replacement. *Acta Orthop. Scand.* **48:** 405–410.

32. Charnley, J. 1972. Postoperative infection after total hip replacement with special reference to air contamination in the operating room air. *Clin. Orthop. Relat. Res.* **87:** 167–187.

33. Cherney, D. L., and H. C. Amstuz. 1983. Total hip replacement in the previously septic hip. *J Bone Jt. Surg. Am. Vol.* **65:**1256–1265.

34. Clegg, J. 1977. The results of the pseudoarthrosis after removal of an infected total hip prosthesis. *J. Bone Jt. Surg. Br. Vol.* **59:**298–301.

35. Coventry, M. B. 1978. Treatment of infections occurring in total hip surgery. *Orthop. Clin. North Am.* **6:**991–1003.

36. Cuckler, J. M., A. M. Star, A. Alavi, and R. B. Noto. 1991. Diagnosis and management of the infected total joint arthroplasty. *Orthop. Clin. North Am.* **22:**523–530.

37. Dajani, A. S., A. L. Bisno, K. J. Chung, D. T. Durack, M. Freed, M. A. Gerber, A. W. Karchmer, H. D. Millard, S. Rahimtoola, S. T. Shulman, C. Watanakunakorn, and K. A. Taubert. 1990. Prevention of bacterial endocarditis: recommendations by the American Heart Association. *JAMA* **264:**2919–2922.

38. Dankert, J., A. H. Hogt, and J. Feijen. 1986. Biomedical polymers: bacterial adhesion, colonization and infection. *Crit. Rev. Biocompat.* **2:**219–301.

39. Dougherty, S. H., and R. L. Simmons. 1982. Infections in bionic man: the pathobiology of infections in prosthetic devices. Part II. *Curr. Probl. Surg.* **19:**265–319.

40. Drinker, H., T. A. Potter, R. H. Turner, and W. H. Thomas. 1979. Arthrodesis for failed total knee arthroplasty. *Orthop. Trans.* **3:**302.

41. Dupont, J. A. 1986. Significance of operative cultures in total hip arthroplasty. *Clin. Orthop. Relat. Res.* **211:**122–127.

42. Eftekhar, N. S. 1987. Long-term results of cemented total hip arthroplasty. *Clin. Orthop. Relat. Res.* **225:**207–217.

43. Eggelmeijer, F., P. Petit, and B. A. Dijkmans. 1992. Total knee arthroplasty infection due to *Gemella haemolysans*. *Br. J. Rheumatol.* **31:**67–69.

44. Ericson, C., L. Lidgren, and L. Lindberg. 1973. Cloxacillin in the prophylaxis of postoperative infections of the hip. *J. Bone Jt. Surg. Am. Vol.* **55:**808–813.

45. Falahee, M. H., L. S. Matthews, H. Kaufer, and A. Arbor. 1987. Resection arthroplasty as a salvage procedure for a knee with infection after a total arthroplasty. *J. Bone Jt. Surg. Am. Vol.* **69:**1013–1021.

46. Fitzgerald, R. H., and D. M. Ilstrup. 1990. A prospective study of unidirectional airflow operating rooms. Presented at the 57th annual meeting of the Academy of Orthopedic Surgeons, New Orleans.

47. Fitzgerald, R. H., Jr., D. R. Nolan, D. M. Ilstrup, R. E. Van Scoy, J. A. Washington, and M. B. Coventry. 1977. Deep wound sepsis following total hip arthroplasty. *J. Bone Jt. Surg. Am. Vol.* **58:**847–855.

48. Foster, M. R., R. B. Heppenstall, Z. B. Friedenberg, and W. J. Hozack. 1990. A prospective assessment of nutritional status and complications in patients with fractures of the hip. *J. Orthop. Trauma* **4:**49–57.

49. Freeman, M. A. R., R. A. Sudlow, M. W. Casewell, and S. S. Radcliff. 1985. The management of infected total knee replacement. *J. Bone Jt. Surg. Br. Vol.* **67:**764–768.

50. Gill, G. S., and D. M. Mills. 1981. Long-term follow-up evaluation of 1000 consecutive cemented total knee arthroplasties. *Clin. Orthop. Relat. Res.* **273:**66–76.

51. Gillespie, W. J. 1990. Infection in total joint replacement. *Infect. Dis. Clin. North Am.* **4:**465–484.

52. **Goksan, S. B., and M. A. Freeman.** 1992. One-stage reimplantation for the salvage of infected total knee arthroplasty. *J. Bone Jt. Surg. Br. Vol.* **74**:78–82.
53. **Gordon, S. M., D. H. Culver, B. P. Simmons, and W. R. Jarvis.** 1990. Risk factors for wound infections after total knee arthroplasty. *Am. J. Epidemiology* **131**:905–916.
54. **Goulet, J. A., P. M. Pellicci, B. D. Brause, and E. M. Salvati.** 1988. Prolonged suppression of infection in total hip arthroplasty. *J. Arthroplasty* **3**:109–116.
55. **Grauer, J. D., H. C. Amstutz, P. F. O'Carroll, and F. J. Dorey.** 1989. Resection arthroplasty of the hip. *J. Bone Jt. Surg. Am. Vol.* **71**:669–678.
56. **Gristina, A. G.** 1987. Biomaterial-centered infection microbial adhesion versus tissue integration. *Science* **237**:1588–1595.
57. **Gristina, A. G., R. A. Jennings, P. T. Naylor, Q. N. Myrvik, and L. X. Webb.** 1989. Comparative in vitro antibiotic resistance of surface colonizing coagulase negative staphylococci. *Antimicrob. Agents Chemother.* **33**:813–816.
58. **Gristina, A. G., and J. Kolkin.** 1986. Total joint replacement and sepsis. *J. Bone Jt. Surg. Am. Vol.* **65**:128–134.
59. **Gristina, A. G., P. T. Naylor, and Q. N. Myrvik.** 1991. Mechanisms of musculoskeletal sepsis. *Orthop. Clin. North Am.* **22**:363–372.
60. **Gristina, A. G., G. D. Rovere, H. Shoji, and J. F. Nicastro.** 1976. An in vitro study of bacterial response to inert and reactive metals and to methyl methacrylate. *J. Biomed. Mater. Res.* **10**:273–281.
61. **Grogan, T. J., F. Dorey, J. Rollins, and H. C. Amstutz.** 1986. Deep sepsis following total knee arthroplasty. Ten-year experience at the University of California at Los Angeles medical center. *J. Bone Jt. Surg. Am. Vol.* **68A**:226–234.
62. **Gruninger, R. P.** 1989. Diagnostic microbiology in bone and joint infections, p. 42–51. *In* R. B. Gustilo (ed.), *Orthopaedic Infection: Diagnosis and Treatment.* The W. B. Saunders Co., Philadelphia.
63. **Hartman, M. B., T. K. Fehring, L. Jordan, and H. J. Norton.** 1991. Periprosthetic knee sepsis. The role of irrigation and debridement. *Clin. Orthop. Relat. Res.* **273**:113–118.
64. **Hill, C., R. Flamant, F. Mazas, and J. Evard.** 1991. Prophylactic cefazolin vesus placebo in total hip replacement. Report of a multicenter double-blind randomized trial. *Lancet* **i**:795–797.
65. **Hope, P. G., K. G. Kristinsson, P. Norman, and R. A. Elson.** 1989. Deep infection of cemented total hip arthroplastices caused by coagulase negative staphylococci. *J. Bone Jt. Surg. Br. Vol.* **71**:851–855.
66. **Horowitz, S. M., J. M. Lane, J. C. Otis, and J. H. Healey.** 1991. Prosthetic arthroplasty of the knee after resection of a sarcoma in the proximal end of the tibia. A report of sixteen cases. *J. Bone Jt. Surg. Am. Vol.* **73**: 286–293.
67. **Inman, R. D., K. V. Gallegos, B. D. Brause, P. B. Redecha, and C. L. Christian.** 1984. Clinical and microbiologic features of prosthetic joint infection. *Am. J. Med.* **77**: 47–53.
68. **Insall, J., W. N. Scott, and C. S. Ranawat.** 1979. The total condylar knee prosthesis. A report of two hundred and twenty cases. *J. Bone Jt. Surg. Am. Vol.* **61**:173–180.
69. **Insall, J. N., F. M. Thompson, and B. D. Brause.** 1983. Two-stage reimplantation for the salvage of infected total knee arthroplasty. *J. Bone Jt. Surg. Am. Vol.* **65**:1087–1098.
70. **Jacobs, M. A., D. S. Hungerford, K. A. Krackow, and D. W. Lennox.** 1989. Revision of septic total knee arthroplasty. *Clin. Orthop. Relat. Res.* **238**:159–166.
71. **Jensen, J. E., T. G. Jensen, T. K. Smith, D. A. Johnston, and S. J. Dudrick.** 1982. Nutrition in orthopaedics. *J. Bone Jt. Surg. Am. Vol.* **64A**:1263–1272.
72. **Johnson, D. P., and G. C. Bannister.** 1986. The outcome of infected arthroplasty of the knee. *J. Bone Jt. Surg. Br. Vol.* **68**:289–291.

73. Johnson, G. M., D. A. Lee, W. E. Regelmann, E. D. Gray, G. Peters, and P. G. Quie. 1986. Interference with granulocyte function by *Staphylococcus epidermidis* slime. *Infect. Immun.* **54:**13–20.

74. Johnson, J. A., M. J. Christie, M. P. Sandler, P. F. Parks, Jr., L. Homra, and J. J. Kaye. 1988. Detection of occult infection following total joint arthroplasty using sequential technetium-99m HDP bone scintigraphy and indium-111 WBC imaging. *J. Nucl. Med.* **29:**1347–1353.

75. Josefsson, G., L. Lindberg, and B. Wiklander. 1981. Systemic antibiotics and gentamicin-containing bone cement in the prophylaxis of post-operative infections in total hip arthroplasty. *Clin. Orthop. Relat. Res.* **159:**194–200.

76. Jupiter, J. B., A. W. Karchmer, J. D. Lowell, and W. H. Harris. 1981. Total hip arthroplasty in the treatment of adult hips with current or quiescent sepsis. *J. Bone Jt. Surg. Am. Vol.* **63:**194–200.

77. Kantor, G. S., J. A. Osterkamp, L. D. Dorr, D. Fischer, J. Perry, and J. P. Conaty. 1986. Resection arthroplasty following infected total hip replacement arthroplasty. *J. Arthroplasty* **1:**83–89.

78. Kaufer, H., and L. S. Matthews. 1986. Resection arthroplasty: an alternative to arthrodesis for salvage of the infected total knee arthroplasty. *Instr. Course Lect.* **35:** 283–289.

79. Knutson, K., L. Hovelius, A. Lindstrand, and L. Lidgren. 1984. Arthrodesis after failed total knee arthroplasty. *Clin. Orthop. Relat. Res.* **191:**202–211.

80. Knutson, K., A. Lindstrand, and L. Lidgren. 1985. Arthrodesis for failed total knee arthroplasty. *J. Bone Jt. Surg. Br. Vol.* **67:**47–52.

81. Lachiewicz, P. F., A. E. Inglis, J. N. Insall, T. P. Sculco, M. W. Hilgartner, and J. B. Bussel. 1985. Total knee arthroplasty in hemophilia. *J. Bone Jt. Surg. Am. Vol.* **67:** 1361–1366.

82. Lidwell, O. M. 1986. Apparent improvement in the outcome of hip or knee-replacement operations over the period of a prospective study. *J. Hyg. Camb.* **97:**501–502.

83. Lidwell, O. M., E. J. L. Lowbury, W. Whyte, R. Blowers, S. J. Stanley, and D. Lowe. 1982. Effect of ultraclean air in operating rooms on deep sepsis in the joint after total hip or knee replacement: a randomized study. *Br Med. J.* **250:**99–102.

84. Lidwell, O. M., E. J. L. Lowbury, W. Whyte, R. Blowers, S. J. Stanley, and D. Lowe. 1983. Airborne contamination of wounds in joint replacement operations: the relationship to sepsis rates. *J. Hosp. Infect.* **4:**111–131.

85. Lindquist, C., and P. Slatus. 1985. Dental bacteremia—a neglected cause of arthroplasty infections. *Acta Orthop. Scand.* **56:**506–508.

86. Lynch, M., M. P. Esser, P. Shelley, and B. M. Wroblewski. 1987. Deep infection in Charnley low-friction arthroplasty. Comparison of plain and gentamicin-loaded cement. *J. Bone Jt. Surg. Am. Vol.* **69:**355–360.

87. Lyons, C. W., T. H. Bergquist, J. C. Lyons, J. A. Rand, and M. L. Brown. 1985. Evaluation of radiographic findings in painful hip arthroplasties. *Clin. Orthop. Relat. Res.* **195:**239–251.

88. Mackowiak, P. A., S. R. Jones, and J. W. Smith. 1978. Diagnostic value of sinus tract cultures in chronic osteomyelitis. *JAMA* **239:**2772–2775.

89. Maderazo, E. G., S. Judson, and H. Pasternak. 1988. Late infections of total joint prostheses: a review and recommendations for prevention. *Clin. Orthop. Relat. Res.* **229:**131–142.

90. Mallory, T. H. 1978. Excision arthroplasty with delayed wound closure for the infected total hip replacement. *Clin. Orthop. Relat. Res.* **137:**106–111.

91. McDonald, D. J., R. H. Fitzgerald, and D. M. Ilstrup. 1989. Two-stage reconstruction of a total hip arthroplasty because of infection. *J. Bone Jt. Surg. Am. Vol.* **71:**828–832.

92. **McElwaine, J. P., and J. Colville.** 1984. Excision arthroplasty for infected total hip arthroplasty. *J. Bone Jt. Surg. Br. Vol.* **66:**168–171.

93. **McQueen, M., A. Littlejohn, and S. P. F. Hughes.** 1987. A comparison of systemic cefuroxime loaded bone cement in the prevention of early infection after total joint replacement. *Int. Orthop.* **11:**241–243.

94. **Miley, G. B., A. D. Scheller, Jr., and R. H. Turner.** 1982. Medical and surgical treatment of the septic hip with one-stage revision arthroplasty. *Clin. Orthop. Relat. Res.* **170:**76–82.

95. **Morrey, B. F., and R. S. Bryan.** 1983. Infection after total elbow arthroplasty. *J. Bone Jt. Surg. Am. Vol.* **65A:**330–338.

96. **Morrey, B. F., F. Westhom, S. Schoifet, J. A. Rand, and R. S. Bryan.** 1989. Long-term results of various treatment options for infected total knee arthroplasty. *Clin. Orthop. Relat. Res.* **248:**120–128.

97. **Murray, R. P., M. H. Bourne, and R. H. Fitzgerald, Jr.** 1991. Metachronous infections in patients who have had more than one total joint arthroplasty. *J. Bone Jt. Surg. Am. Vol.* **73A:**1469–1473.

98. **Murray, W. R.** 1981. Treatment of established deep wound infection after total hip arthroplasty: a report of 65 cases, p. 382–398. *In* R. E. Leach, F. T. Hoaglund, and E. J. Riseborough (ed.), *Controversies in Orthopaedic Surgery.* The W. B. Saunders Co., Philadelphia.

99. **Musher, D., and G. Landon.** 1991. Joint replacement surgery. *N. Engl. J. Med.* **324:**1368. (Letter.)

100. **Myrvik, Q. N., W. Wagner, E. Barth, P. Wood, and A. G. Gristina.** 1989. Effects of extracellular slime produced by *Staphylococcus epidermidis* on oxidative responses of rabbit alveolar macrophages. *J. Invest. Surg.* **2:**381–389.

101. **National Committee for Clinical Laboratory Standards.** 1990. *Methods for Dilution Antimicrobial Susceptibility Tests for Bacteria That Grow Aerobically,* 2nd ed. NCCLS Publication No. M7-A2. NCCLS, Villanova, Pennsylvania.

102. **National Committee for Clinical Laboratory Standards.** 1990. *Performance Standards for Antimicrobial Disk Susceptibility Tests* 4th ed. NCCLS Publication No. M2-A4. NCCLS, Villanova, Pennsylvania.

103. **Naylor, P. T., Q. N. Myrvik, and A. Gristina.** 1990. Antibiotic resistance of biomaterial-adherent coagulase-negative and coagulase-positive staphylococci. *Clin. Orthop. Relat. Res.* **261:**126–133.

104. **Nelson C. L.** 1987. The prevention of infection in total joint replacement surgery. *Rev. Infect. Dis.* **9:**613–618.

105. **Nelson, C. L., T. G. Green, R. A. Porter, and R. D. Warren.** 1983. One day versus seven days of preventive antibiotic therapy in orthopedic surgery. *Clin. Orthop. Relat. Res.* **176:**258–263.

106. **Nelson J. P.** 1982. Total knee arthroplasty infection: a review of 17 cases. *Orthop. Trans.* **6:**477.

107. **Nichols, W. W., S. M. Dorrington, M. P. E. Slack, and H. L. Walmsley.** 1988. Inhibition of tobramycin diffusion by binding to alginate. *Antimicrob. Agents Chemother.* **35:**518–523.

108. **Norden, C. W.** 1991. Antibiotic prophylaxis in orthopedic surgery. *Rev. Infect. Dis.* **13**(Suppl. 10):S842–S846.

109. **Oni, J. A., and T. Kangesu.** 1991. Yersinia enterocolitica infection of a prosthetic knee joint. *Br. J. Clin. Pract.* **45:**225.

110. **Orton, D. W., and W. H. Fulcher.** 1984. *Pasteurella multocida:* bilateral septic knee joint prostheses from a distant cat bite. *Ann. Emerg. Med.* **13:**1065–1067.

111. **Osmon, D. R., J. M. Steckelberg, B. S. P. Ang, A. D. Hanssen, and W. R. Wilson.** 1991. The significance of routine surveillance cultures in predicting primary hip arthroplasty infection. *Program Abstr. 31st Intersci. Conf. Antimicrob. Chemother.*, abstr. 1090.

112. **Osmon, D. R., J. M. Steckelberg, and A. Hanssen.** 1993. Are teeth a risk factor for prosthetic joint infection? Abstract, Musculoskeletal Infection Society Annual Meeting.

113. **Osmon, D. R., J. M. Steckelberg, and A. Hanssen.** 1993. Incidence of prosthetic joint infection due to viridans streptococci. Abstract, Musculoskeletal Infection Society Annual Meeting.

114. **Osmon, D. R., J. M. Steckelberg, M. P. Wilhelm, M. R. Keating, R. C. Walker, A. D. Hanssen, and W. R. Wilson.** 1992. Medical management of total knee arthroplasty, p. 377–392. *In* J. A. Rand (ed.), *Total Knee Arthroplasty.* Raven Press, New York.

115. **Panush, R. S., and R. W. Petty.** 1978. Inhibition of lymphocyte responses by methylmethacrylate. *Clin. Orthop. Relat. Res.* **134:**356–363.

116. **Patton, J. T.** 1989. Bone and joint infection. *Curr. Opin. Radiol.* **1:**324–330.

117. **Petty, W.** 1978. The effect of methylmethacrylate on bacterial inhibiting properties of normal human serum. *Clin. Orthop. Relat. Res.* **132:**266–277.

118. **Petty, W.** 1978. The effect of methylmethacrylate on bacterial phagocytosis and killing by human polymorphonuclear leukocytes. *J. Bone Jt. Surg. Am. Vol.* **60A:**752–757.

119. **Petty, W.** 1978. The effect of methylmethacrylate on chemotaxis of polymorphonuclear leukocytes. *J. Bone Jt. Surg. Am. Vol.* **60A:**492–498.

120. **Petty, W., R. S. Bryan, M. B. Coventry, and L. F. Peterson.** 1975. Infection after total knee arthroplasty. *Orthop. Clin. North Am.* **182:**117–126.

121. **Petty, W., and J. R. Caldwell.** 1977. The effect of methylmethacrylate on complement activity. *Clin. Orthop. Relat. Res.* **128:**354–359.

122. **Petty, W., and S. Goldsmith.** 1980. Resection arthroplasty following infected total hip. *J. Bone Jt. Surg. Am. Vol.* **62:**889–896.

123. **Pollard, J. P., S. P. F. Hughes, J. E. Scott, M. J. Evans, and M. K. D. Benson.** Antibiotic prophylaxis in total hip replacement. *Br. Med. J.* **1:**707–709.

124. **Poss, R., T. S. Thornhill, F. C. Ewald, W. H. Thomas, N. J. Batte, and C. B. Sledge.** 1984. Factors influencing the incidence and outcome of infection following total joint arthroplasty. *Clin. Orthop. Relat. Res.* **182:**117–126.

125. **Powers, K. A., M. S. Terpenning, R. A. Voice, and C. Kaufman.** 1991. Prosthetic joint infections in the elderly. *Am. J. Med.* **88:**5-9N–5-13N.

126. **Pravda, J., and E. Habermann.** 1989. *Hemophilus parainfluenzae* complicating total knee arthroplasty. A case report. *Clin Orthop. Relat. Res.* **243:**169–171.

127. **Pring, D. J., L. Marks, and J. C. Angel.** 1988. Mobility after amputation for failed knee replacement. *J. Bone Jt. Surg Br. Vol.* **70:**770–771.

128. **Rand, J. A.** 1992. Sepsis following total knee arthroplasty, p. 349–376. *In* J. A. Rand (ed.), *Total Knee Arthroplasty.* Raven Press, New York.

129. **Rand, J. A., and M. L. Brown.** 1990. The value of indium 111 leukocyte scanning in the evaluation of painful or infected total knee arthroplasties. *Clin. Orthop. Relat. Res.* **259:**179–182.

130. **Rand, J. A., and R. S. Bryan.** 1983. Reimplantation for the salvage of an infected total knee arthroplasty. *J. Bone Jt. Surg. Am. Vol.* **65:**1081–1086.

131. **Rand, J. A., R. S. Bryan, and E. Y. S. Chao.** 1987. Failed total knee arthroplasty treated by arthrodesis of the knee using the Ace-Fisher apparatus. *J. Bone Jt. Surg. Am. Vol.* **69:**39–45.

132. **Rand, J. A., R. S. Bryan, B. F. Morrey, and F. Westholm.** 1986. Management of infected total knee arthroplasty. *Clin. Orthop. Relat. Res.* **205:**75–85.

133. **Rand, J. A., and R. H. Fitzgerald, Jr.** 1989. Diagnosis and management of the infected total knee arthroplasty. *Orthop. Clin. North Am.* **20**:201–210.

134. **Rand, J. A., B. F. Morrey, and R. S. Bryan.** 1984. Management of the infected total joint arthroplasty. *Orthop. Clin. North Am.* **15**:491–504.

135. **Rosenberg, A. G., B. Haas, R. Barden, D. S. Marquez, G. C. Landon, and J. O. Galante.** 1988. Salvage of infected total knee arthroplasty. *Clin. Orthop. Relat. Res.* **226**:29–33.

136. **Rosenblatt, J. E.** 1991. Laboratory tests used to guide antimicrobial therapy. *Mayo Clin. Proc.* **66**:942–948.

137. **Russotti, G. M., M. B. Coventry, and R. N. Stauffer.** 1988. Cemented total hip arthroplasty with contemporary techniques. A five-year minimum follow-up study. *Clin. Orthop. Relat. Res.* **235**:141–147.

138. **Salvati, E. A., R. P. Robinson, S. M. Zeno, B. L. Koslin, B. D. Brause, and P. D. Wilson, Jr.** 1982. Infection rates after 3175 total hip and total knee replacements performed with and without a horizontal unidirectional filtered air flow system. *J. Bone Jt. Surg. Am. Vol.* **64**:525–535.

139. **Salvati, E. A., K. M. Chekofsky, B. D. Brause, and P. D. Wilson.** 1982. Reimplantation in infection: a twelve year experience. *Clin. Orthop. Relat. Res.* **170**:62–75.

140. **Sanderson, P. J.** 1991. Infection in orthopaedic implants. *J. Hosp. Infect.* **18**(Suppl. A):367–375.

141. **Santavirta, S., Y. T. Konttinenn, D. Nordstrom, V. Bergrtoth, I. Antti Poika, and A. Eskola.** 1989. Immune inflammatory response in infected arthroplasties. *Acta Orthop. Scand.* **60**:116–118.

142. **Santavirta, S., A. Gristina, and Y. T. Konttinen.** 1992. Cemented versus cementless hip arthroplasty. A review of prosthetic biocompatability. *Acta Orthop. Scand.* **63**:225–232.

143. **Sanzen, L., A. K. Carlsson, G. Josefsson, et al.** 1988. Revision operations on infected total hip arthroplasties. Two to nine year follow-up study. *Clin. Orthop. Relat. Res.* **229**:165–172.

144. **Schmalzrie, T. P., H. C. Amstutz, M. K. Au, and F. J. Dorey.** 1992. Etiology of deep sepsis in total hip arthroplasty. The significance of hematogenous and recurrent infections. *Clin. Orthop. Relat. Res.* **280**:200–207.

145. **Schoifet, S. D., and B. F. Morrey.** 1990. Treatment of infection after total knee arthroplasty by debridement with retention of the components. *J. Bone Jt. Surg. Am. Vol.* **72**:1383–1390.

146. **Schultiz, K. P., W. Winkelmann, and B. Schoening.** 1980. The prophylactic use of antibiotics in alloarthroplasty of the hip joint for coxarthrosis. *Arch. Orthop. Trauma Surg.* **96**:79–82.

147. **Smith, T. K.** 1991. Nutrition: its relationship to orthopedic infections. *Orthop. Clin. North Am.* **22**:373–377.

148. **Sneller, M.** 1986. Prosthetic joint infection with *Mycoplasma hominis*. *J. Infect. Dis.* **153**:174–175.

149. **Southwood, R. T., J. L. Rice, P. J. McDonald, P. H. Hakendorf, and M. A. Rozenbilds.** 1985. Infection in experimental hip arthroplasties. *J. Bone Jt. Surg. Br. Vol.* **67**:229–231.

150. **Steckelberg, J. M., L. J. Melton, D. M. Ilstrup, M. S. Rouse, and W. R. Wilson.** 1990. Influence of referral bias on the apparent clinical spectrum of infective endocarditis. *Am. J. Med.* **88**:582–587.

151. **Steckelberg, J. M., and W. R. Wilson.** 1993. Risk factors for infective endocarditis. *Infect. Dis. Clin. North Am.* **7**:9–19.

152. **Stern, S. H., J. N. Insall, R. E. Windsor, A. E. Inglis, and D. M. Dines.** 1989. Total knee arthroplasty in patients with psoriasis. *Clin. Orthop. Relat. Res.* **248:**108–110.
153. **Strazzeri, J. C., and S. Anzel.** 1986. Infected total hip arthroplasty due to *Actinomyces israelii* after dental extraction. *Clin. Orthop. Relat. Res.* **210:**128–131.
154. **Teeny, S. M., L. Door, G. Murata, and P. Conaty.** 1990. Treatment of infected total knee. Irrigation and debridement versus two-stage reimplantation. *J. Arthroplasty* **5:** 35–39.
155. **Trippel, S. B.** 1986. Antibiotic-impregnated cement in total joint arthroplasty. *J. Bone Jt. Surg. Am. Vol.* **68:**1297–1302.
156. **Tsukayama, D. T., B. Wicklund, and R. B. Gustilo.** 1991. Suppressive antibiotic therapy in chronic prosthetic joint infections. *Orthopedics* **14:**841–844.
157. **Tunkel, A. R., C. Y. Thomas, and B. Wispelwey.** 1993. Candida prosthetic arthritis: report of a case treated with fluconazole and review of the literature. *Am. J. Med.* **94:** 100–103.
158. **Turner, R. H., G. B. Miley, and P. Fremont-Smith.** 1982. Septic total hip replacement and revision arthroplasty, p. 291–314. *In* R. H. Turner and A. D. Scheller, Jr. (ed.), *Revision Total Hip Arthroplasty.* Grune and Stratton, New York.
159. **Voutsinas, S., J. Sayakos, and P. Myrnis.** 1987. Echinococcus infestation complicating total hip replacement. A case report. *J. Bone Jt. Surg. Am. Vol.* **69:**1456–1458.
160. **Walker, R. H., and D. J. Schurman.** 1984. Management of infected total knee arthroplasties. *Clin. Orthop Relat. Res.* **186:**81–89.
161. **Wegener, W. A., and A. Alavi.** 1991. Diagnostic imaging of musculoskeletal infection. Roentgenography; gallium, indium-labeled white blood cell, gammaglobulin, bone scintigraphy; and MRI. *Orthop. Clin. North Am.* **22:**401–418.
162. **Weinstein, M. P., C. W. Stratton, H. B. Hawley, A. Ackley, and L. B. Reller.** 1987. Multicenter collaborative evaluation of a standardized serum bactericidal test as a predictor of therapeutic efficacy in acute and chronic osteomyelitis. *Am. J. Med.* **83:** 218–222.
163. **White, R. H., S. A. McCurdy, and R. A. Marder.** 1990. Early morbidity after total hip replacement: rheumatoid arthritis versus osteoarthritis. *J. Gen. Intern. Med.* **5:** 304–309.
164. **Wilde, A. H., and J. T. Ruth.** 1988. Two-stage reimplantation in infected total knee arthroplasty. *Clin. Orthop. Relat. Res.* **236:**23–35.
165. **Wilson, M. G., K. Kelley, and T. S. Thornhill.** 1990. Infection as a complication of total knee-replacement arthroplasty. Risk factors and treatment in sixty-seven cases. *J. Bone Jt. Surg. Am. Vol.* **72:**878–883.
166. **Wilson, P. D., H. C. Amstutz, A. Czerniecki, E. A. Salvati, and D. G. Mendes.** 1972. Total hip replacement with fixation by acrylic cement. A preliminary study of 100 consecutive McKee-Farrar prosthetic replacements. *J. Bone Jt. Surg. Am. Vol.* **54A:** 207–236.
167. **Windsor, R. E., J. N. Insall, W. K. Urs, D. V. Miller, and B. D. Brause.** 1990. Two-stage reimplantation for the salvage of total knee arthroplasty complicated by infection. *J. Bone Jt. Surg. Am. Vol.* **72:**272–278.
168. **Wolfgang, G. L.** 1985. Tuberculosis joint infection following total knee arthroplasty. *Clin. Orthop Relat. Rel.* **201:**162–166.
169. **Woods, G. W., D. R. Lionberger, and H. S. Tullos.** 1983. Failed total knee arthroplasty. *Clin. Orthop. Relat. Rel.* **173:**184–190.
170. **Wroblewski, B. M.** 1986. One-stage revision of infected cemented total hip arthroplasty. *Clin. Orthop. Relat. Res.* **211:**103–107.
171. **Wymenga, A. B., J. R. van Horn, A. Theeuwes, H. L. Muytjens, and T. J. J. H.**

Slooff. 1992. Perioperative factors associated with septic arthritis after arthroplasty. Prospective multicenter study of 362 knee and 2651 hip operations. *Acta Orthop. Scand.* **63:**665–671.

172. **Zimmerli, W., P. D. Lew, and F. A. Waldvogel.** 1984. Pathogenesis of foreign body infections: evidence for a local granulocyte defect. *J. Clin. Invest.* **73:**1191–1200.

Infections Associated with Indwelling Medical Devices, 2nd ed.
Edited by Alan L. Bisno and Francis A. Waldvogel
© 1994 American Society for Microbiology, Washington, DC 20005

Chapter 12

Infections Associated with Foreign Bodies in the Urinary Tract

Donald Kaye and Margaret T. Hessen

Bladder catheterization is by far the most common situation in which infection associated with a foreign body occurs in the urinary tract. The catheter allows bacterial entry into the urinary tract, provides a protected site for organisms to grow, and may alter the intrinsic resistance of bladder epithelial cells to bacterial adherence. Its presence makes the treatment of infection problematic, as eradication of some organisms is difficult and recurrence is common.

Urinary tract infection is the most common nosocomial infection in the United States, and the vast majority of such cases are the result of bladder catheterization (12). Other less common foreign body infections in the urinary tract involve prosthetic devices such as bladder sphincters and penile implants, which will be discussed separately.

BLADDER CATHETERS

Definitions

Classically, "significant" bacteriuria, or bacteriuria indicative of a urinary tract infection, has been defined as a quantitative culture of more than 10^5 CFU/ml (36). Although this definition is based on studies of uncatheterized women, most studies of catheterized patients have followed the same guidelines. It is clear, however, that symptomatic infection with the recovery of fewer than 10^5 CFU/ml is common (78, 80).

Donald Kaye and Margaret T. Hessen • Department of Medicine, The Medical College of Pennsylvania, 3300 Henry Avenue, Philadelphia, Pennsylvania 19129.

Additionally, a number of investigators have found that in catheterized patients, even counts as low as 10^2 CFU/ml are likely to persist and increase and indicate infection (25, 46, 81).

Pathophysiology

Indwelling catheterization may be necessary for a variety of indications: the measurement of urine output, the collection of urine during surgery, urinary retention, and urinary incontinence. Regardless of the indication, placement of the catheter may allow ingress of bacteria. The entry of bacteria may occur in several ways: (i) organisms may be carried into the urethra or bladder as the catheter is inserted; (ii) they may gain entry to the bladder through the sheath of exudate that surrounds the catheter; or (iii) they may travel intraluminally from the inside of the tubing or collecting bag. Clearly, if the catheter is inserted with inadequate aseptic technique, bacteriuria may follow. It has been shown that even with antiseptic preparation, bacteria can be isolated from the urethral meatus in up to 80% of women (56). Guze and Beeson showed that after a single catheterization following an antimicrobial cleansing preparation, bacteria could be cultured from the catheter tips in 6 of 13 women studied (30). Experiments by Kass and Schneiderman demonstrated the development of bacteriuria with organisms colonizing the meatus, implying travel from the perineum along the external surface of the catheter to the bladder (37). This observation has been confirmed by other investigators as well (6, 13, 72). Evidence for the entry of organisms by the intraluminal pathway comes from several sources. Most important, several studies have documented the decrease in infection rate seen with closed systems compared with open drainage (42, 89), the clear implication being that organisms can travel from an unprotected and contaminated drainage vessel intraluminally to the bladder. Additionally, an increase in infection has been observed when the junction between the catheter itself and the connecting tube to the drainage bag is opened, and the trend can be reversed when the junction is made too tight to disconnect easily (65, 96). Finally, several studies have documented bacterial colonization of the drainage bag before the development of bladder bacteriuria with the same organism (71, 89). Presumably this occurs as a result of contamination of the drainage port when the collecting bag is emptied.

Once organisms gain entry to the bladder, they must be able to adhere to mucosal cells in order for infection to be established. Some organisms have particular characteristics that enable them to adhere to, infect, and remain in the urinary tract for long periods. Some strains of *Escherichia coli* may remain in the urinary tract for many months, and the ability to persist seems to correlate with the presence of P fimbriae, which act as adhesins to uroepithelial cells (85, 93). Furthermore, the presence of a catheter may promote the invasion of bladder mucosa and the development of infection. Normally, superficial bladder epithelial cells secrete a layer of mucopolysaccharide that serves as a protective film over the bladder mucosa. When this layer is removed (for example, by dilute acid), the adherence of organisms increases markedly (63). It has also been shown that an indwelling catheter can erode through this mucopolysaccharide layer, exposing bladder epithelial cells and promoting the adherence of bacteria (92). Furthermore, the presence of the catheter as a foreign body provides a protected site for bacterial growth. It is a surface upon which bacteria can deposit a thick glycoprotein matrix that, in combination with host proteins, forms a biofilm that protects organisms from host defenses, antibiotics, and the physical force of urine flow (58, 79).

Microbiology

Infecting organisms may come from the colonic flora of the patient or from the hospital environment. The spectrum of pathogens seen in patients catheterized on a short-term basis differs slightly from that seen in patients catheterized for prolonged periods; this may reflect to some extent differences in the patient populations (general health status, duration of hospitalization, exposure to antibiotics, etc.).

Enteric organisms

Among patients catheterized on a short-term basis, *E. coli* is the most common bacterial pathogen, although *Pseudomonas aeruginosa, Klebsiella* species, *Proteus* species, and enterococci also commonly occur (93). In long-term catheterization, the above-mentioned organisms (other than *E. coli*), *Providencia stuartii,* and *Morganella morganii* are commonly seen. *P. stuartii,* in particular, is able to persist for long periods in the catheterized urinary tract, and some studies suggest that the MR/K hemagglutinin produced by the organism serves as an adhesive factor, enabling the organism to adhere closely to the catheter (93). However, long-term catheterization is characterized in many patients by a turnover of microbiologic flora such that on average a new organism appears in the urine about every 2 weeks (93). These patients are virtually always bacteriuric (79). Polymicrobial bacteriuria is common in patients with long-term catheters (94).

Coagulase-negative staphylococci

As in other nosocomial infections, the role of coagulase-negative staphylococci in producing infection of the urinary tract has been increasingly recognized (59, 74). While novobiocin-resistant *Staphylococcus saprophyticus* is the most common staphylococcus to produce urinary tract infection in sexually active young women, novobiocin-susceptible strains, especially *Staphyloccus epidermidis*, are more commonly found as urinary tract pathogens in older or more debilitated patients, including those with indwelling catheters (59). These organisms are perhaps most frequently seen as urinary tract pathogens in patients who have recently undergone urinary tract surgery (76). The production of a glycoprotein matrix, or "slime," by *S. epidermidis* on plastic intravascular catheters has been well documented (64). It is likely that this occurs on urinary catheters as well and provides a protected site for organisms to grow as outlined above.

Yeasts

Candida and *Torulopsis* species are seen frequently as bladder pathogens in the setting of long-term catheterization. Both occur most commonly in patients who are diabetic or who have been taking antibiotics.

Epidemiology

Various risk factors for the development of catheter-associated urinary tract infection have been identified by multivariate analysis. These include the duration of catheterization, microbial colonization of the drainage bag, female sex, and diabetes mellitus (25). The use of antibiotics and the presence of a urinemeter on the drainage bag correlate inversely with a risk of infection (25, 93). Regardless of these risk factors, the incidence of urinary tract infection differs depending on the type of catheter system used, as does the efficacy of various measures designed to prevent infection. There are two main types of indwelling catheter systems: open and closed.

Open system

The open system consists of a catheter that is connected to a long tube that drains into an open collecting vessel. By 4 days of catheterization, nearly all patients with an open drainage system develop urinary tract infection (36). Several measures have been undertaken to reduce the risk of urinary tract infection in these patients. These measures include the administration of systemic prophylactic antibiotics, the use of local antibiotics either at the urethral meatus or impregnated into the catheter, and the irrigation of the bladder with antimicrobial solutions.

The use of systemic antibiotics for prophylaxis has been studied extensively. Unfortunately, as might be anticipated, systemic antibiotics in this setting do not prevent bacteriuria; they merely determine which organisms will invade, namely, those resistant to the antibiotic administered (4, 36, 48).

The use of local antibiotics in the form of antimicrobial lotions and lubricants has also been studied. This measure was designed to prevent contamination of the catheter as it is inserted into the urethra and to retard colonization of the periurethral area with potential pathogens. This practice has been found to be ineffective with the open drainage system, in which the major source of infection is intraluminal migration of organisms (3).

Several antibacterial bladder rinses have been examined in the setting of open catheter drainage. The solution is administered either as continuous irrigation, using a triple-lumen (three-way) catheter, or as a periodic instillation after which the catheter is clamped, allowing the solution to remain in contact with the bladder mucosa for an hour or so. The use of dilute (0.25%) acetic acid was found to delay the onset of bacteriuria (38, 48). However, the effect occurred only when the urine pH remained under 5, and the solution was not without side effects (bladder irritation, hematuria, and systemic acidosis) (3). A neomycin-polymyxin mixture has also been used as an antimicrobial irrigant for the prevention of infection in open drainage systems. This solution was found to retard the development of bacteriuria and gram-negative bacillus bacteremia. However, when urinary tract infection occurred, it was with resistant organisms (48, 49, 52, 90). This system maintains about 50% of patients free from bacteriuria for 10 days, but it is expensive.

Closed system

By far the most significant improvement in the prevention of catheter-associated bacteriuria came with the development of the closed drainage system. In this system the connecting tube from the catheter drains into a plastic collecting bag, to which it is securely fastened so that there are no open connections between the patient and the environment except for the brief period during which the contents of the collecting bag are emptied. As long as the system is used as designed (i.e., without disconnecting the tubing and with aseptic drainage of the collecting bag), sterility of the urine can be maintained in about 50% of patients for 10 to 14 days (42, 53).

Even with a closed system, the incidence of infection is about 5 to 10%/day (93). Therefore, some of the measures proposed for the prevention of infection in patients with open drainage systems have also been studied as adjunctive measures when closed drainage is used. As with open drainage systems, the use of antimicrobial ointments and lubricants has not been found to add any significant protection from infection (10). Likewise, although bladder instillation or irrigation of antimicrobial solutions was protective in open drainage systems, such measures do not appear to confer any additional protection over the closed system when the two are used together (27, 82). Some investigators have aimed their efforts at preventing colonization of the collected urine by instilling antimicrobial agents into the drainage bag. These efforts have not been particularly successful (26, 86, 88), although one study did show efficacy of hydrogen peroxide in preventing colonization and infection (46).

Other attempts to reduce infection have included impregnating the catheter with antimicrobial materials such as silver oxide. Clinical studies of efficacy have generated conflicting results (35, 43, 79). Other investigators have examined the effect of various structural materials (red rubber, Teflon, etc.) on bacterial adherence, postulating that less adherence will correlate with delayed or less frequent infection (69).

The use of systemic antibiotics for the prophylaxis of infection in patients with closed drainage systems has also been examined. Prospective trials indicate that prophylaxis may be effective in preventing or postponing bacteriuria in the setting of short-term, closed drainage catheterization; i.e., the risk of bacteriuria is reduced for the first 4 days, after which no protective effect is seen (7, 55, 67).

The nosocomial spread of infection from one catheterized patient to another has been documented as the cause of several hospital outbreaks of catheter-associated infection (19, 47, 70). It is presumed that the pathogens are transferred on the hands of hospital personnel or via a contaminated collecting vessel that is not properly cleaned between patients.

Diagnosis and Therapy

The diagnosis of catheter-related urinary tract infection is based on both clinical and laboratory information. Clearly, the catheterized patient with fever, flank pain, and bacteriuria with more than 10^5 CFU/ml should be regarded as having urinary tract infection and should be treated. Often the situation is not so obvious. In more confusing cases (e.g., in the severely ill intensive care unit patient with fever and multiple possible sources of infection) the existence of more than 10^5 CFU/ml in urine does not necessarily indicate a urinary source of fever. As most patients with urinary tract infection (symptomatic or asymptomatic) have pyuria, the absence of pyuria (except in neutropenic patients) should make a urinary source suspect. However, the presence of pyuria does not necessarily indicate a urinary source of fever.

While patients with closed indwelling catheter systems can be cured of their urinary tract infections, reinfection is usually prompt (11, 42). We do not treat catheterized patients with asymptomatic bacteriuria, thus avoiding unnecessary antibiotic exposure and subsequent infection with increasingly resistant organisms.

Once the catheter is removed, therapy is much more likely to result in cure. Often catheter removal alone will result in the clearance of bacteriuria (15, 29, 32). When catheter removal is not feasible but therapy is necessary because of symptoms, antibiotic therapy should be aimed specifically at the organism recovered from the urine. While there is little evidence for any particular duration of therapy, a period of 7 to 10 days seems reasonable. There is no evidence that replacing the old catheter with a new one improves therapy unless the catheter is blocked by concretions or heavy exudate.

Yeasts

The management of candiduria is a difficult and controversial issue. Bladder candiduria occurs frequently and is usually of little consequence (90). However, the possibility of upper tract or systemic infection or both has different implications than those associated with other organisms, as they are often difficult to detect and effective therapeutic options are limited.

Bladder candiduria occurs most frequently in the setting of diabetes or antibiotic administration. When the catheter is removed, the candiduria usually resolves (90). If candiduria continues, the presence of persistent bladder, or even upper tract, infection must be considered (45). *Candida* bladder infection may be diagnosed by the observation of a thrush-like membrane on cystoscopy. Rarely, upper tract infection may occur by the ascending route; more commonly, it is a manifestation of disseminated candidiasis and occurs secondary to hematogenous spread. Fungus balls may be seen in the collecting system when kidney infection occurs and may cause obstruction in the ureter, renal pelvis, or parenchyma.

From a practical (relatively noninvasive) viewpoint, the following approach to the management of candiduria seems reasonable. If the patient is asymptomatic and the catheter can be removed, the patient should be followed clinically and with repeat urinalyses and cultures. If the candiduria persists, or initially if the patient is symptomatic, a 5-day course of amphotericin B bladder washes (100 mg of amphotericin B in 500 ml of 5% glucose instilled over 24 h by a three-way catheter or instilled and left for 1 h with the catheter clamped) may eradicate the candiduria (17). If the candiduria is persistent or recurs promptly, or initially, if the patient is severely or systemically ill and other sources of infection are not apparent, a search for upper tract or systemic infection should be undertaken. Blood cultures, examination of the eye grounds for evidence of *Candida* endophthalmitis, ultrasound of the kidneys for fungus balls, and possibly cystoscopic examination should be done. If renal or systemic involvement is proven or strongly suspected, a course of systemic amphotericin B or fluconazole should be given.

If long-term catheterization cannot be discontinued, an attempt at eradication is reasonable with amphotericin B bladder washes after insertion of a new catheter. However, if this is unsuccessful, the best course is probably to ignore the candiduria unless it becomes symptomatic.

Postcatheterization Follow-Up

Whether the patient has been catheterized for a short or long period, urine should be cultured after catheterization is discontinued. Although bacteriuria will often clear after removal of the catheter, as mentioned, it may not. Indeed, patients who have had catheter-associated bacteriuria, symptomatic or otherwise, are at greater risk the year after catheterization of having symptomatic urinary tract infection (1). It seems warranted to recommend the treatment of even asymptomatic patients who are found to be persistently bacteriuric after catheter removal (93).

Complications

Complications of bladder catheterization are relatively frequent and may be serious. It has been documented that in patients with indwelling catheters, urinary tract infection frequently is not confined to the lower tract but may involve the kidneys as well. In an autopsy study of patients dying in a chronic care facility, those with indwelling catheters at the time of death had a much greater incidence of acute pyelonephritis than did patients without catheters (38 versus 5%) (93). Whether long-term catheterization and frequent infections result in or contribute to chronic inflammation and renal scarring remains unclear, although several studies have attempted to address that issue (16, 61, 87).

Although urinary tract infection is the most common complication of catheterization, bacteremia is the most serious and may be life threatening. Catheter insertion itself may cause transient, and in most cases asymptomatic, bacteremia in up to 8% of patients (18, 84). Approximately 1 to 4% of patients with catheter-associated bacteriuria develop bacteremia (9, 29, 71); in these cases very often the patient is symptomatic, and septic shock and death may occur. In a multivariate analysis of risk factors, some investigators have found that the development of catheter-associated bacteriuria was associated with a threefold-greater risk of mortality than was observed in nonbacteriuric catheterized patients (66).

Various other complications also deserve mention. Urinary tract stones are a common problem in patients with chronic indwelling catheters and may occur in part as a result of chronic or repeated infections with urease-splitting organisms such as *Proteus* species. Such stones may eventually lead to renal failure (91) and may form a nidus for persistent infection that will be refractory to treatment as long as the stone remains. Bladder stones may cause blockage of the catheter, as may concretions composed of bacteria, biofilm, crystals, and Tamm-Horsfall protein. Finally, local periurethral infections such as epididymitis, prostatitis, and scrotal abscess also may occur as complications of bladder catheterization and bacteriuria (95).

Alternatives

Certainly the duration of catheterization should be kept to a minimum whenever possible. In some circumstances, however, it must be recognized that chronic and irremediable difficulties exist and that some method of bladder drainage must be maintained on a long-term basis, e.g., in a chronically ill debilitated patient with a bladder outlet obstruction or neurogenic bladder. Although a chronic indwelling catheter will serve the purpose, alternative methods with fewer complications are often available.

In males, condom catheters may be useful and may avoid urinary infections, as there is no violation of the bladder itself. Nevertheless, bladder bacteriuria may occur occasionally, probably as the result of heavy colonization in the moist enclosed area around the urethral meatus (19, 33, 54, 62). Bacteriuria is most likely to occur in those who manipulate the condom. Additionally, some complications are reported, namely, skin breakdown, urethral diverticuli, and ischemia (28).

Suprapubic catheterization has been enthusiastically endorsed by some as an alternative to the indwelling catheter. Although the bladder is invaded and a foreign body remains in place, the rationale is that entry to the bladder occurs through a relatively clean and dry surface, as opposed to the moist, heavily colonized perineum. The use of suprapubic catheters has been studied extensively in circumstances of short-term catheterization (postsurgical) but has not been studied prospectively in populations requiring long-term drainage (1, 22, 34, 50). In those studies in which the incidence of postoperative bacteriuria with suprapubic drainage was compared with the incidence with Foley catheter drainage, conclusions have been mixed, and several of the studies have methodological flaws. Some authors (1, 22) have found that suprapubic drainage offers considerable protection against infection, but others have been unable to find a significant difference in the rates of bacteriuria (34, 73).

Intermittent straight catheterization has been extensively used as an alternative to chronic indwelling catheterization, particularly in patients who have neurogenic bladders, who are mentally functional, and who have the use of both upper extremities. In most circumstances, catheter insertion occurs under clean, but not sterile, conditions. While bacteriuria occurs in a substantial proportion of patients (31, 83), the incidence of significant bacteriuria is calculated by some to be less than half that associated with chronic indwelling catheterization (93). When infection occurs, it is more easily cured, and the technique provides a less cumbersome and more appealing alternative to some patients. Moreover, some investigators have found that prophylactic antibiotics, administered either locally by bladder instillation or systemically, are effective in reducing the incidence of bacteriuria (2, 41, 51). As indicated previously, however, the chronic or frequent use of antibiotics may ultimately predispose to infections with increasingly resistant organisms.

Recently, an intraurethral catheter has been introduced as an alternative to the standard Foley catheter. This device is a tube measuring several centimeters and is surgically inserted into the bladder neck and prostatic urethra. It may remain in place for several months. Infection rates in one small study were low, but further clinical evaluation is needed (60).

Preventive Measures

Many of the measures designed to prevent or retard the development of bacteriuria have been mentioned already. To summarize, however, the following recommendations should be considered when the use of an indwelling catheter is contemplated.

(i) It should be used only when necessary and for as short a period as possible. Alternative approaches should be considered.

(ii) A stringent aseptic technique must be used when the catheter is inserted.

(ii) Only closed catheter drainage systems should be used, and the system must be kept closed. (a) If it is opened and inadvertently contaminated, it should be replaced. Irrigation should be performed only when obstruction occurs, and in those circumstances, a sterile technique must be used in entering the system. (b) Urine for culture should be aspirated from the proximal port on the drainage tube, using a sterile syringe and needle after carefully preparing the port with antiseptic solution. (c) Urine should be emptied from the drainage port at the bottom of the collecting bag into a sterile vessel. (d) The collecting bag should always be lower than the patient so that "downhill" flow is maintained.

(iv) Catheters should be replaced only if there are obstructing concretions present or if the system is otherwise obstructed.

(v) Catheterized patients should be separated from each other when possible.

(vi) In patients with cardiac lesions predisposing them to endocarditis, prophylactic antibiotics should be given at times of catheter manipulation when the urine is infected, in accordance with the recommendations of the American Heart Association (14).

(vii) Personnel and patients should be instructed in routine catheter care. Some advise perineal care twice daily, consisting of washing gently with soap and water. However, others point out the increased risk of infection associated with manipulation of the catheter, as might occur when this is done.

OTHER PROSTHETIC DEVICES

Prosthetic bladder sphincters and penile devices have been in use since the early 1970s. The prosthetic bladder sphincter has been used for the treatment of urinary incontinence and consists of a periurethral cuff. Two designs are in use. One exerts a fixed periurethral pressure that is overcome when the patient exerts external pressure on the abdominal wall. In the other, the sphincter pressure is exerted by use of a compression pump, and pressure is released manually by decompression of the pump. Likewise, penile prostheses for the treatment of impotence are available in several designs. One type consists of a rod that is hinged or flexible. The other is an inflatable device with a pump, analogous to the bladder sphincter described above. Insertion of any of these foreign bodies may be complicated by infection, although the use of perioperative prophylactic antibiotics has reduced the infection rate significantly (77). The use of special surgical garb, protective tents, HEPA filtration, and similar measures designed to reduce intraoperative contamination may reduce infection rates even further (5).

Even with prophylaxis and meticulous surgical technique, infection of these devices occurs in 1 to 8% of primary implants (5). The most common pathogens are coagulase-negative staphylococci, followed by enteric gram-negative bacteria (5). Gonococcal and fungal infections have been reported (57, 75). The usual route of infection is through the incision at the time of surgery, though the hematogenous route has been implicated in some cases (5). Putative risk factors for infection include paraplegia, neurogenic bladder, presence of a urinary tract infection, repeat implantation, and possibly diabetes mellitus (5, 68). Infection may present promptly or may be delayed for several years, as can happen when organisms such as *S. epidermidis*, which tend to cause indolent infections, are involved. Likewise, infection may be easily detected when fever, pain, erythema, and purulent drainage are present, or it may be more subtly manifested simply by thickening of the surrounding capsule, mild tenderness, malfunction of the device, etc.

Infections may be classified as "superficial" or "deep." The former may be cured by antibiotics alone (40); most deep infections require removal of the device in addition to antibiotic therapy (8, 20, 23, 39, 40). Antibiotic selection should be guided by the susceptibility pattern of the organism(s) isolated. Optimal duration of antibiotic therapy has not been clearly defined. We recommend 10 to 14 days of therapy after the implant has been removed, followed by observation for several months before replacement is considered. Some authors suggest that when infection is mild, a new prosthesis may be reinserted at the same operation, after the cavity has been thoroughly irrigated (21, 24, 44). The rationale for this approach is that if placement of a new prosthesis is delayed, the cavity may become so scarred that replacement is impossible. When a new device is placed at the time the original is removed, long-term (or indefinite) oral antibiotics should be given after an initial course of intravenous therapy, because the risk of infection in the new device is high (5).

SUMMARY

In summary, infections involving foreign bodies in the urinary tract cause significant morbidity, mortality, and cost in the United States and result in a large number of infectious and noninfectious complications. Indwelling catheterization of the urinary tract should be reserved for situations in which it is clearly needed and should be maintained for as short a duration as possible. When an indwelling catheter becomes necessary, a closed drainage system should be used and should be maintained aseptically until it becomes infected. Asymptomatic infection should not be treated. Symptomatic infections should be treated by catheter removal, if possible, and antibiotics. The incidence of infectious complications of permanent implantable devices such as bladder sphincters and penile prostheses may be reduced by the judicious use of prophylactic antibiotics. When infection does occur, removal of the foreign body is often necessary.

REFERENCES

1. Andersen, J. T., L. Heisterberg, S. Hebjorn, K. Petersen, S. S. Sorensen, W. Fisher-Rasmussen, L. M. Pedersen, and N. C. Nielsen. 1985. Suprapubic vs. transurethral bladder drainage after colposuspension/vaginal repair. *Acta Obstet. Gynecol. Scand.* **64:** 139–143.

2. Anderson, R. U. 1980. Prophylaxis of bacteriuria during intermittent catheterization of the acute neurogenic bladder. *J. Urol.* **123:**364–366.

3. Andriole, V. T. 1972. Care of the indwelling catheter, p. 256–266. *In* D. Kaye (ed.), *Urinary Tract Infection and Its Management.* The C. V. Mosby Co., Chicago.

4. Beeson, P. B. 1958. Case against the catheter. *Am. J. Med.* **24:**1–3.

5. Blum, M. D. 1989. Infections of genitourinary prostheses. *Infect. Dis. Clin. North Am.* **3:**259–274.

6. Brehmer, B., and P. O. Madsen. 1972. Route and prophylaxis of ascending bladder infection in male patients with indwelling catheters. *J. Urol.* **108:**719–721.

7. Britt, M. R., R. A. Garibaldi, W. A. Miller, R. M. Hebertson, and J. P. Burke. 1977. Antimicrobial prophylaxis for catheter-associated bacteriuria. *Antimicrob. Agents Chemother.* **11:**240–243.

8. Bruskewitz, R., S. Raz, R. B. Smith, and J. J. Kaufman. 1980. AMS 742 sphincter: UCLA experience. *J. Urol.* **124:**812–814.

9. Bryan, C., and K. Reynolds. 1984. Hospital acquired bacteremic urinary tract infection: epidemiology and outcome. *J. Urol.* **132:**494–498.

10. Butler, H. K., and C. M. Kunin. 1968. Evaluation of polymyxin catheter lubricant and impregnated catheters. *J. Urol.* **100:**560–566.

11. Butler, H. K., and C. M. Kunin. 1968. Evaluation of specific systemic antimicrobial therapy in patients while on closed catheter drainage. *J. Urol.* **100:**567–572.

12. Centers for Disease Control. 1986. Nosocomial infection surveillance, 1984. *Morbid. Mortal. Weekly Rep.* **35:**19SS.

13. Daifuku, R., and W. Stamm. 1984. Association of rectal and urethral colonization with urinary tract infection in patients with indwelling catheters. *JAMA* **252:**2028–2030.

14. Dajani, A. S., A. L. Bisno, K. J. Chung, D. T. Durack, M. Freed, M. A. Gerber, A. W. Karchmer, H. D. Millard, S. Rahimtoola, S. T. Shulman, C. Watanakunakorn, and K. A. Taubert. 1990. Prevention of bacterial endocarditis. Recommendations by the American Heart Association. *JAMA* **264:**2919–2922.

15. Davies, A., and K. Schroff. 1983. When should a urine specimen be examined after removal of a urinary catheter? *J. Hosp. Infect.* **4:**177–180.

16. Dietrick, R. B., and S. Russi. 1958. Tabulation and review of autopsy findings in fifty-five paraplegics. *JAMA* **166:**41–44.

17. Edwards, J. E., Jr. 1991. Candida species, p. 1943–1958. *In* G. L. Mandell, R. G. Douglas, Jr., and J. E. Bennett (ed.), *Principles and Practice of Infectious Disease,* 3rd ed. Churchill Livingstone, New York.

18. Everett, E. D., and J. V. Hirschmann. 1977. Transient bacteremia and endocarditis prophylaxis, a review. *Medicine* **56:**61–77.

19. Fierer, J., and M. Ekstrom. 1981. An outbreak of *Providencia stuartii* urinary tract infections: patients with condom catheters are a reservoir of the bacteria. *JAMA* **245:** 1553–1555.

20. Finney, R. P., J. R. Sharpe, and R. W. Sadlowski. 1980. Finney hinged penile implant: experience with 100 cases. *J. Urol.* **124:**205–207.

21. Fishman, U., F. B. Scott, and A. M. Selim. 1981. Rescue procedure: an alternative to complete removal for treatment of infected penile prostheses. *J. Urol.* **137:**202A.

22. **Frymire, L. J.** 1971. Comparison of suprapubic vs. Foley drains. *Obstet. Gynecol.* **38:** 239–244.
23. **Furlow, W. L.** 1979. Inflatable penile prosthesis: Mayo Clinic experience with 175 patients. *Urology* **13:**166–171.
24. **Furlow, W. L., and B. Goldwasser.** 1987. Salvage of the eroded inflatable penile prosthesis: a new concept. *J. Urol.* **138:**312–314.
25. **Garibaldi, R. A., J. P. Burke, M. R. Britt, W. A. Miller, and C. B. Smith.** 1980. Meatal colonization and catheter-associated bacteriuria. *N. Engl. J. Med.* **303:**316–318.
26. **Gillespie, W., J. Jones, C. Teasdale, R. A. Simpson, L. Nashef, and D. C. E. Speller.** 1983. Does the addition of disinfectant to urine drainage bags prevent infection in catheterized patients? *Lancet* **i:**1037–1039.
27. **Gladstone, J. L., and C. G. Robinson.** 1968. Prevention of bacteriuria resulting from indwelling catheters. *J. Urol.* **99:**458–461.
28. **Golji, H.** 1981. Complications of external condom drainage. *Paraplegia* **19:**189–197.
29. **Gordon, D., A. Bune, B. Grime, P. J. McDonald, V. R. Marshall, J. Marsh, and G. Sinclair.** 1983. Diagnostic criteria and natural history of catheter-associated urinary tract infections after prostatectomy. *Lancet* **i:**1269–1271.
30. **Guze, L. B., and P. B. Beeson.** 1956. Observations on the reliability and safety of bladder catheterization for bacteriologic study of the urine. *N. Engl. J. Med.* **25:**474–475.
31. **Hardy, A. G.** 1966. Experiences with intermittent catheterization in acute paraplegia. *Med. Serv. J. Can.* **22:**538–544.
32. **Harstein, A. L., S. B. Garber, T. Ward, S. R. Jones, and V. H. Morthland.** 1981. Nosocomial urinary tract infections: a prospective evaluation of 108 catheterized patients. *Infect. Control* **2:**380–386.
33. **Hirsch, D. D., V. Fainstein, and D. M. Musher.** 1979. Do condom catheter collecting systems cause urinary tract infections? *JAMA* **242:**340–341.
34. **Hofmeister, F. J., W. E. Martens, and R. L. Strebel.** 1970. Foley catheter or suprapubic tube? *Am. J. Obstet. Gynecol.* **107:**767–769.
35. **Johnson, J. R., P. L. Roberts, R. J. Olsen, K. A. Moyer, W. E. Stamm.** 1990. Prevention of catheter-associated urinary tract infection with a silver oxide-coated urinary catheter: clinical and microbiologic correlates. *J. Infect. Dis.* **162:**1145–1150.
36. **Kass, E. H.** 1956. Asymptomatic infections of the urinary tract. *Trans. Assoc. Am. Physicians* **69:**56–64.
37. **Kass, E. H., and L. J. Schneiderman.** 1957. Entry of bacteria into the urinary tracts in patients with inlying catheters. *N. Engl. J. Med.* **256:**556–557.
38. **Kass, E. H., and H. S. Sossen.** 1959. Prevention of infection of urinary tract in presence of indwelling catheter: description of electromechanical valve to provide intermittent drainage of the bladder. *JAMA* **169:**1181–1183.
39. **Kessler, R.** 1981. Complications of inflatable penile prostheses. *Urology* **18:**470–472.
40. **Kramer, S. A., E. E. Anderson, J. J. Braedael, and D. F. Paulson.** 1979. Complications of Small-Carrion penile prosthesis. *Urology* **13:**49–51.
41. **Krebs, M., R. Halvorsen, I. Fishman, and N. Santos-Merdoza.** 1984. Prevention of urinary tract infection during intermittent catheterization. *J. Urol.* **131:**82–85.
42. **Kunin, C. M., and R. C. McCormack.** 1966. Prevention of catheter-induced urinary tract infections by sterile closed drainage. *N. Engl. J. Med.* **274:**1155–1161.
43. **Liedberg, H., T. Lundeberg.** 1990. Silver alloy coated catheters reduce catheter-associated bacteriuria. *Br. J. Urol.* **65:**379–381.
44. **Light, J. K., and F. B. Scott.** 1986. Salvage of the infected inflatable penile prosthesis, p. 418–419. *In* J. J. Kaufman (ed.), *Current Urologic Therapy*, 2nd ed. The W. B. Saunders Co., Philadelphia.

45. **Louria, D. B., and G. Finkel.** 1965. Candida pyelonephritis, p. 179–184. *In* E. H. Kass (ed.), *Progress in Pyelonephritis.* F. A. Davis, Philadelphia.
46. **Maizels, M., and A. J. Schaeffer.** 1986. Decreased incidence of bacteriuria associated with periodic instillation of hydrogen peroxide into the urethral catheter drainage bag. *J. Urol.* **123:**841–845.
47. **Maki, D. G., C. G. Hennekens, C. W. Phillips, W. V. Shaw, and J. V. Bennett.** 1973. Nosocomial urinary tract infection with *Serratia marcescens:* an epidemiologic study. *J. Infect. Dis.* **128:**579–587.
48. **Martin, C. M., and E. N. Bookrajian.** 1962. Bacteriuria prevention after indwelling urinary catheterization: a controlled study. *Arch. Intern. Med.* **110:**703–711.
49. **Martin, C. M., F. Vaquer, M. S. Meyers, and A. El-Dadah.** 1964. Prevention of gram-negative rod bacteremia associated with indwelling urinary-tract catheterization. *Antimicrob. Agents Chemother.* **3:**617–623.
50. **Mattingly, R. F., D. E. Moore, and D. O. Clark.** 1972. Bacteriologic study of suprapubic bladder drainage. *Am. J. Obstet. Gynecol.* **114:**732–738.
51. **Maynard, F., and A. Diokno.** 1984. Urinary infection and complications during clean intermittent catheterization following spinal cord injury. *J. Urol.* **132:**943–946.
52. **Meyers, M. S., B. C. Schroeder, and C. M. Martin.** 1965. Controlled trial of nitrofurazone and neomycin-polymyxin as constant bladder rinses for prevention of postindwelling catheterization bacteriuria. *Antimicrob. Agents Chemother.* **4:**571–581.
53. **Miller, A., K. B. Linton, W. A. Gillespie, N. Slade, and J. P. Mitchell.** 1960. Catheter drainage and infection in acute retention of urine. *Lancet* **ii:**310–312.
54. **Montgomerie, J. Z., and J. W. Morrow.** 1978. *Pseudomonas* colonization in patients with spinal cord injury. *Am. J. Epidemiol.* **108:**328–336.
55. **Mountokalakis, T., M. Skounakis, and J. Tselentis.** 1985. Short-term versus prolonged systemic antibiotic prophylaxis in patients treated with indwelling catheters. *J. Urol.* **134:**506–508.
56. **Mulla, N.** 1961. Indwelling catheter in gynecologic surgery. *Obstet. Gynecol.* **17:**191–201.
57. **Nelson, R. P., and J. C. Gregory.** 1988. Gonococcal infections of penile prostheses. *Urology* **31:**391–394.
58. **Nickel, J. C., J. A. Downey, and J. W. Costerton.** 1989. Ultrastructural study of microbiologic colonization of urinary catheters. *Urology* **34:**284–291.
59. **Nicolle, L. E., S. A. Hoban, and G. K. M. Hardey.** 1983. Characterization of coagulase-negative staphylococci from urinary tract specimens. *J. Clin. Microbiol.* **17:**267–271.
60. **Nissenkorn, I., and D. Slutzker.** 1991. The intraurethral catheter: long-term followup in patients with urinary retention due to infravesical obstruction. *Br. J. Urol.* **68:**277–279.
61. **Nyren, P., L. Runeberg, A. L. Kostiala, O. V. Renkonen, and R. Roire.** 1981. Prophylactic methenamine hippurate or nitrofurantoin in patients with an indwelling urinary catheter. *Ann. Clin. Res.* **13:**16–21.
62. **Ouslander, J. G., B. A. Greengold, F. J. Silverblatt, and J. P. Garcia.** 1987. An accurate method to obtain urine for culture from men with external catheters. *Arch. Intern. Med.* **147:**286–288.
63. **Parsons, C. L., S. H. Schrom, P. Hanno, and G. Mulholland.** 1978. Bladder surface mucin: examination of possible mechanisms for its antibacterial effect. *Invest. Urol.* **6:**196–200.
64. **Peter, G., R. Locci, and G. Pulverer.** 1982. Adherence and growth of coagulase-negative staphylococci on surfaces of intravascular catheters. *J. Infect. Dis.* **146:**479–482.
65. **Platt, R., B. Murdock, B. J. Polk, and B. Rosner.** 1983. Reduction of mortality associated with nosocomial urinary tract infection. *Lancet* **i:**1893–1897.

66. **Platt, R., B. F. Polk, B. Murdock, and B. Rosner.** 1982. Mortality associated with nosocomial urinary tract infection. *N. Engl. J. Med.* **307**:637–642.
67. **Polk, B. F., M. Shapiro, P. Goldstein, I. B. Tager, B. Goren-White, and S. C. Schoenbaum.** 1980. Randomized clinical trial of perioperative cefazolin in preventing infection after hysterectomy. *Lancet* **i**:437–440.
68. **Radomski, S. B., and S. Herschorn.** 1992. Risk factors associated with penile prosthesis infection. *J. Urol.* **147**:383–385.
69. **Roberts, J. A., E. N. Fussell, and M. B. Kaack.** 1990. Bacterial adherence to urethral catheters. *J. Urol.* **144**:264–269.
70. **Schaberg, D. R., R. W. Haley, A. K. Highsmith, R. L. Anderson, and J. E. McGowan.** 1980. Nosocomial bacteriuria: a prospective study of case clustering and antimicrobial resistance. *Ann. Intern. Med.* **93**:420–424.
71. **Schaeffer, A. J.** 1986. Catheter-associated bacteriuria. *Urol. Clin. North Am.* **13**:735–747.
72. **Schaeffer, A. J., and J. Chmiel.** 1983. Urethral colonization in the pathogenesis of catheter-associated bacteriuria. *J. Urol.* **130**:1096–1099.
73. **Schiotz, H. A., P. A. Malme, and T. G. Tanbo.** 1989. Urinary tract infections and asymptomatic bacteriuria after vaginal plastic surgery: a comparison of suprapubic and transurethral catheters. *Acta Obstet. Gynecol. Scand.* **68**:453–455.
74. **Sewell, C. M., J. E. Clarridge, E. L. Young, and R. K. Guthrie.** 1982. Clinical significance of coagulase-negative staphylococci. *J. Clin. Microbiol.* **16**:236–239.
75. **Shabsigh, R., I. J. Fishman, D. L. Kessler, and F. B. Scott.** 1986. Experience with fungal infection of genitourinary prostheses. *J. Urol.* **135**:359A.
76. **Shrestha, T. L., and J. H. Darrell.** 1979. Urinary infection with coagulase negative staphylococci in a teaching hospital. *J. Clin. Pathol.* **32**:299–302.
77. **Small, M. P.** 1978. The Small-Carrion penile prosthesis. *Urol. Clin. North Am.* **5**:549–562.
78. **Stamey, T. A., D. E. Govan, and J. M. Palmer.** 1965. The localization and treatment of urinary tract infections: the role of bactericidal urine levels as opposed to serum levels. *Medicine* **44**:1–36.
79. **Stamm, W. E.** 1991. Catheter-associated urinary tract infections: epidemiology, pathogenesis, and prevention. *Am. J. Med.* **91**(Suppl. 3B):65S–71S.
80. **Stamm, W. E., G. W. Counts, K. R. Running, S. Fihn, M. Turck, and K. K. Holmes.** 1982. Diagnosis of coliform infection in acutely dysuric women. *N. Engl. J. Med.* **307**:463–468.
81. **Stark, R. P., and D. G. Maki.** 1984. Bacteriuria in the catheterized patient: what quantitative level is relevant? *N. Engl. J. Med.* **311**:560–564.
82. **Stickler, D.J.** 1990. The role of antiseptics in the management of patients undergoing short-term indwelling bladder catheterization. *J. Hosp. Infect.* **16**:89–108.
83. **Stickler, D. J., C. B. Wilmot, and J. D. O'Flynn.** 1970. The mode of development of urinary infections in intermittently catheterized male patients. *Paraplegia* **8**:243–252.
84. **Sullivan, N. M., V. L. Sutter, M. M. Mims, V. H. Marsh, and S. M. Finegold.** 1973. Clinical aspects of bacteremia after manipulation of the genitourinary tract. *J. Infect. Dis.* **127**:49–55.
85. **Svanborg-Eden, C., and H. A. Hansson.** 1978. *Escherichia coli* pili as possible mediators of attachment to human urinary tract epithelial cells. *Infect. Immun.* **21**:229–237.
86. **Sweet, D. E., H. C. Goodpasture, K. Hill, S. Smart, H. Alexander, and A. Hedari.** 1985. Evaluation of H_2O_2 prophylaxis of bacteriuria in patients with long-term indwelling Foley catheters: a randomized controlled study. *Infect. Control* **6**:263–266.
87. **Talbot, H. S.** 1966. Renal disease and hypertension in paraplegics and quadriplegics. *Med. Serv. J. Can.* **22**:570–575.

88. Thompson, R. C., C. E. Hally, M. A. Searcy, S. M. Guenther, D. L. Kaiser, D. H. M. Groschel, Y. Gillenwater, and R. P. Wenzel. 1984. Catheter-associated bacteriuria: failure to reduce attack rates using periodic instillations of a disinfectant into urinary drainage systems. *JAMA* **251:**747–751.

89. Thornton, G. F., and V. T. Andriole. 1970. Bacteriuria during indwelling catheter drainage. II. Effect of a closed sterile drainage system. *JAMA* **214:**339–342.

90. Thornton, G. F., B. Lytton, and V. T. Andriole. 1966. Bacteriuria during indwelling catheter drainage. *JAMA* **195:**179–183.

91. Tribe, C. R., and J. R. Silver. 1969. *Renal Failure in Paraplegia,* p. 51. Pitman Medical Publishing Co., London.

92. Vardi, Y., T. Meschulam, N. Obedeanj, D. Merzbach, and J. D. Sobel. 1983. In vivo adherence of *Pseudomonas aeruginosa* to rat bladder epithelium. *Proc. Soc. Exp. Biol. Med.* **172:**449–456.

93. Warren, J. W. 1987. Catheter-associated urinary tract infections. *Infect. Dis. Clin. North Am.* **1:**823–854.

94. Warren, J. W. 1991. The catheter and urinary tract infection. *Med. Clin. North Am.* **75:** 481–493.

95. Warren, J. W., H. L. Muncie, Jr., E. J. Bergquist, and J. M. Hoopes. 1981. Sequelae and management of urinary infection in the patient requiring chronic catheterization. *J. Urol.* **125:**1–8.

96. Warren, J. W., R. Platt, R. J. Thomas, B. Rosner, and E. H. Kass. 1978. Antibiotic irrigation and catheter-associated urinary-tract infections. *N. Engl. J. Med.* **299:**570–573.

Infections Associated with Indwelling Medical Devices, 2nd ed.
Edited by Alan L. Bisno and Francis A. Waldvogel
© 1994 American Society for Microbiology, Washington, DC 20005

Chapter 13

Infections Associated with the Peritoneum and Hemodialysis

Stephen I. Vas

End-stage renal disease, the complete failure of the ultrafiltering capacity of the kidneys, is a complication of many diseases. The development of this complication results in the accumulation of metabolic by-products, the loss of the controlling function of the kidney on electrolytes, the disturbance of several of the endocrine functions of the kidney, and ultimately death. The definitive solution of end-stage renal disease is transplantation of a kidney from a donor (live or cadaver). Not all patients are suitable for transplantation, however, and others reject the transplant.

Therefore, patients with end-stage renal disease require the constant removal of accumulating metabolic degradation products from the bloodstream. The methods of choice are dialysis procedures. They are based on circulating blood on one side of a semipermeable membrane against a solution (dialysis solution) on the other.

Hemodialysis uses an artificial membrane, while peritoneal dialysis uses the peritoneal membrane of the body. Both modalities predispose the patient to infections because of the need for connections between the bloodstream or peritoneal cavity of the patient and extracorporeal devices and the need for frequent manipulations.

Early attempts to remove the toxic molecules through the skin or the intestinal mucous membrane failed. In the early 1940s an extracorporeal device was constructed by Kolff (156), and thus practical hemodialysis was born. In the mid-1940s attempts were made (40, 43, 131) to use

Stephen I. Vas • Departments of Microbiology and Medicine, University of Toronto, Toronto, Ontario M5T 2S8, Canada.

the peritoneal cavity for dialysis. These attempts, though short-term, resulted in high rates of peritoneal infections (5.2 to 7.5 episodes per patient year). Palmer and associates (108) started prolonged peritoneal dialysis (12 to 16 h every 2 to 3 days) with an improved silastic peritoneal catheter (142), and home peritoneal dialysis could be performed (141) with an infection rate of 0.23 to 1.2 episodes per patient year.

In 1976 Popovich and colleagues (117, 118) described a modification of the method, using small volumes of fluid (usually 2 liters) kept in the peritoneal cavity and changing the fluid every 6 h. This was accomplished by using sterile bottles of fluid and filling the peritoneal cavity every 6 h. Oreopoulos and colleagues (107) further modified the technique by using plastic bags instead of bottles and draining the fluid into the original load bag, thus reducing the number of disconnections necessary. Also, the system became truly portable, hence the name continuous ambulatory peritoneal dialysis (CAPD).

HEMODIALYSIS

Access to the vascular space is a prerequisite for hemodialysis. The search for an acceptable access is an ongoing process (37, 101, 145).

Permanent Access Sites

Arteriovenous shunt

The "Scribner shunt," first introduced in 1960 in Seattle, revolutionized hemodialysis access (138). The shunt is an external conduit connecting the radial artery and the cephalic vein at the wrist. It was made first from Teflon and later from silicone rubber. Insertion requires a surgical procedure, and maintenance requires a rigorous sterile technique. Its useful life is limited to 8 to 10 months. It is also sometimes used for temporary dialysis while an arteriovenous fistula is maturing (see below). A modification of the Scribner shunt is the Thomas femoral shunt. It is rarely used now because of a high infection rate.

Arteriovenous fistula

Introduced in 1966 by Brescia and Cimino, the arteriovenous fistula (60) is the mainstay of hemodialysis. It consists of a surgical autologous graft between the radial and cephalic veins. The graft requires maturation for about 30 days. During this period alternative dialysis methods have to be established (temporary hemodialysis access, peritoneal dialysis). At the present time, the most commonly used graft material is polytetrafluoroethylene. Bovine heterografts are also widely employed, and Dacron has been tried recently with some success.

Temporary Access Sites

Femoral vein catheterization

Rapid temporary access can be gained for hemodialysis by femoral vein catheterization. This is achieved by using a standard Teflon catheter (Angiocath) through a needle introduced into the femoral vein and removing it at the end of the dialysis session. While this procedure has a relatively low complication rate, it requires a puncture for each cycle. It is preferred for patients who will not require frequent dialysis as well as for septic patients, in whom a plastic central vein canula may become secondarily infected.

Subclavian vein catheters

Temporary access for hemodialysis for longer periods is usually achieved through the subclavian vein (75, 133, 143, 144). There are single-lumen and double-lumen catheters available. They differ in that double-lumen catheters permit better hemodialysis mechanics. The word "temporary" is a euphemism, since hemodialysis has been continued through these lines for several months. It mainly refers to the fact that they are relatively easy to insert, remove, or change and do not require surgical manipulation.

The insertion of hemodialysis catheters is done by the modified Seldinger technique. The process should be performed under sterile conditions by a trained operator. The delegation of this procedure to inexperienced persons leads to unacceptably high complication and infection rates.

Antimicrobial Prophylaxis

Antibiotic prophylaxis for the establishment of temporary access is not warranted. Standard vascular surgical prophylaxis should be used, however, at the time when a permanent access site is established. This consists of 1 g of a cephalosporin antibiotic 30 min before the operation and 1 g of the same antibiotic 6 to 12 h postoperatively. In randomized prospective studies (11, 17), infections were significantly lower in patients who received cefamandole than in those who received a placebo. For patients hypersensitive to cephalosporins, vancomycin (1 g intravenously 30 min before the operation) is appropriate. Continuous antibiotic prophylaxis for hemodialysis is not generally used. However, in one study, weekly injections of vancomycin were reported to decrease infections in pediatric patients on chronic hemodialysis (41).

Development of Infections

The development of infections on hemodialysis grafts depends on several factors, including the infecting organism, the structure of the graft material, and the route of infection.

The majority of graft infections are caused by coagulase-positive and coagulase-negative staphylococci. Bacteremia during hemodialysis has been reported with an incidence of 0.15 episode per patient dialysis year (32, 120). Seventy-three percent of bacteremias were due to access site infections.

No graft material studied to date is infection proof. The surface of all materials contains microscopic irregularities that may trap fibrin, platelets, and bacteria. Well-endothelialized autografts are the least offending surface. Teflon (polytetrafluoroethylene), by its hydrophobic nature, is more resistant to the attachment of blood coagulation components. Its colonization, therefore, is slower than that of other grafts.

Infections may become established by one of two routes: intraluminal, in which the organism enters the path of dialysis from the blood compartment, and extraluminal, in which bacteremia occurs by infection of the access site. The cause of intraluminal infection may be rarely the dialysis fluid or a distant nidus causing bacteremia, e.g., bacteremia from an intestinal source. These events usually manifest themselves in a transient pyrogenic reaction, and blood cultures taken at the time of reaction are usually positive. Such infections, however, do not colonize the access site and are usually of no consequence. Comorbid conditions may also increase the risk infections. Patients infected with human immunodeficiency virus (HIV) may show a higher risk for access site infections (33). A lower serum albumin level was also identified as a risk factor for infections (19).

Temporary access sites carry with them the same infectious risks as do other central venous lines (75, 144); such infections are usually relatively easy to manage (144). In a 2-year study (33), it was found that with a Quinton double-lumen Dacron cuff catheter, the exit site infection rate was 1 per 7.4 patient-months while bacteremia occurred at a rate of 1 per 66 patient-months. Infection of permanent access sites can be divided into two groups, immediate and late.

Immediate graft infections are perioperative infections affecting the site. They are usually caused by skin organisms, and the incidence is below 1% in most centers. They require conventional types of postoperative infection management, including drainage of localized collections of pus. Because the infection is extraneous to the graft, removal of the graft is rarely necessary. Such infections may, however, delay the maturation of the graft.

Late graft infections are more serious. They are usually caused by staphylococci (70%) or gram-negative organisms (25%). When bacteremia ensues, especially with *Staphylococcus aureus*, complications (6, 26, 96) may include osteomyelitis, endocarditis (4%), and metastatic abscesses. Mortality has been reported to be between 8 and 18%, as a result of a wide range of complications and the state of the underlying disease. Patients with metastatic foci have experienced a higher incidence of treatment failure and a higher mortality rate (42, 120). Removal of infected grafts is essential, and replacement should be attempted only after bacteremia has been effectively controlled.

Fungal infections in grafts have also been reported (105). The removal of such infected grafts may be essential before antifungal therapy can be successful.

Clinical Presentation and Laboratory Diagnosis

The clinical appearance of the access site is important. Erythema, induration, edema, and exudate confirm the presence of infection. Standard blood culture methodology is the mainstay of laboratory diagnosis. For the establishment of bacteremia, samples for cultures should be drawn from a distant site and not from the access device. Samples for cultures that are drawn through the access site may help to document the fact that the device is colonized and, especially in central venous line dialysis, may help in deciding whether to remove the catheter. Culturing specimens from the access site is nonproductive because of the easy contamination of site swabs with skin flora.

Therapy

The therapy of access site infections should follow the well-established principles of therapy of prosthetic device infections.

(i) Microbiological diagnosis of the infection should be pursued.

(ii) Intravenous treatment with appropriate antibiotics should be initiated on clinical grounds, even without microbiological proof.

(iii) Treatment with antibiotics should be continued for a prolonged period.

(iv) If an abscess is present at the access site, it should be drained immediately.

(v) If clinical improvement is not evident within 2 to 3 days, the prosthetic device should be removed.

(vi) An aggressive search should be conducted for metastatic sites, and these should be drained whenever possible.

Preservation of the access site is of paramount importance. Surgical exposure of the graft (140) may lead to the salvage of infected sites.

Infections associated with central venous dialysis catheters require the removal of the catheter. After 24 to 48 h of adequate treatment, the central line catheter can be reestablished at an alternate site.

The antibiotics most commonly used for the initiation of therapy are semisynthetic penicillins, cephalosporins (including broad-spectrum ones), and vancomycin. While penicillin and cephalosporins may need to be administered in reduced dosage, they still require injection several times a day. Vancomycin is an obvious choice since it can be given once a week (6). With the increase in methicillin resistance among staphylococci, the use of vancomycin may become increasingly important.

The concomitant use of rifampin or fusidic acid for synergy with the above antibiotics has been established in other prosthetic device infections. Careful monitoring of liver functions in dialysis patients on these antibiotics is advised.

If the infection is caused by relatively antibiotic-resistant gram-negative organisms, the use of aminoglycosides may be necessary. These antibiotics are given after hemodialysis because they dialyze out of the blood compartment. Careful monitoring of the level in blood is necessary to prevent vestibular and ototoxicity, since a slow retention of aminoglycosides is possible. It is advisable to assay predialysis, postdialysis, and 30-min-postdose levels in blood to make an informed dosage adjustment. It is important to remember that the use of amidopenicillins with aminoglycosides may lead to the inactivation of the latter, and therapeutic concentrations of aminoglycosides may be difficult to reach. For an extensive review that provides a detailed dosage adjustment for all antibiotics, refer to reference 12.

Prevention of Infections

Access site infections in a well-organized dialysis unit are infrequent. The following principles are useful in preventing infections.

(i) The hemodialysis unit is a restricted site. Personnel and visitors should change and wear protective clothing.

(ii) All access site punctures should be performed with meticulous sterile techniques. Disinfection of the site with 3% iodine tincture followed by a 70% ethyl alcohol wipe is preferred. Sterile gloves and a mask should be worn.

(iii) The space between dialysis chairs should be generous.

(iv) A regular cleaning schedule for the dialysis unit, with appropriate disinfectants, should be established. Two percent hypochlorite is a commonly used disinfectant.

(v) The dialysate supply system should be operated at "near-sterile" conditions.

The role of skin colonization of patients and personnel in the genesis of access site infections has been investigated (50, 165). There were significantly more isolates of S. *aureus* from patients on hemodialysis than from personnel. Such differences could not be shown for coagulase-negative staphylococci, streptococci, or gram-negative bacilli. Skin and nasal carriage of S. *aureus* was positively correlated in patients. The possibility of autoinoculation of access sites by the flora of the patient is suggested.

Recently, a prospective controlled study (165) showed the importance of nasal carriage of S. *aureus* in access site infections. Those carrying S. *aureus* were subject to significantly more frequent infections with the same phage type. Prophylactic treatment with rifampin for 5 days resulted in a decrease in nasal carriers, but colonization recurred frequently after 3 months. It appears from the study that although inconvenient and complex, regular rifampin prophylaxis and nasal screening can reduce access site infections with S. *aureus*. Limitations imposed by the possible development of resistance to rifampin remain to be assessed. Recently the use of mupirocin ointment has been investigated both as regular treatment of access sites and as nasal ointment for preventing S. *aureus* colonization. The natural history of nasal carriers indicates that the colonization is intermittent and recolonization is frequent. Furthermore, recolonization may be acquired from family members and fellow patients in the dialysis unit as well as health personnel. My personal view is that treatment of all patients at regular intervals will be the effective prophylaxis. Further studies will have to prove the most suitable interval for such an approach.

PERITONEAL DIALYSIS

The solutions used for peritoneal dialysis are basically balanced salt solutions containing various concentrations (0.5 to 4.5%) of glucose for achieving ultrafiltration by hyperosmolality. The solutions contain either acetate or lactate, they are hyperosmolar, and the starting pH of the solutions is 5.5 to 6.0. During dialysis the pH increases to close to 7.0 in 2 to 3 h and the hyperosmolality decreases.

Types of Peritoneal Dialysis

Acute peritoneal dialysis

Acute peritoneal dialysis is performed on patients with acute renal failure, when the length of peritoneal dialysis is expected to be a few days only. The dialysis is performed through an acute (stylet) catheter or temporary catheter, with manual exchanges every 2 to 3 h as needed. While the efficiency of dialysis is adequate, there is a high risk of infection both on the insertion of the catheter (stylet) and through the exit site.

Intermittent peritoneal dialysis (IPD)

The principle of IPD is that patients are dialyzed for prolonged periods (16 to 20 h) with usually 2 days between sessions. The dialysis can be achieved manually by using bags with a 2-h dwell time, but this requires the continuous presence of an operator. Machines are available to perform the dialysis. Earlier machines utilized solute concentrates, making the dialysis solution in the machine. More recently, machines have been developed on the reverse-osmosis principle, making the machines smaller and safer to operate. While this treatment modality is mainly used in dialysis centers, home dialysis with dedicated machines is possible. The patients selected for this treatment are usually those who do not want to participate in their own treatment. Generally, the rates of peritonitis are lower than in CAPD.

CAPD

CAPD is preferred by most patients. It provides mobility and can be performed at home or at the place of work. It consists of placing 2 to 3 liters of dialysis fluid into the abdominal cavity through the catheter. The delivery bag is rolled up and carried until the 6-h cycle of dialysis ends. At this point, this bag becomes the drainage bag and is exchanged with a fresh full bag, and the cycle repeats. All manipulations are performed under strict sterile conditions to reduce the danger of external contamination. Recently introduced techniques (flush-before-refill) have reduced the incidence of peritonitis to once every 24 months (14, 87).

Continuous-cycling or night (NIPD) peritoneal dialysis

The need to reduce the frequency of manipulations in CAPD led to the combination of continuous-cycling peritoneal dialysis with IPD. The method (29) provides continuous automated dialysis at night, with a prolonged dwell time dialysis in the abdomen during the daytime. Its advantages are claimed to be fewer connections, a reduced chance for infections, and less work for the patient. Its disadvantage is that it is partially machine oriented. If the patient is on a machine that provides continuous automated exchanges with long dwell time at night, it is usually referred to as NIPD.

Peritoneal Access Devices

Peritoneal catheters (49) are used for access to the peritoneal cavity. These can be temporary or permanent. Temporary catheters are sometimes made of stainless steel (stylet) or from silicone rubber. They are usually inserted at the bedside and used for a few days. Permanent catheters are of silicone rubber, they have one or two Dacron cuffs for stabilization subcutaneously and at the peritoneum, and they are usually surgically inserted. They may be used for several years. The cutaneous entry is called the exit site; the subcutaneous path to the peritoneum is called the tunnel.

Pathogenesis of Peritonitis

Initially the pathogenesis of peritonitis in dialysis patients was considered to be similar to that of surgical peritonitis (58). This was a reasonable assumption until it became evident that considerable differences exist. In surgical peritonitis, small amounts of contamination are usually of no clinical significance, as evidenced by the large numbers of laparotomies with no infectious consequences. Minor contaminations, on the other hand, may lead to serious peritonitis in dialysis patients. Surgical peritonitis is usually caused by major soils of the peritoneal cavity. Such major soils are rare in dialysis, except for intestinal perforations. Finally, in surgical peritonitis about 30% of cases have bacteremia as part of the disease (58), while in dialysis patients bacteremia is a rare event and is usually the result of an infection elsewhere in the body rather than the consequence of a local infection at the dialysis site (147).

Portals of entry

It is not known how frequently bacterial penetration occurs through or around the dialysis catheter, but from studies of the use of in-line filters during peritoneal dialysis (4) and other studies (136), there is reason to believe that it occurs frequently, without leading to peritonitis.

Patients appear to acquire most infections from their endogenous flora. When skin surveillance cultures of patients are analyzed, the distribution of organisms is the same as the distribution of bacteria during their peritonitis episodes. Furthermore, an analysis of cutaneous and peritoneal organisms from the same subjects by biotype or phage type strengthens this hypothesis (64).

It is possible to devise a distribution frequency of probable causes of infection and portals of entry (106). While this distribution is admittedly speculative, it is logical, and it provides a helpful framework upon which the approaches to prophylaxis may be constructed.

Table 1. Routes of infection in peritoneal dialysis patients

Route	Organisms	%
Transluminal	Coagulase-negative staphylococci *S. aureus* *Acinetobacter* spp. *Pseudomonas* spp.	30–40
Periluminal	Coagulase-negative staphylococci *S. aureus* Fungi *Pseudomonas/Xanthomonas* spp. Diphtheroids	20–30
Transmural	Enteric organisms Anaerobic organisms	25–30
Hematogenous	*Streptococcus* spp. *M. tuberculosis*	5–10
Ascending (vaginal)	*Candida* spp. Enteric organisms	2–5

Intraluminal infections. Intraluminal infections (Table 1) occur when bacteria enter the peritoneal cavity through touch contamination of the spike, through discontinuities in the tubing, or from the dialysis fluid. Although the question frequently arises, there are no recent instances in which bacterial contamination of commercial fluid has been implicated in peritonitis cases. Touch contaminations are reduced by developing strict sterile protocols for bag changing, and material failure is minimized by frequent inspections and the regular replacement of the tubing and spike.

Periluminal infections. While improvements in the placement of the peritoneal catheter have reduced peritoneal leaks (49), the catheter itself never forms a sealed junction with the skin, permitting bacteria to establish themselves in the exit site or the tunnel. Catheters have single or double Dacron cuffs to increase stability. It is believed that the cuff plays a major role in preventing the penetration of bacteria. There is no difference in the use of single- or double-cuff catheters and the incidence of peritonitis.

Established exit site or tunnel infections are frequently, although not necessarily, associated with peritonitis due to the same organism that is cultured from the infected site. Since the organisms isolated from periluminal and intraperitoneal infections both reflect prevailing skin flora, the causal relationship between the former and the latter remains speculative.

Transmural (intestinal) infections. The isolation of enteric organisms from peritoneal dialysis fluid, especially if more than one species is isolated or anaerobic organisms are present, is indicative of fecal contamination. The chances of becoming infected by more than one organism simultaneously from the environment are very small, especially since the carriage of enteric organisms on the skin of the hands or the abdomen is infrequent (146).

Bacteria may penetrate through the intestinal wall without obvious discontinuity (130), or ischemic damage to the intestine may lead to leakage (7). More frequently though, preexisting diverticulosis is the cause of peritonitis, since diverticular disease is more frequent in the elderly and in those with polycystic disease (163, 164).

Hematogenous infections. It has been observed that hematogenous peritonitis develops frequently in cirrhotic ascites (22). We have observed several patients with peritonitis due to viridans group streptococci in whom the peritonitis was preceded by positive blood cultures. This implies that the peritonitis developed secondarily to the bacteremia.

Ascending (vaginal) infections. Ascending (vaginal) infections are a rare complication in which the communication between the vagina and the peritoneum through the fallopian tubes or through a fistula leads to peritonitis (25, 28, 72, 139).

Environmental infections. Rarely, peritonitis has been observed from which *Pseudomonas maltophilia, Acinetobacter calcoaceticus* (1), or other environmental bacteria are isolated. It is possible that these infections develop by contact with water (86) (showering, swimming pool) entering through the exit site. Episodes of infections with *Mycobacterium chelonae* (8, 116) have been described in which the source was ascribed to tap water entering the peritoneal cavity.

Pathogenetic factors

Biofilm. It is a general property of certain organisms (62) to form a glycocalyx on surfaces (see chapters 2 and 3). Biofilms on peritoneal catheters have been described (27, 89, 91, 97, 100, 111). The biofilm appears to be present on catheter surfaces regardless of the peritonitis history of the patient (27). The role of the biofilm in initiating peritonitis is questioned (154). It appears that the presence of biofilm on the catheters does not necessarily lead to peritonitis, and an added injury (decrease in defense mechanism, chemical injury, etc.) is needed.

Inflammatory mediators. The entrance of microorganisms into the peritoneal cavity in the presence of opsonins and complement will result in the release of chemotactic factors. The consequent invasion of polymorphonuclear phagocytes increases the cell number present in the peritoneal cavity and changes it from a predominantly mononuclear cell (58, 161) to a polymorphonuclear cell population. The release of a variety of other inflammatory mediators results in vasodilation, an increase in the protein content of the peritoneal fluid, and the development of typical peritoneal pain.

Fibrin. Normal peritoneal cavity fluid contains fibrinogen and fibrinolysin (36). The latter substance degrades fibrin and maintains the shiny slippery surface of the peritoneum. During inflammation, increased amounts of fibrinogen enter the peritoneal cavity, and fibrinolysis is defective (45). The net result is the formation of fibrin filaments and fibrin clots, a process that likely contributes to the formation of intraperitoneal adhesions (12, 35, 45, 58).

Fibronectin. Fibronectin, a normal constituent of biological fluids, has been studied in CAPD patients (52, 70). While its concentration increases in the peritoneal fluid of CAPD patients during peritonitis, it has no predictive value for susceptibility to peritonitis.

Cell migration. The normal peritoneal cell population consists primarily of mononuclear cells, probably of bone marrow origin (51), and some mesothelial cells from the peritoneal lining. On inflammation, a rapid migration of polymorphonuclear cells occurs (162). Indeed, it may take only a few hours for a completely clear peritoneal fluid to turn cloudy. The estimation of the peritoneal cell population is a useful tool in the diagnosis of peritonitis. A cell decrease follows the improvement of peritonitis on therapy and is a good clinical sign to follow therapeutic success. Occasionally, eosinophilic cells enter the peritoneal cavity (see below).

Abscess formation is a complication of peritonitis in peritoneal dialysis patients. Onderdonk et al. (104) demonstrated that intra-abdominal abscess formation appeared to be related to synergy between anaerobes and gram-negative aerobic bacteria. Since the isolation of anaerobes is a rare occurrence in peritonitis of peritoneal dialysis patients, abscess formation in peritonitis due to fecal flora should be suspected. Also, *S. aureus* is associated with the frequent formation of abscesses (66).

Defense mechanisms of the peritoneum

The peritoneum is a thin membrane lining the interior of the abdominal wall (parietal peritoneum) and the abdominal viscera (visceral peritoneum), forming a potential space, the peritoneal cavity. The peritoneal membrane consists of a surface layer of mesothelial cells that lie on a basement membrane with deeper layers of capillaries and lymphatics. Transport across the peritoneal membrane moves from the capillaries through the basement membrane via intercellular junctions. Small particles may traverse the membrane through cellular junctions or through pinocytosis by mesothelial cells (23, 85). Small particles are removed from the peritoneum via the lymphatics, primarily through those below the diaphragmatic surface (15). The exact mechanism of this movement is not clear, although Courtice and Simmonds (24) have postulated that openings exist between the peritoneal cavity and the diaphragmatic lymphatics. The primary flow, however, is toward the peritoneal cavity during peritonitis episodes. This may explain the extremely low rate of bacteremia of 15% in peritoneal dialysis patients during peritonitis (20), as opposed to secondary surgical peritonitis (30%) (83) and spontaneous peritonitis in cirrhotic patients (39 to 76%) (157). We have not observed a single positive blood culture in several hundred episodes of bacterial peritonitis in CAPD patients, except (as noted above) when the bacteremia preceded peritonitis.

Humoral factors. It has been shown that immunoglobulins and complement are present in the peritoneal fluid, although the normal level of these components is not established (81, 82). The serum immunoglobulin levels of these patients are not severely compromised (47). Certain patients may, however, have a decreased level of opsonins and probably other factors needed for immunological reactions in the peritoneal cavity (121, 153). The relative lack of opsonins has been proposed as a cause of repeated episodes of peritonitis in the peritoneal dialysis fluid of so-called high-risk patients (78, 153). The lack of ability to produce adequate amounts of interleukin-1 and the release of large amounts of prostaglandin E_2 by the macrophages of certain patients have also been postulated as causes of recurrent peritonitis (77).

Cellular factors. While the normal self-clearing mechanism of the peritoneum is primarily dependent on mesothelial cells and mononuclear cells in the peritoneal cavity, during inflammation a large number of active phagocytic polymorphonuclear cells enter the peritoneal cavity, participating in the removal of bacteria. Whether these cells have a reduced bactericidal capacity is subject to controversy (65, 81, 90, 112, 122, 158). Under the conditions of peritoneal dialysis, patients have, instead of the normal few milliliters of fluid, 2 liters of dialysis fluid with a low pH and high osmolality. We have shown that a low pH and high osmolality decrease the efficiency of phagocytic cells, which may not be fully functional at least during the initial periods of peritoneal dialysis (2, 34, 57, 62, 92, 99). In addition, urea, creatinine, and other low-molecular-weight substances enter the peritoneal cavity during peritoneal dialysis. We have examined the effect of these molecules and did not find them deleterious to phagocytosis in the concentrations present in the peritoneal dialysis fluid. Similarly, heparin, which is added to reduce fibrin formation, did not appear to inhibit phagocytosis.

The large volume of fluid present in the peritoneal cavity during peritoneal dialysis diminishes the chance of interaction between bacteria and phagocytic cells. It is therefore suggested that smaller volumes of peritoneal dialysis fluid be used during the therapy of acute peritonitis.

The role of the eosinophils in peritoneal dialysis fluid is not established. While some phagocytosis is performed by eosinophilic cells, they probably represent a reaction to inflammatory agents rather than a primary defense mechanism. While it is known that end-stage renal failure inhibits cellular immune functions, the importance of such inhibition in peritoneal infections is not established (21, 46, 52).

Patients with renal failure are considered to exhibit increased susceptibility to infections (93), which may be due to lack of inflammatory mediators or production of inhibitors (77). At present, however, a subset of patients at high risk of peritonitis has not been identified.

Diagnosis

Clinical manifestations and course of peritonitis

Incubation period. The incubation period of peritonitis in peritoneal dialysis is not well established. It can be estimated from touch contamination incidents that the incubation period usually is 24 to 48 h. Occasionally, incubation periods may be as short as 6 to 12 h. The appearance of the symptoms may be very rapid (147), developing during one peritoneal dialysis period. The incubation period of endogenous infections is unknown but is probably much shorter than that of exogenous infections, since the initial number of infecting organisms is larger.

Presenting signs and symptoms. We have reviewed presenting symptoms and signs in 103 episodes of peritonitis in CAPD patients. Fever of more than 37.5°C was present in 53%, abdominal pain was present on admission in 79%, 31% experienced nausea, and 7% complained of diarrhea. All but one patient had cloudy fluid before admission, but only 78% had cloudy fluid on admission; 70% showed abdominal tenderness, and 50% showed rebound tenderness. Besides the above-mentioned signs and symptoms, patients sometimes present with profound hypotension and shock. This presentation is usually a sign of either *S. aureus* peritonitis or fecal peritonitis. On the other hand, many patients will have only very mild symptoms and do not require hospitalization.

Clinical features of exit site and tunnel infections. Exit site infections are frequent. The 1987 report of the U.S. CAPD Registry of the

National Institutes of Health shows that about 31% of the patients develop exit site infections within year 1, and probably about half of these patients will require catheter replacement during this period (95). Exit site and tunnel infections rarely cause symptoms. Usually they are discovered on routine investigation of the exit site, or the patient notices a purulent discharge. The exit site is inflamed, with a serous or purulent discharge, and at times local tenderness and induration may be present. Tunnel infections are much more difficult to diagnose if they are present without exit site infections, and radioactive scanning has been recommended as a diagnostic procedure. Exit site and tunnel infections may be present for prolonged periods without leading to peritonitis, but they always represent a potential source for the development of peritonitis (97, 119).

Relapse, recurrence, and reinfection. The concepts of relapse, recurrence, and infection are not well defined in the peritoneal dialysis population. Relapse is considered to be present if there is a reappearance of symptoms, an appearance of positive cultures after cultures have become negative during therapy, or an increase in the polymorphonuclear cell number in the peritoneal dialysis fluid after the cell number has declined. It indicates either inadequate treatment or, rarely, the opening of an abscess cavity that was previously inaccessible to treatment.

Recurrence is the term used for the reappearance of symptoms of infection within 2 weeks after cessation of antimicrobial therapy. It may indicate either inadequate therapy or the presence of an endogenous focus, such as an exit site or tunnel infection, from which reseeding occurred.

Reinfection is a new peritonitis episode beyond the 2-week period, with either the same organism or a different organism. If reinfection happens with the same organism, an internal focus should be suspected (e.g., colonization of catheter [see below]).

Complications. As a consequence of peritonitis, fibrous adhesions may develop between the peritoneal membranes (92, 126). This is especially frequent as a consequence of S. aureus peritonitis or fecal peritonitis. A small prospective study (164) from our unit has demonstrated that diverticulosis is a risk factor for development of fecal peritonitis.

An alarming condition, called sclerosing peritonitis (44, 75a, 129), in which the peritoneum develops thick fibrinous organizing exudate, making the exchange of fluid and solutes impossible, has been described in peritoneal dialysis patients. The etiology of this condition is presently unclear. It may possibly be due to repeated injuries to the peritoneum by processes such as frequent peritonitis and chemical injury.

Mortality. It is difficult to establish accurately the mortality due to peritonitis. The mortality associated with peritonitis is estimated to be 2 to 3%. While this is certainly high, it is not surprising, since the patients with peritonitis suffer from an ultimately fatal disease. Many of the deaths during peritonitis are attributable not directly to the infection but to complications of the underlying disease of the patient (myocardial infarction, metabolic imbalance, etc.) (163).

Laboratory diagnosis of peritonitis

Microbiologic studies. For an accurate microbiological diagnosis in CAPD peritonitis (12a, 39, 74, 125, 152, 155), attention should be directed to the following points.

(i) Specimens for cultures should be taken as early as possible from suspected cases of peritonitis and processed expeditiously. Prompt identification of the infecting organism and its susceptibility pattern greatly facilitates rational antibiotic therapy (148).

(ii) Large volumes should be concentrated for improving the recovery rate.

(iii) Washing of the specimens with sterile saline may be necessary when patients are on antibiotic therapy.

Cell count. The normal peritoneal drainage fluid after a 6-h dwell time contains 50 to 100 cells per mm^3, most of which are mononuclear (124). The cell count is a function of the peritoneal fluid volume and the length of dwell time. An increase in cell count indicates inflammation of the peritoneal membrane and is usually accompanied by a shift to predominantly neutrophils. Routine cell counts, as well as differential counts, are very helpful in establishing the diagnosis of peritonitis (159). Cell counts rapidly decrease on successful treatment of peritonitis. A subsequent increase in cell count may indicate a recurrence or treatment failure. An increase in cell count and a mononuclear cell predominance may indicate unusual organisms, e.g., *Mycobacterium tuberculosis* infection (102), while an increase in eosinophils indicates a noninfectious cause (peritoneal eosinophilia [see below]). We find that the use of centrifugal smears (Cytospin) in establishing differential counts is very helpful (161).

Organisms Causing Peritonitis

The overwhelming majority of peritonitis episodes are caused by bacteria (Tables 2 and 3). A small number (4 to 8%) of peritonitis episodes are caused by fungi, most of them belonging to *Candida* species. Occasionally *Torulopsis* spp. and some filamentous fungi (e.g., *Dermatophyton*,

Table 2. Bacteria isolated from CAPD patients with peritonitis[a]

Acinetobacter spp.	*Micrococcus mucilaginosus*
Actinomyces israelii	*Mycobacterium chelonae*
Aeromonas hydrophila	*Mycobacterium fortuitum*
Alcaligenes faecalis	*Mycobacterium tuberculosis*
Bacillus cereus	*Neisseria* spp.
Bacteroides fragilis	*Neisseria gonorrhoeae*
Bordetella bronchiseptica	*Pasteurella multocida*
Campylobacter fetus	Propionibacteria
Campylobacter jejuni	*Proteus* spp.
Citrobacter spp.	*Pseudomonas aeruginosa*
Corynebacteria	*Pseudomonas cepacia*
Corynebacterium aquaticum	*Pseudomonas maltophilia*
Clostridium difficile	*Pseudomonas stutzeri*
Clostridium perfringens	*Serratia* spp.
Escherichia coli	*Staphylococcus aureus*
Enterobacter agglomerans	*Staphylococcus epidermidis*
Enterococcus spp.	*Stomatococcus mucilaginosus*
Gardnerella vaginalis	*Streptococcus faecalis*
CDC group IV c-2	*Streptococcus pneumoniae*
CDC group Ve-1	*Streptococcus pyogenes*
CDC group Ve-2	Viridans group streptococci
Klebsiella spp.	*Vibrio alginolyticus*
Listeria monocytogenes	

[a] While an attempt has been made to make the listing comprehensive, it may not be complete. From reference 146.

Table 3. Distribution of organisms isolated from peritonitis episodes

Organism(s)	%
Coagulase-negative staphylococci	30–40
Staphylococcus aureus	10–20
Streptococcus spp.	10–15
Neisseria spp.	1–2
Diphtheroids	1–2
Escherichia coli	5–10
Pseudomonas spp.	5–10
Enterococci	3–6
Klebsiella spp.	1–3
Proteus spp.	3–6
Acinetobacter spp.	2–5
Anaerobic organisms	2–5
Fungi	2–10
Other (mycobacteria, etc.)	2–5
Culture negative	0–30

Table 4. Yeasts, fungi, and algae isolated from CAPD patients with peritonitis[a]

Yeasts	Filamentous fungi (continued)
Candida albicans	Aspergillus flavus
Candida guillermondii	Curvularia lunata
Candida krusei	Drechslera spicifera
Candida parapsilosis	Exophiala jenselmei
Candida tropicalis	Fusarium moniliforme
Coccidioides immitis	Fusarium oxysporum
Pityrosporum ovale	Fusarium verticilloides
Pityrosporum pachydermatis	Lecythophora mutabilis
Cryptococcus neoformans	Mucor spp.
Rhodotorula rubra	Penicillium spp.
Torulopsis glabrata	Trichosporon cutaneum
Algae	Trichoderma koningii
Prototheca wickerhamii	Trichoderma viride
Filamentous fungi	
Alternaria alternans	
Aspergillus fumigatus	

[a] While an attempt has been made to make the listing comprehensive, it may not be complete. From reference 146.

Mucor, Penicillium, and *Fusarium* species) (3, 71) are involved (Table 4). Peritonitis due to viruses has not been reliably confirmed.

Coagulase-negative staphylococci

Coagulase-negative staphylococci are the most frequent cause of peritonitis. Infections caused by these organisms are generally benign. Their origin is the skin, and they reach the peritoneum by the transluminal or periluminal route. They respond well to appropriate antibiotic treatment and are, therefore, suitable for home treatment with oral antibiotics. When coagulase-negative staphylococci isolated in our hospital were biotyped (73), *Staphylococcus epidermidis* sensu stricto was the leading cause of peritonitis in these patients (5, 55, 152), with other types occasionally isolated. The distribution of types follows the distribution of coagulase-negative staphylococci on the skin.

S. aureus

S. aureus peritonitis is a much more alarming infection. Patients with this infection usually are hypotensive, some of them in outright shock, and they complain of severe abdominal pain. Patients with *S. aureus* peritonitis showing symptoms of toxic shock syndrome have been reported (54, 147). While the acute infection is alarming, it usually responds well to antibiotic treatment, albeit more slowly than do *S. epider-*

midis infections. We have found that it is useful to treat these patients with a combination including a penicillin-type antibiotic (penicillin or cloxacillin, depending on the susceptibility of the organisms) or the combination of vancomycin and rifampin (147).

The infection subsides slowly, and sometimes residual abscesses are found (66). Patients with exit site infections and tunnel infections due to *S. aureus* will frequently have recurrent peritonitis, and catheter removal may be necessary.

Streptococci

Streptococcal peritonitis is a milder form of peritonitis, although patients often complain of severe pain. The organisms most commonly causing peritonitis in these patients belong to the alpha-hemolytic group. We assume that this infection is caused by hematogenous spread as well as by direct intraluminal infection from the oral flora (oral aerosol). Bacteremia secondary to dental manipulations may play a role in the pathogenesis of these infections. Therefore, prophylactic antibiotic recommendations applicable to prosthetic devices in cardiac patients should be followed.

Enterococci

Other groups of streptococci may also cause peritonitis in dialysis patients. Enterococci clearly are fecal organisms and indicate transmural infection. Peritonitis caused by these organisms has no distinguishing features from gram-negative peritonitis (see below).

Diphtheroids

Diphtheroids are skin organisms indicating intraluminal or periluminal infections. While some of them are quite resistant to antibiotics, most of them respond to appropriate antibiotic treatment. The isolation of the JK bacterium (113) requires the use of vancomycin. Propionibacteria, organisms similar to diphtheroids but growing under anaerobic conditions, are occasionally isolated from peritoneal dialysis fluid. Since most of the organisms belonging to this group are slow growing, a prolonged incubation period (10 to 12 days) is needed to isolate them. The organisms are isolated from CAPD, as well as IPD, patients, who usually are asymptomatic (136). While the isolation of these organisms clearly indicates contamination with skin flora, the pathogenic significance of this group is unknown.

Gram-negative organisms

While a small number of members of the family *Enterobacteriaceae* occur on the skin, it is more likely that peritonitis with these organisms indicates direct fecal contamination. The presence of more than a single gram-negative species in the peritoneal fluid is a strong indication of a perforation. Peritonitis due to a single species of the *Enterobacteriaceae* usually responds well to appropriate treatment with aminoglycosides or cephalosporins.

Pseudomonas/Xanthomonas infections are usually more resistant to treatment, often cause multiple abscesses, and therefore require careful evaluation. Patients with these infections are usually hypotensive on admission. These organisms may be resistant to multiple antibiotics and may require treatment with a combination of agents (see Tables 6 and 7). Also, since pseudomonads may form a biofilm on the catheter, early catheter removal may be indicated.

Acinetobacter peritonitis (1), while having no special distinguishing features, may be an indication of environmental contamination, usually from water. It is usually readily amenable to treatment.

Miscellaneous organisms

Single episodes of peritonitis caused by any of a large number of microorganisms (e.g., *Haemophilus, Neisseria,* and *Campylobacter* species) have been described, indicating that most organisms have the capability to cause infections if inoculated into the peritoneal cavity of CAPD patients.

Because anaerobic bacteria have been isolated from only a small percentage of peritoneal fluids in patients on dialysis (123), some workers question the importance of doing anaerobic cultures on peritoneal fluids (134). Despite their relative rarity, anaerobic peritoneal infections are very severe, usually requiring laparotomy, and there is a high propensity for abscess formation (113). Aggressive surgical management is necessary (123, 135, 148, 163, 164); therefore, we consider that it is important to culture peritoneal fluids for these organisms.

M. tuberculosis, another organism causing peritonitis in peritoneal dialysis patients only rarely, requires special consideration. It usually reaches the peritoneum from a distant site by hematogenous spread. It occurs in patients who have had a previous primary infection with this organism and whose disease was inadequately treated. It is therefore a disease to be considered in high-risk groups (128). Tuberculosis may be difficult to diagnose because the organism grows relatively slowly on artificial media, and microbiology laboratories may not be of much help initially. The index of suspicion should be high if a patient has pain and cloudy fluid which is predominantly mononuclear in composition and repeated cultures do not yield a bacteriological answer (94, 102). If tuberculosis is suspected, peritoneal biopsy through direct laparotomy or laparoscopy is indicated (31, 162). A histological diagnosis of caseous granulomas with or without the presence of acid-fast organisms is an indication for antituberculous chemotherapy and catheter removal. Antituberculosis prophylactic therapy should be considered for patients with a positive tuberculin skin test (149). This consideration is even more important in view of the fact that many patients on peritoneal dialysis will later enter a transplant program and therefore are at high risk for reactivation of tuberculosis.

Peritoneal infections with *M. chelonae* have been observed in intermittent peritoneal dialysis units from the contamination of dialysers from water sources (116). *Mycobacterium fortuitum* infection has also been observed (76).

Viruses have not been confirmed to cause peritonitis in dialysis patients, although virus infections have been implicated in predisposing dialysis patients to bacterial peritonitis (53). The presence of hepatitis B surface antigen has been demonstrated in peritoneal dialysis fluid (127, 151), although not in association with peritonitis. Human immunodeficiency virus may be present in peritoneal dialysis fluids. The implications of this virus for dialysis are beyond the scope of this chapter. For a discussion of this issue, see other reviews (15a, 38, 132).

Yeasts are the most common fungal organisms causing peritonitis in peritoneal dialysis patients (9, 69). They most often enter the peritoneal cavity intraluminally or periluminally, although in a few cases vaginal infection has been noted (71, 72).

The clinical course of yeast peritonitis is not different from that of any other peritonitis except for its resistance to treatment with antibacterial antibiotics. This is often the diagnostic clue calling attention to the disease, although the organisms are relatively easy to culture with the methods usually used for processing peritoneal dialysis fluids. Gram stains often show yeast elements in the peritoneal fluid on direct smear, calling early attention to the condition.

The reason for yeast peritonitis is not clear. Diabetics do not appear to have a higher incidence. Prolonged treatment of previous bacterial peritonitis with conventional antibiotics—especially combinations covering a wide range of microorganisms—leads to colonization with yeasts, which in turn may be the source of yeast infections.

Yeast infections of the peritoneal cavity are very difficult to treat with antifungal agents (69, 71). These agents do not show good penetration into the peritoneal cavity and cannot be administered intraperitoneally because they are very irritating and painful. 5-Fluorocytosine, an antifungal agent often used in the treatment of *Candida* cystitis, is not suitable for treatment as a single agent, because resistance to it emerges fairly rapidly. Treatment with amphotericin, miconazole, ketoconazole, and fluconazole—with or without 5-fluorocytosine—has been reported to be successful, but convincing comparative studies are lacking (16, 61, 79). Moreover, fungi, including *Candida* spp., may colonize the surface of the silastic material of the catheter, greatly hindering eradication of the infection. Catheter removal, therefore, has to be considered early in these patients (71, 72, 79, 150). After catheter removal the symptoms subside rapidly with or without chemotherapy. If the patient cannot be considered for catheter removal and antifungal therapy has to be attempted, peritoneal lavage with antifungal agents may be considered. Placing the patient on IPD may improve peritoneal host defenses, as discussed above.

Filamentous fungi rarely cause peritoneal infections (3, 72, 110). Since most filamentous fungi are resistant to antifungal antibiotics early, catheter removal has to be considered.

Failure to identify an infecting microorganism is usually due to inappropriate culture procedures or the suppressive effects of concomitantly administered antibiotics. The incidence of sterile peritonitis varies among units from 2 to 20% (147), depending on the methods used in the laboratory. Chemical peritonitis was described early in the peritoneal dialysis experience (67). More recently, chemical peritonitis due to intraperitoneal vancomycin has been observed (114).

Treatment of Peritonitis

Antimicrobial therapy

Therapy often has to be initiated empirically in the absence of definitive diagnostic information. Antibiotics selected for the initial treatment should be effective against the organisms most frequently observed in peritonitis, keeping in mind local epidemiologic patterns of antimicrobial resistance. The kinetics of antibiotic absorption have been well studied (10, 13, 88). Recommended antibiotic dosages, modified for peritoneal use, are listed in Table 5.

Most centers use intraperitoneal vancomycin as the initial therapy in view of the increasing incidence of infections with methicillin-resistant staphylococci, but cephalothin or cefazolin may also be used (Tables 5 and 6). These cephalosporin antibiotics are effective against methicillin-susceptible *S. epidermidis* and *S. aureus*, as well as a limited spectrum of

Table 5. Antibiotic administration in peritoneal dialysis

Drug	Dose/route of administration[a]	
	Loading[b]	Maintenance
Antibacterial antibiotics		
Penicillin[c]	1 mU/liter i.p.	50,000 U/liter i.p.
Cloxacillin[c]	1,000 mg/liter i.p.	100 mg/liter i.p.
Ampicillin[c]	500 mg/liter i.p.	50 mg/liter i.p.
Piperacillin[c]	1,000 mg/liter i.p.	100 mg/liter i.p.
Cephalothin[c]	500 mg/liter i.p.	250 mg/liter i.p.
Cefazolin	500 mg/liter i.p.	250 mg/liter i.p.
Cefamandole	1,000 mg/liter i.p.	250 mg/liter i.p.
Cefoxitin	1,000 mg/liter i.p.	250 mg/liter i.p.
Ceftazidime	500 mg/liter i.p.	125 mg/liter i.p.
Cefuroxime	1,000 mg/liter i.p.	250 mg/liter i.p.
Ceftizoxime	1,000 mg/liter i.p.	125 mg/liter i.p.
Cefoperazone	2,000 mg/liter i.p.	500 mg/liter i.p.
Moxalactam	1,000 mg/liter i.p.	250 mg/liter i.p.
Cephalexin[c]	500 mg p.o.	250 mg p.o./6 h
Cephradine	500 mg p.o.	250 mg p.o./6 h
Gentamicin	1.5 mg/kg/bag i.p.	6.0 mg/liter i.p.
Tobramycin[c]	1.7 mg/kg/bag i.p.	8.0 mg/liter i.p.
Netilmycin	1.7 mg/kg/bag i.p.	8.0 mg/liter i.p.
Amikacin[c]	5 mg/kg/bag i.p.	25 mg/liter i.p.
Vancomycin[c]	1,000 mg/liter i.p.	30 mg/liter i.p.
Rifampin	N/A	150 mg q6h p.o.
Trimethoprim-sulfamethoxazole	80 mg/liter i.p. 400 mg/liter i.p.	5 mg/liter i.p. 25 mg/liter i.p.
Clindamycin[c]	300 mg/liter i.p.	150 mg/liter i.p.
Metronidazole[c]	500 mg p.o.	500 mg p.o./6 h
Antifungal antibiotics[d]		
Amphotericin B[c]		25 mg/24h i.v.
5-Fluorocytosine[c]	2,000 mg p.o.	1,000 mg p.o.
Fluconazole[c]		150 mg i.p. every 2nd day

[a] Abbreviations: i.p., intraperitoneally; p.o., orally; N/A, not available; q6h, every 6 h; i.v., intravenously.
[b] Loading doses can be given intravenously or intramuscularly if achievement of rapid blood concentration is desired.
[c] Dosages used by author. Other dosages compiled from pharmacokinetic data in the literature.
[d] The use of antifungal antibiotics is controversial (see text).

gram-negative organisms. If one wants to cover the more highly resistant gram-negative organisms, the addition of an aminoglycoside is justified. After the organisms have been identified and an antibiotic susceptibility is available, adjustments should be made to the therapy.

The penetration of antibiotics from the peritoneal cavity to serum is good and rapid (88, 160). It is, therefore, unnecessary in most cases to give an intravenous loading dose.

Table 6. Treatment of CAPD peritonitis[a,b]

Culture: no growth in 2–3 days	Culture: gram positive	Culture: gram negative
Continue vancomycin for 2 more doses every 7 days 2 g i.p. if BW > 40 kg 1 g i.p. if BW < 40 kg Stop aminoglycoside[c]	Continue vancomycin for 2 more doses every 7 days 2 g i.p. if BW > 40 kg 1 g i.p. if BW < 40 kg Stop aminoglycoside	Continue ceftazadime, 125 mg/liter each exchange or Aminoglycoside, 8 mg/liter each exchange for 7 days then 6 mg/liter each exchange or Aminoglycoside, 20 mg/liter, one exchange/day
Oral therapy depending on antibiotic sensitivity	Culture: *S. aureus*	Fecal peritonitis
Ciprofloxacin 750 mg b.i.d. or Ofloxacin 300 mg/day or Trimethoprim-sulfamethoxazole 1 DS tablet b.i.d. or Cephalexin 250 mg t.i.d. plus Rifampin 300 mg b.i.d. p.o.	Continue vancomycin for 2 more doses every 7 days 2 g i.p. if BW > 40 kg 1 g i.p. if BW < 40 kg add Rifampin 300 mg b.i.d. p.o. Stop aminoglycoside	As in gram-negative peritonitis add Metronidazole 500 mg/8 h p.o. or i.v. or rectal suppository Consider surgery

Fungal peritonitis	Patient sensitive to vancomycin	Pseudomonas/Xanthomonas peritonitis
Fluconazole 150 mg i.p. in one bag every 2nd day and Flucytosine Loading dose: 2,000 mg p.o. Maintenance: 1,000 mg p.o./day or Amphotericin B 25 mg/day i.v. and Flucytosine as above	Clindamycin 150 mg/liter in each exchange	Aminoglycoside 8 mg/liter each exchange for 7 days, then 6 mg/liter each exchange for 14 days or Aminoglycoside 20 mg/liter one exchange/day for 21 days add Antipseudomonas antibiotic (see Table 7)

a Initial treatment
Vancomycin   2 g i.p. if BW > 40 kg
                    1 g i.p. if BW < 40 kg
            and
Ceftazidime   Loading dose: 500 mg/liter i.p.
                Maintenance: 125 mg/liter i.p.
        or
Aminoglycoside Loading dose: 1.7 mg/kg BW i.p.
                Maintenance: 8 mg/liter
        or
Aminoglycoside 20 mg/liter in one exchange/day
    and
heparin   1000 U/liter each exchange while fluid is cloudy

b BW, body weight; i.p., intraperitoneally, usually in 2 liter exchange, 6 h dwell time; b.i.d., twice a day; p.o., orally; i.v., intravenously.

c Aminoglycoside includes netilmycin < amikacin < tobramycin < gentamicin in increasing order of toxicity. For amikacin, multiply dosage by 3. (Example: tobramycin 8 mg = amikacin 24 mg).

Recently an expert committee (68) made therapeutic recommendations. The innovations in these recommendations focus on once-weekly vancomycin use and consideration of once-a-day high-dose aminoglycoside. For aminoglycosides, the principle of intermittent therapy is based on two experimental observations. The first is the fact that the bactericidal action of aminoglycosides is proportionate to their concentration. This does not apply to penicillin or cephalosporin-type antibiotics. The second observation is the so-called "postantibiotic effect" (80a). This means that after the application of an appropriate concentration of aminoglycoside, the majority of susceptible bacteria are killed while the remaining ones have an increased susceptibility to the antibiotic.

On the basis of the above, once-a-day aminoglycoside therapy for a localized infection like CAPD peritonitis becomes feasible. This approach, besides being cheaper and easier to use, has also been shown to reduce toxic side effects. Although limited experiences with intermittent dosing for peritonitis have been reported, its success in other closed-space infections suggests a useful role in the treatment of peritonitis.

A simplified scheme adopted from reference 68 is shown in Tables 6 and 7. All treatments should be guided by the antibiotic susceptibility of the causative organisms. If there is no clinical improvement or decrease in cell count in dialysis fluid within 3 to 4 days, the culture should be repeated. If cultures are consistently positive after 5 days, catheter removal should be considered, especially in the presence of exit site infection with the same organism. The suggested duration of treatment is as follows: gram-positive peritonitis, 14 days (3 doses of vancomycin); gram-negative peritonitis, 21 days; *Pseudomonas/Xanthomonas* peritonitis, 28 days. An initial attempt at chemotherapy of fungal peritonitis may be made. If no improvement occurs in clinical course, cell count, or cultures, however, the catheter should be removed.

Table 7. Antibiotics for treatment of peritonitis

Antibiotic	Dosage[a]
Ceftazidime	125 mg/liter i.p. each exchange
Piperacillin	4 g every 12 h i.v.
Ciprofloxacin	750 mg b.i.d. p.o.
Aztreonam	Load 500 mg/liter; maint 250 mg/liter i.p.
Imipenem	Load 500 mg/liter; maint 100 mg/liter i.p.
Sulfamethoxazole-trimethoprim[b]	Load 1,600/320 mg i.p.; maint 200/40 mg i.p.
Minocycline[b]	100 mg b.i.d. p.o.

[a] Abbreviations: i.p., intraperitoneally; i.v., intravenously; b.i.d., twice a day; p.o., orally; maint., maintenance dosage.
[b] Antibiotics with anti-*Pseudomonas/Xanthomonas* activity.

Side effects. Hypersensitivity reactions against antibiotics have been observed from peritoneal application only, and should this occur, the use of such drugs must be discontinued. Eosinophilia in the peritoneal fluid may occur as a manifestation of drug allergy. Recently, chemical peritonitis after the use of a preparation of vancomycin (Vancoled) has been reported (114).

Aminoglycosides are known to have nephrotoxic and ototoxic effects as well as vestibular toxicity. With the concentrations used in our hospital (8 mg/liter of peritoneal dialysis fluid), we have not observed nephrotoxicity, although the evaluation of nephrotoxicity in patients with little residual renal function is difficult. All attempts should be made to preserve residual function, because the loss of such function may necessitate one extra peritoneal dialysis cycle per day (48).

Ototoxicity and vestibular toxicity have been observed in patients receiving intraperitoneal gentamicin. Tobramycin, netilmicin, and amikacin are believed to exhibit less otic and vestibular toxicity. We have rarely observed such toxicity except in patients who accidentally overdose themselves severalfold with intraperitoneal antibiotics (18, 98).

The use of rifampin occasionally results in an elevation in liver enzymes or nausea, necessitating the discontinuation of the drug. In our hospital we use a dose of 600 mg of rifampin per day, which, if divided into 300 mg twice a day, may have less adverse effects.

Pseudomembranous enterocolitis due to *Clostridium difficile* may occur in patients receiving intraperitoneal antibiotics (134). This serious complication necessitates the discontinuation of antibiotic therapy and, in many cases, the institution of oral agents such as vancomycin, metronidazole, and cholestyramine.

Response to therapy. In most cases of peritonitis, the symptoms become less pronounced rapidly after the initiation of therapy and disappear within 2 to 3 days. During this period, the cell counts decrease and bacterial cultures become negative. In the majority of cases, peritoneal cultures remain positive for only 3 to 4 days (147). Any prolongation of symptoms is indicative of complications or an organism that does not respond well to antibiotic therapy.

Other modalities of therapy

Peritoneal lavage. Peritoneal lavage has been utilized in the treatment of "surgical" peritonitis to remove detritus and fecal contamination from the peritoneal cavity (11a). It has been shown, however, that the effect of lavage may reduce peritoneal defenses and remove necessary phagocytic cells (34). Peritoneal lavage with added iodine has been advocated (137), but the efficacy of such treatment has not been clinically substantiated (109). Studies show that peritoneal antibiotic treatment with the CAPD protocol is clinically efficacious and less costly than peritoneal lavage (30, 161).

Heparin. Heparin should be added to the peritoneal dialysis fluid during peritonitis to inhibit the formation of fibrin and to reduce subsequent adhesions of the peritoneal membrane (103).

Treatment of exit site infections

Exit site infections are a major problem of peritoneal dialysis (114). Their treatment is not very successful and often requires the removal of the catheter. Most commonly, exit sites are infected with *S. epidermidis* or *S. aureus*, although occasionally *Pseudomonas* or *Proteus* infections can be observed. The exit site is erythematous and elevated, draining pus or serous fluid, but generally not painful. In tunnel infections, an abscess can sometimes be palpated under the skin along the cannula tract. To establish a microbiological diagnosis, a culture swab should be taken carefully from the depths of the exit site, not touching adjoining skin.

The treatment of exit site infections can be attempted with local disinfectants or oral antibiotics. The use of neomycin ointment should be discouraged, since its effectiveness is questionable and it may lead to the emergence of resistant organisms. In addition, the ointment forms a crust over the exit site, making cleaning difficult. With daily cleaning and local care, exit site infections sometimes can be cured. If the outer cuff (double-cuffed catheters) appears in the exit site or is extruded, catheter shaving (59, 98, 108, 115) can be attempted, although with no great success.

Catheter removal. The most common reason for catheter removal is a persistently infected exit site or tunnel (150). Catheter replacement at a different site can be done on these patients usually 1 to 2 weeks after catheter removal. If the catheter has to be removed because of frequent recurrence of peritonitis with the same organism or other infectious causes, it can usually be replaced 3 weeks after the termination of successful treatment of peritonitis. Paterson et al. recommend replacement of catheters at the same time as removal (109). This approach appears to be successful in patients who show improvement on antimicrobial therapy, with a decrease in cell count and no organisms in the peritoneal fluid.

Other infectious causes for catheter removal include fungal peritonitis, tuberculous peritonitis, and fecal peritonitis that required laparotomy. Catheter replacement can be considered after the successful treatment of peritonitis or the complete healing of the operative wound. If peritonitis is not responding adequately to appropriate therapy, catheter removal should also be considered.

Prevention of Peritonitis

The risks of infection are minimized when the necessary environmental precautions are taken (masks, handwashing, etc.). In addition, a number of sterile connecting devices have been developed (4, 56, 63, 80, 100). These devices may reduce peritonitis rates in high-risk individuals but are not suitable for widespread use.

Previous clinical studies have examined the use of prophylactic antibiotics primarily in patients on IPD. It is difficult to draw conclusions from these studies because of the low incidence of peritonitis in these patients. We have instituted a double-blind prospective study (84) to investigate the use of oral cephalexin twice daily for peritonitis prophylaxis. We have found that this approach did not decrease the number of infections. More recently, sulfamethoxazole-trimethoprim prophylaxis has been examined in a blind prospective study (18a), with similar negative results. Antibiotic prophylaxis to prevent wound infections during catheter implantations should be used according to the surgical protocol of each hospital. If perioperative antibiotic prophylaxis is employed during surgical implantation, the wound infection rate due to catheter insertions is exceedingly low.

It appears that a certain plateau in the frequency of peritonitis has now been reached, and a peritonitis rate of 1 every 2 patient-years may be acceptable (95). One will have to consider what is the acceptable cost and risk of peritonitis in peritoneal dialysis patients. A further reduction in the peritonitis rate awaits major progress in one or more of a number of areas, including new developments in catheter technology, improved connections, better understanding of patient selection and training programs, improved diagnostic and therapeutic methods in the management of peritonitis, the development of effective chemical or drug prophylaxis of peritonitis, and fresh insights into the infectious and immune processes underlying peritonitis.

REFERENCES

1. **Abrutyn, E., G. L. Goodhart, K. Roos, R. Anderson, and A. Buxton.** 1978. Acinetobacter calcoaceticus outbreak associated with peritoneal dialysis. *Am. J. Epidemiol.* **107:**328–335.
2. **Alobaidi, H. M., G. A. Coles, M. Davies, and D. Lloyd.** 1986. Host defense in continuous ambulatory peritoneal dialysis: the effect of dialysate on phagocyte function. *Nephrol. Dial. Transplant.* **1:**16–21.
3. **Arfania, D., E. D. Everett, K. Nolph, and J. Rubin.** 1981. Uncommon causes of peritonitis in patients undergoing peritoneal dialysis. *Arch. Intern. Med.* **141:**61–64.

4. **Ash, S. R., R. Hoswell, E. M. Heefer, and R. Bloch.** 1983. Effect of the Peridex filter on peritonitis rates in a CAPD population. *Perit. Dial. Bull.* **3**:89–93.

5. **Baddour, L. M., D. L. Smalley, A. P. Kraus, W. J. Lamoreaux, and G. D. Christensen.** 1986. Comparison of microbiologic characteristics of pathogenic and saprophytic coagulase negative staphylococci from patients on continuous ambulatory peritoneal dialysis. *Diagn. Microbiol. Infect. Dis.* **5**:197–205.

6. **Barcenas, G., T. J. Fuller, J. Elms, R. Cohen, and M. G. White.** 1976. Staphylococcal sepsis in patients on chronic hemodialysis regimens. Intravenous treatment with vancomycin given once weekly. *Arch. Intern. Med.* **136**:1131–1134.

7. **Bar-Meir, S., and H. O. Conn.** 1976. Spontaneous bacterial peritonitis induced by intraarterial vasopressin therapy. *Gastroenterology* **70**:418–421.

8. **Baud, J. D., J. Ward, D. W. Fraser, N. J. Peteroon, V. A. Silcox, R. C. Good, P. R. Ostroy, and J. Kennedy.** 1982. Peritonitis due to a Mycobacterium chelonei like organism associated with intermittent chronic peritoneal dialysis. *J. Infect. Dis.* **145**:9–17.

9. **Bayer, A. S., M. Y. Blumenkrantz, J. Z. Montgomerie, J. E. Galpin, J. W. Coburn, and L. B. Gruze.** 1976. Candida peritonitis. *Am. J. Med.* **61**:832–840.

10. **Bennett, W. M., G. R. Aronoff, G. Morrison, T. A. Golper, J. Pulliam, W. Wolfson, and I. Singer.** 1983. Drug prescribing in renal failure: dosing guidelines for adults. *Am. J. Kidney Dis.* **3**:155–193.

11. **Bennion, R. S., J. R. Hiatt, R. A. Williams, and S. E. Wilson.** 1985. A randomized prospective study of perioperative antimicrobial prophylaxis for vascular access surgery. *J. Cardiovasc. Surg.* **26**:270–274.

11a.**British Medical Journal.** 1979. Antibiotic lavage for peritonitis. *Br. Med. J.* **1979**:691–692.

12. **Buckman, R. F., M. Woods, L. Sargent, and A. S. Gervin.** 1976. A unifying pathogenetic mechanism in the etiology of intraperitoneal adhesions. *J. Surg. Res.* **20**:1–5.

12a.**Buggy, B. P.** 1986. *Clin. Microbiol. Newsl.* **8**:12–14.

13. **Bunke, C. M., G. R. Aronoff, and C. Luft.** 1983. Pharmacokinetics of common antibiotics used in continuous ambulatory peritoneal dialysis. *Am. J. Kidney Dis.* **3**:114–117.

14. **Canadian CAPD Clinical Trials Group.** 1989. Peritonitis in continuous ambulatory peritoneal dialysis (CAPD): a multi-center randomized clinical trial comparing the Y connector disinfectant system to standard systems. *Perit. Dial. Int.* **9**:159–163.

15. **Casley-Smith, J. R.** 1967. An electron microscopical study of the passage of ions through the endothelium of lymphatic and blood capillaries, and through the mesothelium. *Q. J. Exp. Physiol.* **52**:105–113.

15a.**Centers for Disease Control.** 1986. Recommendations for providing dialysis treatment to patients infected with human T-lymphotropic virus type III/lymphadenopathy-associated virus. *Morbid. Mortal. Weekly Rep.* **35**:376–378, 383.

16. **Chapman, J. R., and D. W. Warnoch.** 1983. Ketoconazole and fungal CAPD peritonitis. *Lancet* **ii**:510–511.

17. **Cheesebrough, J. S., R. G. Finch, and R. P. Burden.** 1986. A prospective study of the mechanism of infection associated with hemodialysis catheters. *J. Infect. Dis.* **154**:579–589.

18. **Chong, T. K., B. Piraino, and J. Bernardini.** 1991. Vestibular toxicity due to gentamicin in peritoneal dialysis patients. *Perit. Dial. Int.* **11**:152–155.

18a.**Churchill, D. N., D. G. Oreopoulos, D. W. Taylor, S. I. Vas, M. A. Manuel, and G. Wu.** 1987. *Abstr. 20th Annu. Meet. Am. Soc. Nephrol.*, p. 97A.

19. **Churchill, D. N., D. W. Taylor, R. J. Cook, P. LaPlante, P. Cartier, W. P. Fay, M. B. Goldstein, J. K. Jindal, H. Mandin, J. K. Mckenzie, N. Muirhead, P. S. Parfrey, G. A. Posen, D. Slaughter, R. A. Ulan, and T. Werb.** 1992. Canadian Hemodialysis Morbidity Study. *Am. J. Kidney Dis.* **19**:214–234.

20. **Cohen, S. L., and A. Percival.** 1968. Prolonged peritoneal dialysis in patients awaiting renal transplantation. *Br. Med. J.* **1:**409–413.

21. **Collart, F., C. Tielemaus, L. Schandene, E. Dupont, Y. Wybrau, and M. Dratwe.** 1983. CAPD and cellular immunity: no different than hemodialysis patients. *Perit. Dial. Bull.* **3:**163–164.

22. **Conn, H. O., and J. M. Fessel.** 1971. Spontaneous bacterial peritonitis in cirrhosis: variations on a theme. *Medicine* (Baltimore) **50:**161–197.

23. **Cotran, R. S., and M. J. Karnowsky.** 1968. Ultrastructural studies on the permeability of the mesothelium to horse radish peroxidase. *J. Cell Biol.* **37:**123–137.

24. **Courtice, F. C., and W. J. Simmonds.** 1954. Physiological significance of lymph drainage of the serous cavities and lungs. *Physiol. Rev.* **34:**419–448.

25. **Coward, R. A., R. Gokal, and N. P. Mallick.** 1983. Recurrent peritonitis associated with vaginal leak. *Perit. Dial. Bull.* **3:**164–165.

26. **Cross, A. S., and R. T. Steigbigel.** 1976. Infective endocarditis and access site infections in patients on hemodialysis. *Medicine* (Baltimore) **55:**453–466.

27. **Dasgupta, M. K., K. B. Bettcher, R. A. Ulan, V. Burns, K. Lam, J. B. Dossetor, and J. W. Costerton.** 1987. Relationship of adherent bacterial biofilms to peritonitis in chronic ambulatory peritoneal dialysis. *Perit. Dial. Bull.* **7:**168–173.

28. **Dias-Bruxo, J. A., P. Burgess, and P. J. Walker.** 1983. Peritoneovaginal fistula—unusual complication of peritoneal dialysis. *Perit. Dial. Bull.* **3:**142–143.

29. **Dias-Bruxo, J. A., P. J. Walker, C. D. Farmes, J. T. Chandler, and K. L. Holt.** 1983. Continuous cyclic peritoneal dialysis—the Nalle Clinic experience, pp. 23–25. *In* J. D. E. Price (ed.), *Peritoneal Dialysis. The State of the Art.* Communications Media for Education, Princeton, N.J.

30. **Digenis, G. E., R. Khanna, A. Pierratos, and S. Vas.** 1982. Morbidity and mortality after treatment of peritonitis with prolonged exchanges and intraperitoneal antibiotics. *Perit. Dial. Bull.* **2:**45–46.

31. **Dineen, P., W. P. Hornan, and W. R. Grafe.** 1976. Tuberculous peritonitis: 43 years experience in diagnosis and treatment. *Am. Surg.* **184:**712–717.

32. **Dobkin, J. F., M. H. Miller, and N. H. Steigbiegel.** 1978. Septicemia in patients on chronic hemodialysis. *Ann. Intern. Med.* **88:**28–33.

33. **Dryden, M. S., A. Samson, H. A. Ludlam, A. J. Wing, and I. Phillips.** 1991. Infective complications associated with the use of the Quinton "Permcath" for long term central vascular access in haemodialysis. *J. Hosp. Infect.* **19:**257–262.

34. **Duwe, A., S. I. Vas, and J. W. Weatherhead.** 1981. Effect of composition of peritoneal dialysis fluid on chemiluminescence, phagocytosis and bactericidal activity in vitro. *Infect. Immun.* **33:**130–135.

35. **Ellis, H.** 1962. The etiology of post-operative abdominal adhesions. An experimental study. *Br. J. Surg.* **50:**10–16.

36. **Ellis, H.** 1971. The cause and prevention of post-operative intraperitoneal adhesions. *Surg. Gynecol. Obstet.* **133:**497–511.

37. **Fan, P. Y.** 1992. Vascular access: concepts for the 1990s. *J. Am. Soc. Nephrol.* **3:**1–11.

38. **Favero, M. S.** 1985. Recommended precautions for patients undergoing hemodialysis who have AIDS or non-A non-B hepatitis. *Infect. Control* **6:**301–305.

39. **Fenton, P.** 1982. Laboratory diagnosis in patients undergoing continuous ambulatory peritoneal dialysis. *J. Clin. Pathol.* **35:**1181–1184.

40. **Fine, J., H. A. Frank, and A. M. Seligman.** 1946. The treatment of acute renal failure by peritoneal irrigation. *Ann. Surg.* **124:**857–878.

41. **Fivush, B. A., G. H. Bock, P. C. Guzzetta, J. R. Salcedo, and E. J. Ruley.** 1985. Vancomycin prevents polytetrafluoroethylene graft infections in pediatric patients receiving chronic hemodialysis. *Am. J. Kidney Dis.* **5:**120–123.

42. **Francioli, P., and H. Masur.** 1982. Complications of Staphylococcus aureus bacteremia. Occurrence in patients undergoing long-term hemodialysis. *Arch. Intern. Med.* **142:**1655–1658.
43. **Frank, H. A., A. M. Seligman, and J. Fine.** 1984. Further experiences with peritoneal irrigation for acute renal failure. *Ann. Surg.* **128:**561–608.
44. **Gandhi, V. C., H. M. Humayun, T. S. Ing, J. T. Daugirdas, V. R. Jablokow, S. Iwantsuki, W. P. Geis, and J. E. Hano.** 1980. Sclerotic thickening of the peritoneal membrane in maintenance peritoneal dialysis patients. *Arch. Intern. Med.* **140:**1201–1203.
45. **Gervain, A. S., C. L. Puckett, and D. Silver.** 1973. Serosal hypofibrinolysis. A cause of post-operative adhesions. *Am. J. Surg.* **125:**80–88.
46. **Giaccino, F., S. Alloatti, F. Guarello, R. Coppo, M. Pellerey, and G. Piccoli.** 1982. The influence of peritoneal dialysis on cellular immunity. *Perit. Dial. Bull.* **2:**165–168.
47. **Gilmour, J., R. Tymiansky, A. Pierratos, S. Vas, M. Klein, R. Khanna, G. Digenis, S. Cuff, and D. G. Oreopoulos.** 1983. Changes in some inflammatory proteins during peritonitis in CAPD patients. *Perit. Dial. Bull.* **3:**201–204.
48. **Gokal, R., and S. I. Vas.** 1982. Risk of tobramycin use in CAPD patients with peritonitis. *Perit. Dial. Bull.* **2:**139–141.
49. **Gokal, R., S. R. Ash, G. B. Helfrich, C. L. Holmes, P. Joffe, K. Nichols, D. G. Oreopoulos, M. C. Riella, A. Slingeneyer, Z. J. Twardowski, and S. I. Vas.** 1993. Peritoneal catheters and exitsite practices: toward optimum peritoneal access. *Perit. Dial. Int.* **13:**29–39.
50. **Goldblum, S. E., J. A. Ulrich, R. S. Goldman, and W. P. Reed.** 1982. Nasal and cutaneous Staphylococcus among patients receiving hemodialysis and attending personnel. *J. Infect. Dis.* **145:**396.
51. **Goldstein, C. S., J. S. Bomalaski, R. B. Zurier, E. G. Neilson, and S. D. Douglas.** 1984. Analysis of peritoneal macrophages in continuous ambulatory peritoneal dialysis patients. *Kidney Int.* **26:**733–740.
52. **Goldstein, C. S., R. E. Garrik, R. A. Polin, J. S. Gerdes, G. B. Kolski, E. G. Neilson, and S. D. Douglas.** 1986. Fibronectin and complement secretion by monocytes and peritoneal macrophages in vitro from patients undergoing continuous ambulatory peritoneal dialysis. *J. Leukocyte Biol.* **39:**457–464.
53. **Goodship, T. H. J., A. Heaton, R. S. C. Rodger, M. K. Ward, R. Wilkinson, and D. N. S. Kerr.** 1984. Factors affecting development of peritonitis in continuous ambulatory peritoneal dialysis. *Br. Med. J.* **289:**1485–1486.
54. **Gregory, M. C., and D. P. Duffy.** 1983. Toxic shock following staphylococcal peritonitis. *Clin. Nephrol.* **20:**101–104.
55. **Gruer, L. D., R. Bartlett, and A. J. Aycliffe.** 1984. Species identification and antibiotic sensitivity of coagulase negative staphylococci from CAPD peritonitis. *J. Antimicrob. Chemother.* **13:**577–583.
56. **Hamilton, R. W., B. A. Disher, S. A. Dillingham, and A. F. Nicholas.** 1983. The sterile weld: a new method for connections in continuous ambulatory peritoneal dialysis. *Perit. Dial. Bull.* 3(Suppl. 4):8–10.
57. **Harvey, D. M., K. J. Sheppard, A. G. Morgan, and J. Fletcher.** 1987. Effect of dialysate fluids on phagocytosis and killing by normal neutrophyls. *J. Clin. Microbiol.* **25:**1424–1427.
58. **Hau, T., D. H. Ahrenholz, and R. I. Simmons.** 1979. Secondary bacterial peritonitis: the biologic basis of treatment. *Curr. Probl. Surg.* **16:**1–65.
59. **Helfrich, G. B., and J. F. Winchester.** 1982. Shaving of external cuff or peritoneal catheter. *Perit. Dial. Bull.* **2:**183.

60. **Hickman, R., G. I. Thomas, and B. H. Scribner.** 1984. The arteriovenous shunt, p. 85–94. *In* W. C. Waltzer and F. T. Rapaport (ed.), *Angioaccess. Principles and Practice.* Grune and Stratton, Orlando, Fla.

61. **Holdsworth, S. R., R. C. Atkins, D. F. Scott, and R. Jackson.** 1975. Management of Candida peritonitis by prolonged peritoneal lavage containing 5-fluorocytosine. *Clin. Nephrol.* **4:**157–159.

62. **Holmes, C. J., and R. Evans.** 1986. Biofilm and foreign body infection—the significance to CAPD associated peritonitis. *Perit. Dial. Bull.* **6:**168–177.

63. **Holmes, C. J., C. Miyake, and W. Kubey.** 1984. In vitro evaluation of an ultraviolet germicidal connection system for CAPD. *Perit. Dial. Bull.* **3:**215–218.

64. **Horsman, G. B., L. Macmillan, Y. Amatnieks, O. Rifkin, and S. I. Vas.** 1986. Plasmid profile and slime analysis of coagulase negative staphylococci from CAPD patients with peritonitis. *Perit. Dial. Bull.* **6:**195–198.

65. **Huttunen, K., E. Lampainen, S. Silvennoinen-Kassinen, and A. Tiilikainen.** 1984. The neutrophil function of uremic patients treated by hemodialysis or CAPD. *Scand. J. Urol. Nephrol.* **18:**167–172.

66. **Kapral, F. A., J. R. Godwin, and E. S. Dye.** 1980. Formation of intraperitoneal abscesses by *Staphylococcus aureus. Infect. Immun.* **30:**204–211.

67. **Karanicolas, S., D. G. Oreopoulos, S. H. Frath, A. Shiminer, R. F. Manning, H. Sepp, G. A. deVeber, and T. Darby.** 1972. Epidemic of aseptic peritonitis caused by endotoxin during chronic peritoneal dialysis. *N. Engl. J. Med.* **296:**1336–1337.

68. **Keane, W. F., E. D. Everett, T. A. Golper, R. Gokal, C. Halstenson, Y. Kawaguchi, M. Riella, S. Vas, and H. A. Verburgh.** 1993. Peritoneal dialysis related peritonitis treatment recommendations: 1993 update. *Perit. Dial. Bull.* **13:**14–28.

69. **Kerr, C. M., J. R. Perfect, P. C. Craven, J. H. Jorgensen, D. J. Drutz, J. D. Shelburne, H. A. Gallis, and R. A. Gutman.** 1983. Fungal peritonitis in patients on continuous ambulatory peritoneal dialysis. *Ann. Intern. Med.* **99:**334–337.

70. **Khan, R. H., M. Klein, and S. Vas.** 1987. Fibronectin in the normal peritoneal fluids of patients on chronic ambulatory peritoneal dialysis and during peritonitis. *Perit. Dial. Bull.* **7:**69–73.

71. **Khanna, R., D. J. McNeeley, D. G. Oreopoulos, S. I. Vas, and W. McCready.** 1980. Treating fungal infections: fungal peritonitis in CAPD. *Br. Med. J.* **280:**1147–1148.

72. **Khanna, R., D. G. Oreopoulos, S. I. Vas, W. McCready, and N. Dombros.** 1980. Fungal peritonitis in patients undergoing chronic intermittent or continuous peritoneal dialysis. *Proc. Eur. Dial. Transplant. Assoc.* **17:**291–296.

73. **Kloos, W. E., and K. H. Schleifer.** 1975. Simplified scheme for the routine identification of human staphylococcus species. *J. Clin. Microbiol.* **1:**82–88.

74. **Knight, K. R., A. Polak, J. Crump, and R. Maskell.** 1982. Laboratory diagnosis and oral treatment of CAPD patients. *Lancet* **ii:**1301–1304.

75. **Lally, K. P., L. P. Brennan, N. J. Sherman, C. Grushkin, E. Lieberman, and J. B. Atkinson.** 1987. Use of a subclavian venous catheter for short- and long-term hemodialysis in children. *J. Pediatr. Surg.* **22:**603–605.

75a. **Lancet.** 1983. Sclerosing peritonitis. Letter. July 9, Aug. 13, Sept. 3, Sept. 24, Nov. 5.

76. **LaRocco, M. T., J. E. Moortensen, and A. Robinsson.** 1986. Mycobacterium fortuitum peritonitis in a patient undergoing chronic peritoneal dialysis. *Diagn. Microbiol. Infect. Dis.* **4:**161–164.

77. **Lamperi, S., and S. Carozzi.** 1986. Suppressor resident peritonitis macrophages and peritonitis incidence in continuous ambulatory peritoneal dialysis. *Nephron* **44:**219–225.

342   Vas

78. **Lamperi, S. and S. Carozzi.** 1986. Defective opsonic activity of peritoneal effluent during continuous ambulatory peritoneal dialysis (CAPD): importance and prevention. *Perit. Dial. Bull.* **6:**87–92.

79. **Lempert, K. D., and J. M. Jones.** 1982. Flucytosine micronazole treatment of Candida peritonitis: its use during continuous ambulatory peritoneal dialysis. *Arch. Intern. Med.* **142:**577–578.

80. **Lempert, K. D., J. A. Kolb, R. D. Swartz, V. Campese, T. A. Golper, J. F. Winchester, K. D. Nolph, F. E. Husserl, S. W. Zimmerman, and S. B. Kurtz.** 1986. A multicenter trial to evaluate the use of the CAPD "O" set. *ASAIO Trans.* **32:**557–559.

80a.**Levison, M. E.** 1992. New dosing regimens for aminoglycoside antibiotics. *Ann. Intern. Med.* **117:**693–694.

81. **Lewis, S., and C. Holmes.** 1992. Host defense mechanisms in the peritoneal cavity of continuous ambulatory peritoneal dialysis patients. Part 1. *Perit. Dial. Int.* **11:**14–21.

82. **Lewis, S., and C. Holmes.** 1992. Host defense mechanisms in the peritoneal cavity of continuous ambulatory peritoneal dialysis patients. Part 2. *Perit. Dial. Int.* **11:**112–117.

83. **Lorber, B., and R. M. Swenson.** 1975. The bacteriology of intra-abdominal infections. *Surg. Clin. North Am.* **55:**1349–1354.

84. **Low, D. E., S. I. Vas, D. G. Oreopoulos, R. A. Manuel, C. S. Saiphoo, C. Finer, and N. Dombros.** 1980. Randomized clinical trial of prophylactic cephalexin in CAPD. *Lancet* **ii:**753–754.

85. **MacCallum, W. G.** 1903. On the mechanism of absorption of granular materials from the peritoneum. *Bull. Johns Hopkins Hosp.* **14:**105–110.

86. **Mader, J. T., and J. A. Reinarz.** 1978. Peritonitis during peritoneal dialysis. The role of the preheating water bath. *J. Chron. Dis.* **31:**635–664.

87. **Maiorca, R., A. Cantaluppi, G. C. Cancarini, A. Scalamogna, R. Broccoli, G. Graziani, S. Brasa, and C. Ponticelli.** 1983. Prospective controlled trial of a Y connector and disinfectant to prevent peritonitis in continuous ambulatory peritoneal dialysis (CAPD). *Lancet* **ii:**642–644.

88. **Manuel, M. A., T. W. Paton, and W. R. Cornish.** 1983. Drugs and peritoneal dialysis. *Perit. Dial. Bull.* **3:**117–125.

89. **Marrie, T. J., M. A. Noble, and J. W. Costerton.** 1983. Examination of the morphology of bacteria adhering to peritoneal dialysis catheters by scanning and transmission electron microscopy. *J. Clin. Microbiol.* **18:**1388–1398.

90. **McGregor, S. J., J. H. Brock, J. D. Briggs, and B. J. Junor.** 1987. Bactericidal activity of peritoneal macrophages from continuous ambulatory peritoneal dialysis patients. *Nephrol. Dial. Transplant.* **2:**104–108.

91. **McNeely, D., S. I. Vas, N. Dombros, and D. G. Oreopoulos.** 1981. Fusarium peritonitis: an uncommon complication. *Perit. Dial. Bull.* **1:**94–96.

92. **Mion, C. M., S. T. Boen, and P. Scribner.** 1965. Analysis of factors responsible for the formation of adhesions during chronic peritonitis dialysis. *Am. J. Med. Sci.* **250:**675–679.

93. **Montgomery, Y. Z., G. R. Kalmanson, and L. B. Guze.** 1968. Renal failure and infection. *Medicine* (Baltimore) **47:**1–32.

94. **Morford, D. W.** 1982. High index of suspicion for tuberculous peritonitis in CAPD patients. *Perit. Dial. Bull.* **2:**189–190.

95. **National Institutes of Health.** 1987. *National CAPD Registry.* Characteristics of participants and selected outcome measures for the period January 1, 1981 through August 31, 1986. National Institutes of Health, Bethesda, Md.

96. **Nicholls, A., N. Edward, and G. R. D. Catto.** 1980. Staphylococcal septicemia, endocarditis and osteomyelitis in dialysis and renal transplant patients. *Postgrad. Med. J.* **56:**642–648.

97. **Nichols, W. K., and K. D. Nolph.** 1983. A technique for managing exit site and cuff infection in Tenckhoff catheters. *Perit. Dial. Bull.* **3**(Suppl.):S4–S5.

98. **Nicolaidis, P., S. Vas, V. Lawson, L. Kennedy-Vosu, A. Bernard, G. Abraham, S. Izatt, S. Khanna, J. M. Bargman, and D. G. Oreopoulos.** 1991. Is intraperitoneal tobramycin ototoxic in CAPD patients? *Perit. Dial. Int.* **11**:156–161.

99. **Nolph, K. D.** 1980. Round table discussion, p. 272. *In* M. Legrain (ed.), *Continuous Ambulatory Peritoneal Dialysis.* Excerpta Medica, New York.

100. **Nolph, K. D.** 1985. Randomized multicenter clinical trial to evaluate the effects of an ultraviolet germicidal system on peritonitis rates in continuous ambulatory peritoneal dialysis. *Perit. Dial. Bull.* **5**:19–24.

101. **Nolph, K. D.** 1993. Access problems plague both peritoneal dialysis and hemodialysis. *Kidney Int. Suppl.* **40**:S81–S84.

102. **O'Connor, J., and M. MacCormick.** 1981. Tuberculous peritonitis in patients on CAPD: the importance of lymphocytosis in the peritoneal fluid. *Perit. Dial. Bull.* **1**: 106.

103. **O'Leary, J. P., F. S. Malik, R. R. Donahoe, and A. D. Johnston.** 1979. The effects of a minidose of heparin on peritonitis in rats. *Surg. Gynecol. Obstet.* **148**:571–575.

104. **Onderdonk, A. B., J. G. Bartlett, T. Louie, N. Sullivan-Seigler, and S. L. Gorbach.** 1976. Microbial synergy in experimental intra-abdominal abscess. *Infect. Immun.* **13**: 22–26.

105. **Onorato, I. M., J. L. Axelrod, J. A. Lorch, J. M. Brensilver, and V. Bokkenheuser.** 1979. Fungal infections of dialysis fistulae. *Ann. Intern. Med.* **91**:50–52.

106. **Oreopoulos, D., S. Vas, and R. Khanna.** 1983. Prevention of peritonitis during continuous ambulatory peritoneal dialysis. *Perit. Dial. Bull. Suppl.* **3**:S18–S20.

107. **Oreopoulos, D. G., M. Robson, S. Izatt, S. Clayton, and G. A. deVeber.** 1978. A simple and safe technique for continuous ambulatory peritonealialysis (CAPD). *Trans. Am. Soc. Artif. Intern. Organs* **24**:484–487.

108. **Palmer, R. A., W. E. Quinton, and J. E. Gray.** 1964. Prolonged peritoneal dialysis for chronic renal failure. *Lancet* **i**:700–702.

109. **Paterson, A. D., M. C. Bishop, A. G. Morgan, and R. P. Burden.** 1986. Removal and replacement of Tenckhoff catheter at a single operation: successful treatment of resistant peritonitis in continuous ambulatory peritoneal dialysis. *Lancet* **ii**:1245–1247.

110. **Pearson, J. G., T. D. McKinney, and W. J. Stone.** 1983. Penicillium peritonitis in a CAPD patient. *Perit. Dial. Bull.* **3**:20–21.

111. **Peter, G., R. Locci, and G. Pulverer.** 1982. Adherence and growth of coagulase negative staphylococci on surfaces of intravenous catheters. *J. Infect. Dis.* **146**:479–482.

112. **Peterson, P. K., E. Gaziano, H. J. Suh, M. Devalon, L. Peterson, and W. F. Keane.** 1985. Antimicrobial activities of dialysate-elicited and resident human peritoneal macrophages. *Infect. Immun.* **49**:212–218.

113. **Pierard, D., S. Lauwers, M. C. Monton, J. Sennesael, and D. Verbeelen.** 1983. Group JK Corynebacterium peritonitis in a patient undergoing continuous ambulatory peritoneal dialysis. *J. Clin. Microbiol.* **18**:1011–1014.

114. **Piraino, B., J. Bernardini, J. Johnston, and M. Sorkin.** 1987. Chemical peritonitis due to intraperitoneal vancomycin (Vancoled). *Perit. Dial. Bull.* **7**:156–159.

115. **Piraino, B., J. Bernardini, A. Peitzman, and M. Sorkin.** 1987. Failure of peritoneal cuff shaving to eradicate infection. *Perit. Dial. Bull.* **7**:179–182.

116. **Poisson, M., V. Beromicide, C. Falardeau, C. Vega, and R. Morisset.** 1983. Mycobacterium chelonei peritonitis in a patient undergoing continuous ambulatory peritoneal dialysis (CAPD). *Perit. Dial. Bull.* **3**:86–88.

117. **Popovich, R. P., J. W. Moncrief, J. B. Decherd, J. B. Bomar, and W. K. Pyle.** 1976. *Abstr. Am. Soc. Artif. Intern. Organs* **5**:64–68.

118. **Popovich, R. P., J. W. Moncrief, K. D. Nolph, A. J. Ghods, Z. J. Twardowski, and W. K. Pyle.** 1978. Continuous ambulatory peritoneal dialysis. *Ann. Intern. Med.* **88:** 449–456.

119. **Prowant, B. F., B. A. Warady, and K. D. Nolph.** 1993. Peritoneal dialysis exit site care: results of an international survey. *Perit. Dial. Int.* **13:**149–154.

120. **Quarles, L. D., E. A. Rutsky, and S. G. Rostand.** 1985. Staphylococcus aureus bacteremia in patients on chronic hemodialysis. *Am. J. Kidney Dis.* **6:**412–419.

121. **Rubin, J., L. M. Lin, R. Lewis, J. Cruse, and J. D. Bower.** 1983. Host defense mechanisms in continuous ambulatory peritoneal dialysis. *Clin. Nephrol.* **20:**140–144.

122. **Rubin, J., J. Humphries, G. Smith, and J. Bower.** 1983. Antibiotic activity in peritoneal dialysate. *Am. J. Kidney Dis.* **3:**205–208.

123. **Rubin, J., D. G. Oreopoulos, T. T. Lio, R. Mathews, and G. A. deVeber.** 1976. Management of peritonitis and bowel perforation during chronic peritoneal dialysis. *Nephron* **16:**220–225.

124. **Rubin, J., W. A. Rodgers, H. M. Taylor, E. D. Everett, B. F. Prowant, L. U. Fruto, and K. D. Nolph.** 1980. Peritonitis during continuous ambulatory dialysis. *Ann. Intern. Med.* **92:**7–13.

125. **Rubin, S. J.** 1984. *Clin. Microbiol. Newsl.* **6:**3–5.

126. **Ryan, G. B., J. Grobety, and G. Majno.** 1971. Post-operative peritoneal adhesions. A study of the mechanisms. *Am. J. Pathol.* **65:**117–138.

127. **Salo, R. J., A. A. Salo, W. J. Fahlberg, and J. T. Ellzey.** 1980. Hepatitis B surface antigen (HB(s)Ag) in peritoneal fluid of HB(s)Ag carriers undergoing peritoneal dialysis. *J. Med. Virol.* **6:**29–35.

128. **Sasaki, S., T. Aliba, M. Suenaga, S. Tornura, N. Yoobiyama, S. Nakagawa, T. Shoji, T. Sasavka, and J. Takenchi.** 1979. Ten year survey of dialysis associated tuberculosis. *Nephron* **24:**141–145.

129. **Schmidt, R. W., and M. Blumenkrantz.** 1981. Peritoneal sclerosis. A sword of Damocles for peritoneal dialysis. *Arch. Intern. Med.* **141:**1265–1267.

130. **Schweinburg, F. B., A. M. Seligman, and J. Fine.** 1950. Transmural migration of intestinal bacteria. A study based on the use of radioactive Escherichia coli. *N. Engl. J. Med.* **242:**747–751.

131. **Seligman, A. M., H. A. Frank, and J. Fine.** 1946. Treatment of experimental uremia by means of peritoneal irrigation. *J. Clin. Invest.* **25:**211–219.

132. **Sewell, D. L., and T. A. Golper.** 1982. Stability of antimicrobial agents in peritoneal dialysate. *Antimicrob. Agents Chemother.* **21:**528–529.

133. **Sherertz, R. J., R. J. Falk, K. A. Huffman, C. A. Thomann, and W. D. Mattern.** 1983. Infections associated with subclavian Uldall catheters. *Arch. Intern. Med.* **143:** 52–56.

134. **Silva, J., and R. Fekety.** 1981. Clostridia and antimicrobial enterocolitis. *Am. Rev. Med.* **32:**327–333.

135. **Simkin, E. P., and F. K. Wright.** 1968. Perforating injuries of the bowel complicating peritoneal catheter insertion. *Lancet* **i:**64–66.

136. **Sombolos, K., S. Vas, O. Rifkin, A. Ayomamitis, P. McNamee, and D. G. Oreopoulos.** 1986. Propionibacteria isolates and asymptomatic infections of the peritoneal effluent in CAPD patients. *Nephrol. Dial. Transplant.* **1:**175–178.

137. **Stephen, R. L., C. Kablitz, M. Kitahara, J. A. Welson, D. P. Duffin, and W. J. Kolff.** 1979. Peritoneal dialysis: peritonitis: saline iodine flush. *Dial. Transpl.* **8:** 584–595.

138. **Sterioff, S.** 1984. Arteriovenous fistula for hemodialysis, p. 95–106. *In* W. C. Waltzer and F. T. Rapaport (ed.), *Angioaccess. Principles and Practice.* Grune and Stratton, Orlando, Fla.

139. **Swartz, R. D., D. A. Campbell, D. Stone, and C. Dickinson.** 1983. Recurrent polymicrobial peritonitis from a gynecological source as a complication of CAPD. *Perit. Dial. Bull.* **3:**32–33.

140. **Tanchajja, S., A. H. Mohaiden, M. M. Avram, and M. M. Eisenberg.** 1985. Management of infection associated with prosthetic graft exposure in angioaccess. *Vasc. Surg.* **19:**117–121.

141. **Tenckhoff, H., and F. K. Curtis.** 1970. Experience with maintenance peritoneal dialysis in the home. *Trans. Am. Soc. Artif. Intern. Organs* **16:**90–95.

142. **Tenckhoff, H., and H. Schecter.** 1968. A bacteriologically safe peritoneal access device. *Trans. Am. Soc. Artif. Intern. Organs* **14:**181–187.

143. **Uldall, P. R.** 1984. Use of the subclavian cannula in vascular access, p. 65–83. *In* W. C. Waltzer and F. T. Rapaport (ed.), *Angioaccess. Principles and Practice.* Grune and Stratton, Orlando, Fla.

144. **Uldall, P. R., N. Merchant, F. Woods, U. Yaworski, and S. Vas.** 1981. Changing subclavian hemodialysis cannulas to reduce infection. *Lancet* **i:**1373.

145. **Uldall, R., M. DeBruyne, M. Besley, J. McMillan, M. Simons, and R. Francoeur.** A new vascular access catheter for hemodialysis. *Am. J. Kidney Dis.* **21:**270–277.

146. **Vas, S. I.** 1986. Peritonitis of peritoneal dialysis patients: pathogenesis and treatment, p. 21–63. *In* C. S. F. Easmon and J. Jeljaszewicz (ed.), *Medical Microbiology,* vol. 5. Academic Press, London.

147. **Vas, S. I.** 1983. Microbiologic aspects of chronic ambulatory peritoneal dialysis. *Kidney Int.* **23:**83–92.

148. **Vas, S. I., D. E. Low, S. Layne, R. Khanna, and N. Dombros.** 1981. Microbiological diagnostic approach to peritonitis in CAPD patients, p. 269–271. *In* R. C. Atkins et al. (ed.), *Peritoneal Dialysis.* Churchill Livingstone, Edinburgh.

149. **Vas, S. I.** 1982. Editorial comment. *Perit. Dial. Bull.* **2:**190.

150. **Vas, S. I.** 1981. Indications for removal of peritoneal catheter. *Perit. Dial. Bull.* **1:**145–46.

151. **Vas, S. I., and D. G. Oreopoulos.** 1981. Handle with care: hepatitis B antigen carriers in peritoneal dialysis units. *Nephron* **29:**105–106.

152. **Vas, S. I., and L. Low.** 1985. Microbiological diagnosis of peritonitis in patients on continuous ambulatory peritoneal dialysis. *J. Clin. Microbiol.* **21:**522–523.

153. **Verbrugh, H. A., W. F. Keane, J. R. Hoidal, M. R. Freiberg, G. R. Elliott, and P. K. Peterson.** 1983. Peritoneal macrophages and opsonins: antibacterial defense in patients undergoing chronic peritoneal dialysis. *J. Infect. Dis.* **147:**1018–1029.

154. **Verger, C., A. M. Chesneau, M. Thibault, and N. Bataille.** 1987. Biofilm on Tenckhoff catheters: a negligible source of contamination. *Perit. Dial. Bull.* **6:**174–178.

155. **Von Graevenitz, A., and D. Amsterdam.** 1992. Microbiological aspects of peritonitis associated with continuous ambulatory peritoneal dialysis. *Clin. Microbiol. Rev.* **5:**26–48.

156. **Waltzer, W. C., and F. T. Rapaport (ed.).** 1984. *Angioaccess. Principles and Practice.* Grune and Stratton, Inc., Orlando, Fla.

157. **Weinstein, M. P., P. B. Iannini, C. W. Stratton, and T. L. Eickhoff.** 1978. Spontaneous bacterial peritonitis. A review of 28 cases with emphasis on improved survival and factors influencing prognosis. *Am. J. Med.* **64:**592–598.

158. **Wierusz-Wysocka, B., H. Wysocki, G. Michta, A. Wykretowicz, R. Czarneckiand, and K. Baczyk.** 1984. Phagocytosis and neutrophil bactericidal capacity in patients with uremia. *Folia Haematol.* **111:**589–594.

159. **Williams, P., D. Pantalony, S. I. Vas, R. Khanna, and D. G. Oreopoulos.** 1981. The value of dialysate cell count in the diagnosis of peritonitis in patients on continuous ambulatory peritoneal dialysis. *Perit. Dial. Bull.* **1:**59–62.

160. **Williams, P., R. Khanna, H. Simpson, and S. I. Vas.** 1982. Tobramycin blood levels of CAPD patients during peritonitis. *Perit. Dial. Bull.* **2**:48.

161. **Williams, P., R. Khanna, S. Vas, S. Layne, D. Pantalony, and D. G. Oreopoulos.** 1980. Treatment of peritonitis in patients on CAPD: to lavage or not. *Perit. Dial. Bull.* **1**:14–17.

162. **Wolfe, J. H. N., A. R. Behn, and B. T. Jackson.** 1978. Tuberculous peritonitis and role of diagnostic laparoscopy. *Lancet* **i**:852–853.

163. **Wu, G.** 1983. Review of peritonitis episodes that caused interruption of CAPD. *Perit. Dial. Bull. Suppl.* **3**:S11–S13.

164. **Wu, G., R. Khanna, S. Vas, and D. G. Oreopoulos.** 1983. Is extensive diverticulosis of the colon a contraindication to CAPD. *Perit. Dial. Bull.* **3**:180–183.

165. **Yu, V. L., A. Goetz, M. Wagener, P. B. Smith, J. D. Rihs, J. Hanchett, and J. Zuravleff.** 1986. Staphylococcus aureus nasal carriage and infection in patients on hemodialysis. Efficacy of antibiotic prophylaxis. *N. Engl. J. Med.* **315**:91–96.

Infections Associated with Indwelling Medical Devices, 2nd ed.
Edited by Alan L. Bisno and Francis A. Waldvogel
© 1994 American Society for Microbiology, Washington, DC 20005

Chapter 14

Infections of the Female Genital Tract

P. Joan Chesney

Over the last quarter of a century, the use of intrauterine devices (IUDs) and tampons by millions of women worldwide has introduced four previously rare and unrecognized infections. The morbidity and mortality associated with toxic shock syndrome (TSS), spontaneous septic midtrimester abortion, pelvic actinomycosis, and IUD-associated pelvic inflammatory disease (PID) have been significant. These events have focused badly needed attention on the composition of these devices and pathogenesis of these infections. The impact of these infections is particularly important as these foreign bodies, the products of modern technology, are not placed to improve or cure a disease process but for modification of normal physiological processes.

INTRAUTERINE DEVICES

History and Importance

Hippocrates wrote about the use of IUDs, but the first recorded descriptions came from Germany in the 1920s with the use of IUDs made of silkworm gut. Reports of subsequent associated severe pelvic infections discouraged further experimentation until two reports in the late 1950s by Oppenheimer and Ishihama suggested that intrauterine rings were safe, providing they were inserted aseptically and in women with no history of PID (64, 145). The subsequent development of inert and

P. Joan Chesney • Department of Pediatrics, University of Tennessee, Memphis, and LeBonheur Children's Medical Center, 848 Adams Avenue, Memphis, Tennessee 38103.

chemically modified plastic IUDs led to a new era of IUD investigation and use.

Clinical studies in the mid-1960s reported PID rates of 0.6 to 3.5% per year in IUD users. The study by Mishell et al. in 1969, in which IUDs removed surgically directly through the uterine fundus were cultured, suggested that IUDs and the uterine cavity were sterile within 30 days of insertion (84, 85). Thus, it was assumed that episodes of PID occurring more than 30 days after insertion were due to a sexually transmitted disease and unrelated to the IUD. Reports of midtrimester spontaneous septic abortions and death in women using the Dalkon Shield in the mid-1970s led to a reexamination of this assumption (19, 68).

Subsequent clinical studies in the United States presented a less optimistic view of the association of PID and IUD use. In 1977 these studies culminated in a recommendation by the Conception Control Sub-committee of the Panel on Review of Obstetrical-Gynecological Devices of the Food and Drug Administration (FDA). They recommended that IUD labeling contain the statement that "IUD use is associated with a 3–5 fold increase in infection rate" and further that IUDs be replaced every 3 years (145). Recent studies and commentaries have cast doubt on whether IUDs are associated with an increased risk of PID (74). Although the FDA has not withdrawn approval of IUDs, most types are no longer manufactured in the United States as a result of the lawsuit costs for manufacturers.

Worldwide, the IUD continues to be used in many countries, including China, Taiwan, South Korea, Indonesia, India, Pakistan, Turkey, and Egypt. In 1984 it was estimated that over 40 million women in China were using IUDs, accounting for about 70% of the 60 million users worldwide (145).

Types of IUDs

IUDs are generally of two types: inert devices made of a nonabsorbable material, such as polyethylene, impregnated with barium sulfate for radiopacity and those from which there is continuous elution of a chemically active substance, primarily copper or a progestational agent (96, 140). In order to determine the location of the IUD and to facilitate easy removal, most IUDs have a tail. These tails are composed of a plastic monofilament surrounded by a nylon sheath. The Dalkon Shield had a tail composed of a bundle of 200 to 400 monofilaments surrounded by a sheath. The shapes of IUDs vary from that of the Copper T or 7 (with the copper wire wound around the lower "leg") to curved or shieldlike, pliable, easily deformable devices (96, 140).

Advantages of IUDs

IUDs are second only to oral contraceptives in terms of contraceptive effectiveness and far more convenient than barrier or oral contraceptives. Recent studies have shown that extended use is safe for modern IUDs. The Copper T 380 series, multiload 375, and 20 μg/day levonorgestrel devices can safely remain in place at least 8 years (90). Five years is recommended for the Nova T, as the pregnancy rate increases subsequently (138). Although the levonorgestrel devices can cause amenorrhea and other hormonal side effects (127), they are not nearly as significant as for oral contraceptives, and overall, the mortality associated with oral contraceptives is twice that of IUDs. Cardiovascular disorders are 3 to 5 times more common with oral contraceptives, and deaths from pregnancy far exceed those associated with IUDs (96, 140).

Mechanism of Action of IUDs

The mechanism of action of the IUD is unclear. Although they may touch less than 20% of the surface area of the endometrium, they prevent implantation of the blastocyst on areas of the endometrium not in contact with the IUD.

In all mammals, intrauterine foreign bodies evoke an endometrial and tubal inflammatory response of macrophages, neutrophils, multinucleated giant cells, edema, and vascular dilatation (14, 52, 89, 103, 111, 129). Initial insertion of the IUD is associated with bacterial colonization of the normally sterile uterine cavity. Within 20 to 30 days, the uterus may again be sterile (85), although this has been disputed (117, 142). The sterile-foreign-body-induced inflammation may persist in both the endometrium and the endosalpinx, as demonstrated by histopathology and the presence of neutrophils and macrophages in uterine washes. Involvement of the endosalpinx in this sterile inflammatory foreign body response is suggested by the studies of Beerthuizen et al., who found histologic signs of tubal inflammation in 53.5% of IUD wearers compared with 6.4% of controls. No bacteria were found in the oviducts, and the incidence of lesions was not correlated with duration of IUD use (6). Similar findings were reported by Smith and Soderstrom, who also found that the noninfectious tubal inflammation was most extensive with IUDs with large surface areas in contact with the endometrium (116).

Numerous hypotheses have been proposed to explain how this sterile inflammatory response of the endometrium and endosalpinx prevents pregnancy. These hypotheses include a failure of implantation, lysosomal enzyme destruction of the blastocyst and spermatozoa, phagocytosis of spermatozoa by macrophages, and inhibition of sperm transport. It has been suggested that any or all of these effects may be mediated by uterine prostaglandin or cytokine release by the sheets of macrophages that surround IUDs soon after insertion (89). The repeated failure of IUDs to prevent pregnancy in women taking anti-inflammatory drugs further supports the role of chronic inflammation and/or prostaglandin release in preventing nidation (14).

Zipper et al. were the first to observe the antifertility effect of intrauterine copper (147). The effect of copper appears to be a local one, as a short metallic copper wire placed in one uterine horn of a rabbit prevents blastocyst implantation there but not in the adjacent horn. Devices containing copper not only greatly enhance the contraceptive action of the same device without copper but also are effective when inserted up to 7 days after intercourse. An antibacterial action of copper has also been described in vitro against *Neisseria gonorrhoeae* (118).

In order to combine the beneficial effects of both intrauterine and hormonal contraception, the levonorgestrel IUD was developed. Studies have shown that the slow release of this hormone from a polydimethylsiloxane polymer "sleeve" is a highly effective contraceptive agent and may significantly lower the incidence of PID (127).

Disadvantages of IUDs

The disadvantages of IUDs include a discontinuation rate of about 10% because of expulsion or heavy bleeding, hormonal side effects with the levonorgestrel device (127), a possible increased incidence of PID, and a potentiation of the risk that pelvic infection will result in tubal infertility and ectopic pregnancies (74).

Infectious Complications of IUDs

The infectious complications that have been associated with IUD use include spontaneous septic midtrimester abortions, vaginitis and vaginosis, pelvic actinomycosis, *Candida* chorioamnionitis, HIV infections, and PID with tubal infertility, tubo-ovarian abscesses, and peritonitis. Whereas other contraceptive methods offer protection against sexually transmitted PID, the IUD does not. TSS has only rarely been reported as a complication of IUD use.

Spontaneous Septic Midtrimester Abortions

An increase in the incidence of spontaneous septic midtrimester abortions occurring in women with the Dalkon Shield in place was the first warning that some IUDs were not as safe as anticipated. Although the outcome of this infection, often due to anaerobes, was serious and could be fatal, the true risk and incidence with Dalkon Shield use are not known. The incidence of IUD-related spontaneous septic abortion deaths peaked in 1973 and virtually disappeared from 1974 on, as the coincident PID epidemic of sexually transmitted PID receded and the FDA recommended the removal of any IUD when patients became pregnant (74, 130).

The woman who elects to continue her pregnancy with an IUD in place and in whom the tail is not visible for early IUD removal must be warned of the potential for a septic abortion. If signs of sepsis develop, it is suggested that the products of conception and the device be removed immediately and antibiotic and supportive therapy be given to prevent fulminant and fatal infection of the mother.

Vaginitis/Vaginosis

About 20% of women with an IUD have a malodorous, homogeneous, grey, thin, and nonpurulent discharge resembling a nonspecific vaginitis and composed primarily of anaerobes (1, 53, 58, 62, 102). This incidence is four times greater than that in non-IUD users. In women using IUDs, the normal lactobacillus-dominated microbial vaginal flora present in women using barrier contraception is replaced by a flora rich in anaerobes and *Gardnerella vaginalis*. Thus the IUD in some way changes the normal cervicovaginal flora to one that contains more virulent microorganisms.

Pelvic Actinomycosis

In 1976 Gupta and associates first described a strong association between the use of IUDs and the presence of anaerobic actinomyceslike organisms and sulfur granules in cervicovaginal Papanicolaou (Pap) smears. Also, significant clinical disease due to actinomycetes and the closely related *Eubacterium nodatum* has been well described in women using IUDs (28, 42, 56, 60).

The prevalence of these organisms on Pap smears varies with the population studied, type of IUD, duration of IUD use, and reliability in reading the smears. Of women wearing IUDs, the prevalence in public clinic populations has varied from 5.3 to 25.5%, compared with that in private patients of 1.6 and 8%, respectively, in two studies (17). The prevalence of positive smears clearly increases with duration of use (17).

Much controversy has been raised regarding the significance of finding these actinomyceslike organisms on Pap smears (17, 32, 107). On one hand, it has been suggested that these organisms may be part of the normal vaginal flora, with their presence increased in the presence of an IUD or lower genital tract foreign body. In one study of 50 randomly selected women, 27% without an IUD and 44% of IUD users had positive cervical smears that stained with fluorescent antibody to *Actionomyces israelii* (17). Another study, in which culture techniques were used, detected actinomycetes in cervicovaginal cultures of 20.7% of 58 women who were not using an IUD (17). In support of these findings, another study demonstrated no statistical difference in symptoms for IUD users, regardless of whether actinomyceslike organisms were detected on Pap smear (94). On the basis of these types of data, the association of British Family Planning Doctors has recommended that asymptomatic women with positive smears should only be followed with repeat smears. No active form of therapy is recommended for asymptomatic women (17).

Other groups have taken a more aggressive stance, recommending that all IUD users should have periodic screening for these organisms. Those women who are asymptomatic but have a positive smear should have the IUD removed and be restudied in 4 to 6 weeks. If the smear is negative, reinsertion could be considered. This more aggressive approach is based on a finding, not well substantiated, that 25% of women with actinomycetes on Pap smears had PID. The Centers for Disease Control (CDC) estimates that the risk is probably very low, citing only 200 cases of actinomycosis among an estimated 20 to 30 million patient-years of risk (32).

Most important, as actinomyceslike organisms are usually found in association with other anaerobic bacteria, their presence may simply serve as a marker for colonization or infection by these other organisms (17).

Although the clinical manifestations of actinomycosis are not different from those of PID, women who are symptomatic and have a positive smear should probably have the IUD removed and be treated for at least 2 weeks with either penicillin or tetracycline. If there is no response to this conservative management, surgery and 2 months or more of antibiotics may be necessary (17).

Candida Chorioamnionitis

Candida albicans is frequently found in the normal flora of the female genital tract. Recently it has been reported in association with amniotic fluid infection in women with preterm labor, premature deliveries, and midtrimester abortions. Several cases were associated with retained IUDs or cervical cerclage sutures (25, 37).

HIV Infection

In three family planning clinics in Dar-es-Salaam, Tanzania, 2,009 women were interviewed regarding contraceptive use history and other potential risk factors for HIV infection. Of the 2,009 women enrolled, 252 (25%) were HIV antibody positive. In multivariable analyses, women who were using or who had ever used an IUD were at a threefold increased risk of HIV infection. This unique report clearly requires confirmation and further investigation (69).

Pelvic Inflammatory Disease

Many epidemiologic studies have examined the association between PID, infertility, and IUD use. In order to interpret these often conflicting studies, it is important to clarify several aspects of PID. PID is an inflammation of the organs of the upper genital tract, which are normally sterile (18, 39–41, 62). Infection may include endometritis, salpingitis, oophoritis, inflammation of the parametrial supporting structures, and peritonitis. Organisms can ascend to the uterus. Once inert particles and spermatozoa have reached the uterus, they are quickly transmitted to the fallopian tubes, and presumably this is also true of bacteria (73).

PID may be due to sexually (gonococcus or chlamydia) or non-sexually transmitted organisms. It is estimated that 25–65% of all cases of PID are non-sexually transmitted. These latter cases of polymicrobial PID, believed to occur in a compromised genital tract, are caused by both aerobes (*Streptococcus* species, *Escherichia coli*, and *Haemophilus influenzae*) and anaerobes (*Peptococcus*, *Peptostreptococcus*, and *Bacteroides* species), with anaerobes predominating (18, 39–41, 62).

The clinical diagnosis of PID is difficult in the vast majority of cases that do not manifest the classical clinical presentation. Numerous studies have documented the diagnosis as being incorrect (false positive or negative) in 17 to 63% of cases without laparoscopy. In addition, up to 6% of women who are asymptomatic have been found to have tubal inflammation when laparoscopy was performed for other reasons. Tubal and endometrial histology is the most definitive technique (144). Laparoscopy may be diagnostic, allowing the fallopian tubes to be directly visualized and specimens for culture and/or histology to be taken directly.

Complications of PID include the acute problems of peritonitis, pelvic abscess, tubo-ovarian abscess with or without sepsis or rupture, and the need for hysterectomy and oophorectomy (119, 126). The long-term or chronic complications of PID are called residues and include chronic abdominal pain, recurrent PID, periadventitial adhesions, and tubal occlusion with resulting infertility and ectopic pregnancies (18, 39–41, 62, 136).

Numerous epidemiologic studies with both case-control and prospective cohort studies performed in the 1970s and early 1980s suggested that IUDs increased the risk of PID and its sequelae. More recent studies and reevaluations of older studies, eliminating certain biases, have suggested that there are a limited number of risk factors that increase the risk for PID in women using IUDs (74). Those at highest risk include young (<25 years) nulliparous women (121), those with several partners, and those with a preceding episode of PID (86).

Varying numbers of factors have been examined in each study, including different populations, type of device, duration of use prior to development of PID, age, race, marital status, parity, number of sexual partners, frequency of intercourse, number of prior episodes of PID and/ or gonorrhea, hospitalization versus outpatient diagnosis, prior pregnancy or abortion, and criteria used for the diagnosis of PID. In addition, the control groups have varied, including either non-contraceptive users or non-IUD contraceptive users. As all other contraceptive methods, including tubal ligation, provide protection against PID, studies using non-IUD contraceptive users as controls suggest that IUDs are a greater risk factor than do studies in which non-contraceptive users serve as controls.

With so many variables involved, it is not surprising that the results have been divergent. One risk factor on which all studies are in agreement is that there is an increased risk of PID during the 20 to 30 days following IUD insertion or replacement (15, 16, 38, 44, 73, 80). This increased risk is felt to be due to the introduction of bacteria into the uterus following transient contamination of the IUD by cervical-vaginal flora. Studies of intrauterine flora after removal of IUDs from the fundus within 1 to 3 days after insertion have documented this transient colonization in humans (61, 85, 117, 142), as have similar studies of primates (115). IUD insertions in women with undiagnosed cervical infections, including chlamydial (86, 101, 128) and gonococcal infections, which are frequently asymptomatic, could be a common cause of these early cases of PID (74). Replacement of an IUD has been associated with a 13% rate of transient bacteremia (88). Studies examining the use of doxycycline prophylaxis at the time of IUD insertion have been inconclusive (78, 113). Ideally, women should be screened and treated for asymptomatic sexually transmitted diseases before IUD insertion (44).

The studies, however, are not in agreement about the risk of PID occurring more than 1 month following insertion. For example, as part of the Women's Health Study, Lee and associates compared the relative risk of PID in IUD users and control women using no contraceptives (80). The Women's Health Study is a concurrent case-control study at 16 hospitals in 9 cities across the United States. The relative risk was 3.1 for women who used their IUDs for less than 5 months and only 1.1 (not significantly different from 1) for women who used their IUDs for more than 4 months. These data suggested an elevated risk of PID attributable to the insertion procedure itself but no increased risk with continued IUD use.

Eschenbach and associates found the risk of acute salpingitis to be 4.4 times higher in IUD users than in nonusers. In IUD users, the risk of salpingitis was greater in nulligravid than in previously gravid women (40). Westrom and associates found the risk of salpingitis increased 6.9 times in nulligravid women and 1.7 times in previously pregnant women, compared with controls (137). In a prospective study through the British Family Planning Association, Vessey et al. followed 3,162 IUD users over a 4-year period and compared them with a group of 13,838 non-IUD contraceptive users (132). They found that IUD users had a 3- to 3.5-fold increased rate of PID, compared with non-IUD users.

Several studies have examined the risk of IUD use and PID severe enough to require hospitalization. Burkman and associates, as part of the Women's Health Study, examined 1,447 hospitalized patients with PID and 3,453 patients as controls. For all IUD users, the estimated risk of hospitalization for PID for IUD users was 1.6 (95% confidence limits, 1.4 to 1.9) (15, 16). They found also, however, that the relative risk varied from 1.6 to 4.5, depending on the control group used for comparison.

In another study examining risk factors in women hospitalized for PID, Kaufman et al. compared 155 women with a control group of 305 women with nongynecologic diagnoses (70). The relative risk of 8.6 was highest, for women who had had an IUD inserted within the preceding month, compared with women who had never had an IUD. For women who had had an IUD inserted more than a month earlier, the relative risk was 1.6. Finally, Flesh et al. compared 163 hospitalized patients with acute salpingitis with 220 control patients seen in the minor trauma section of the emergency room (46). They found that black race, IUD use, multiple sexual partners, and previous salpingitis each independently increased the risk of PID. For both black and nonblack patients, the use of an IUD increased the risk ratio twofold above that for controls for each group.

A recent reassessment of IUDs as a risk factor for PID compares results from prospective cohort studies and from case-control studies. In the cohort studies, the risk of PID in women with IUDs was similar to estimates of PID in sexually active women from industrial countries who were not using IUDs. In the case-control studies, removal of the oral contraceptive users generally reduced the reported odds ratio, "frequently to borderline statistical significance for studies with a high accuracy of PID diagnosis" (74).

When the relative risk of PID is examined for the different IUDs, several studies suggest an increased risk for the Dalkon Shield (31, 70, 80, 134), although this finding has been refuted (38, 87). An antibacterial action of copper has been described in vitro against *Neisseria gonorrhoeae* (118). A recent prospective study compared the rates of PID for a copper-releasing IUD (the Nova-T) with the 20 µg/day levonorgestrel IUD. A significantly decreased rate of PID was found in the levonorgestrel users (13, 127), although this finding has been disputed (63, 114).

Thus, overall, the case control and cohort studies have shown that the relative risk of PID for IUD users varies greatly, depending on which risk factors are examined. In general, the risk is higher for the first 20 to 30 days after insertion, for nulliparous women, for those with several partners, for those under 25 years of age, and for those with a preceding episode of PID.

Risk of Infertility

A recent reassessment of the association between IUDs and tubal infertility suggests that "IUD use alone does not increase the risk of infertility or ectopic pregnancy" (74). However, perhaps as a result of the presence of the noninfectious foreign body-mediated inflammatory reaction in the endosalpinx, IUD use appears to potentiate the risk of pelvic infection for tubal infertility (29, 33). "This potentiating effect is greatest for IUD's with a large surface area in contact with the endometrium. The effect is minimal, if it exists for small copper devices."

Pathogenesis of Infectious Complications

The upper genital tract is normally sterile, as the cervix provides an effective physical and chemical barrier to bacteria (73, 141). The closed internal os, resistant squamous epithelium, and bacteriostatic endocervical mucus maintain the barrier. Infection is more likely to occur when this barrier is interrupted, as occurs when the endometrial cavity is exposed following delivery, abortion, menses, dilation and curettage, and placement of an IUD with a tail projecting into the vagina and with scarring following an episode of PID.

It is unclear how bacteria ascend into the uterus, but several theories have been proposed. They may be directly deposited during IUD placement (51) or may ascend the tails of the IUD. Trichomonads and spermatozoa often carry bacteria on their surfaces and are readily found in the oviducts. Despite the cervical barrier, passive movement of carbon or carmine particles from the cervix or vagina into the uterus and oviducts within minutes following intercourse has been well documented (73). Uterine contractile activity or pressure differentials may account for some of this "passive" movement (73).

The most pathogenic organisms, such as *Neisseria gonorrhoeae* and *Chlamydia trachomatis*, may produce factors such as immunoglobulin A proteases that allow them to directly break down the cervical barrier and enter the uterus. The pathogenicity of the normal endogenous microflora is low, however, and in order for these organisms to cause disease, there must be an alteration of the local defense mechanisms described above. In an in vitro gel system, bacteria were unable to migrate through the gel except in the presence of a monofilament thread (139). Another in vitro experiment demonstrated that bacteria could grow throughout the length of both mono- and multifilament tails that had been coated with cervical mucus (97). This finding suggested a route of access for bacteria, even with single-filament IUD tails.

Colonization of IUDs In Vivo

Evidence supporting bacterial colonization of IUDs in vivo is conflicting. Mishell et al. cultured the uterus of hysterectomy specimens from IUD wearers. They found a definite bacterial presence in the first 24 h, which decreased and disappeared from the 30th day of insertion onward (85). Sparks and coworkers, however, found that the uterine cavities and half the endocervical canals in 50 controls and 2 women wearing a tailless IUD were sterile (117). Bacteria were found in all uterine cavities containing a tailed IUD.

Wolf and Krieger removed 152 IUDs either through the transcervical route or through a sterile fundal incision in the uterus following hysterectomy (142). The population included the following: 70 women who were asymptomatic IUD wearers, 13 who had dysfunctional bleeding, 23 with PID, 31 in whom the IUD tail was no longer visible, and 17 who were pregnant with an IUD in situ.

The IUDs of all groups of patients were densely colonized by a variety of organisms, with a predominance of coagulase-negative staphylococci, enterococci, and anaerobic lactobacilli. Of 16 IUDs removed transfundally from asymptomatic women, only 4 (25%) were sterile. Almost half (48%) of the IUDs without a tail were sterile. When pregnancy occurred in the presence of an IUD, only 29% were sterile. Bacteria of low pathogenicity predominated, except from the IUDs of patients with PID. Pathogenic organisms, especially beta-hemolytic streptococci,

Staphylococcus aureus, and *E. coli,* in addition to anaerobes, grew from these devices.

Extensive in vitro evidence has accumulated to support the concept that the "tail" on an IUD may permit the ascent of cervicovaginal organisms into the normally sterile uterus. Studies by Tatum et al. in 1975 provided dramatic evidence that the multifilament tail of the Dalkon Shield could serve as a wick in vitro. Five different IUDs, including the Dalkon Shield, were suspended on a glass rod, with the tails immersed in an aqueous dye solution. Dye ascended the tail of the Dalkon Shield within 2 h, whereas no dye ascended the monofilament tails of the other four IUDs (124). In addition, tails of IUDs removed electively from women were examined by transmission electron microscopy (TEM) and were cultured carefully both aerobically and anaerobically. By TEM, the spaces between the monofilaments in the Dalkon Shield tail were found to be filled with bacteria (see Fig. 3). Culture of these spaces after sterilization of the outer surface of the tail revealed that 42% were positive for a variety of aerobes and 86% were positive for anaerobes. Cultures of monofilament IUD tails were all negative, presumably because the surface was sterilized prior to culture (123, 124). Tatum et al. suggested that ascent of the colonized tail into the uterus after the first 8 to 10 weeks of pregnancy might be responsible for the increased incidence of midtrimester septic abortions associated with the Dalkon Shield.

Bank et al. used scanning electron microscopy (SEM) to examine Dalkon Shield tails from IUDs removed from asymptomatic women after at least 2 years of use (2). They also found extensive cellular debris and numerous bacteria in the spaces between filaments. As noted by the authors, these bacteria are inaccessible to cellular host defenses.

Despite this evidence for bacterial colonization of tails with the postulated access of organisms into the uterus, the epidemiologic evidence from clinical studies is not conclusive with respect to the PID risk being higher in patients using IUDs with tails, although sample sizes have been small (5, 49, 92, 145, 146). One study, however, did show a difference in incidence of PID of 18.8 versus 0.8% when devices with and without tails were compared (145). In addition, several reports by Sparks and colleagues document bacteria in the uterus of users of IUDs with tails and sterile uterine cavities in those using tailless IUDs (117). A recent prospective controlled study confirmed that infectious complications of IUDs are more frequent if the threads lead from the uterine cavity to the vagina than if they are contained within the uterine cavity (92).

Where are the bacteria that have been isolated from these devices found histologically in vivo? A great deal of evidence now confirms the

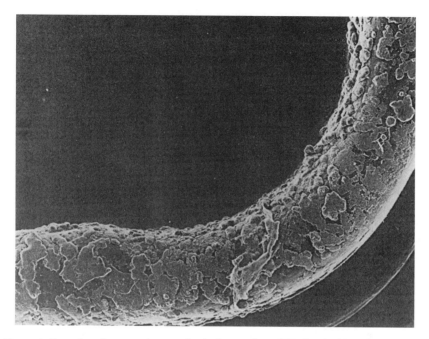

Figure 1. Scanning electron micrograph of a Lippes loop IUD that had been in place for 8 years. The rounded granules on the concave side are compatible with bioapatite, which is similar to dental plaque. Magnification, × 100. (Reprinted with permission from reference 106.)

fact that IUDs removed after more than 6 months in utero are covered with a thick calcified biofilm (Fig. 1 to 3).

IUDs removed from 24 h to 15 years following insertion have been examined using routine cultures, SEM, TEM, and electron microprobe analysis. The predominant cell type covering the IUD in sheets even within 2 days of insertion is the macrophage. Scattered neutrophils, lymphocytes, and plasma cells are present, giving the appearance of a granulomatous reaction. Within the first 6 months of insertion, the macrophages continue to surround the IUD in sheets, showing, in addition, many mitotic figures, giant cells, and much phagocytosed material including spermatozoa. Also within 1 to 6 months following insertion, numerous fibroblasts with mitotic figures are found along with sheets of fibrin threads, occasional platelets, and much cell debris, including degenerating spermatozoa and a few bacteria. Thus, within the first 6 months of insertion, within the uterine cavity and surrounding the IUD

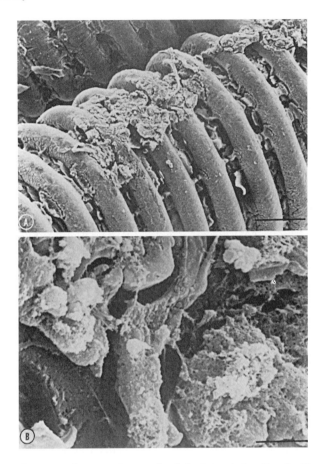

Figure 2. (A) Scanning electron micrograph of the intrauterine tip of a Copper 7 IUD. Note the moderate amount of biofilm on the surface. Bar = 500 μm. (B) Greater detail of the biofilm seen in panel A. Bar = 5 μm. (Reprinted with permission from reference 83.)

is a foamlike collection of cells, fibrin, mucus, and cellular debris (103, 112, 129).

Six months after insertion, the character of this material begins to change to that of a thick (up to 200 μm), tightly adherent biofilm or encrustation around the IUD, composed of fibrinous material and a polysaccharide glycocalyx resembling dental plaque (2, 3, 54, 55, 72, 75, 83, 106, 108, 112, 123, 129, 134) (Fig. 1–3). Within this biofilm or crust are embedded many different morphologic types of bacteria (Fig. 3) and actinomyceslike organisms (83), cellular debris, and, with time, a pro-

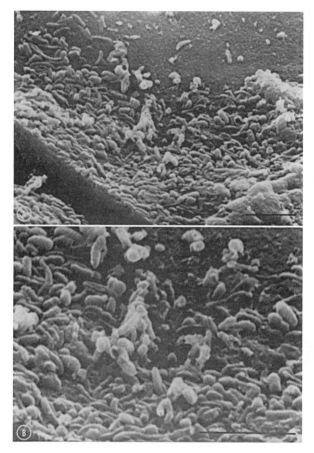

Figure 3. (A) Higher magnification of the biofilm seen in Fig. 2. Note the presence of bacteria on the surface. (B) Greater detail of the bacteria seen in panel A. Both bars = 5 μm. (Reprinted with permission from reference 83.)

gressive increase in the amount of calcium. The copper wires may become corroded and blackened, with coils obscured, resembling a rusty nail. Outside, these biofilms are surrounded by macrophages, neutrophils, and lymphocytes, with neutrophils predominant around the copper devices.

This encrustation has the effect of making the device rigid and of decreasing the ability of the copper or progestational agent to leave the device (55, 145).

Surface aerobic cultures of 10 such biofilms had growth primarily

of gram-positive organisms, including coagulase-negative staphylococci
(83). Extensive aerobic and anaerobic cultures of decalcified and homoge-
nized crusts have not been reported.

BARRIER CONTRACEPTIVES

Barrier contraceptives act to mechanically or chemically prevent
spermatozoa from reaching the cervix (95, 122). Of these contraceptives,
TSS has been reported to follow the use of both diaphragms (7, 27, 77,
100, 109) and sponges (23, 35, 43, 67, 99). The limited number of case
reports associated with barrier contraceptives, compared with their
widespread use, suggests that TSS is a rare complication (109). In most
cases, TSS developed following prolonged retention or fragmentation of
the sponge with difficult removal. In vitro, the sponge, which contains
1 g of the spermicide nonoxynol-9, appears to inhibit production of TSS
toxin-1 (TSST-1) (109).

Cervical lacerations following use of the Vimule cervical cap raised
concerns that these patients might be at increased risk for TSS (11). Thus
far, no cases following cervical cap use have been reported.

Urinary tract infections have also been reported as a complication
of diaphragm use (62a). They may result from misplacement of the diaphragm with urethral and bladder irritation and/or partial urethral obstruction.

TAMPON-INDUCED ULCERATIONS

Vaginal ulcerations have followed both short- and long-term use of
super-absorbent tampons (4, 9, 34, 48, 66, 135). Vaginal drying, epithelial
peeling or layering, microulcerations, and macroulcerations were observed by colposcopy. Although tampon fibers could be seen embedded
in the ulcerations, no infectious complications of these foreign bodies
were described. Initial reports suggested that these ulcers might permit
growth of S. aureus and/or entry of toxin in TSS, but it now seems most
likely that the toxin(s) associated with TSS caused mucosal membrane
ulcerations throughout the body, including in the vagina (79).

TAMPON-ASSOCIATED TSS

Intravaginal tampons of varying formulations have been used for
centuries. Until the late 1970s, most tampons were composed of cotton
or cotton and rayon mixtures. In the late 1970s, tampon absorbencies

were increased by most manufacturers by increasing the size of the tampon, changing its geometry, and/or introducing new components, such as polyacrylate fibers, carboxymethyl cellulose chips, and polyester foam.

Epidemiology

In 1978 an apparently new disease caused by presumed *S. aureus* toxins was described by Todd et al. (125). Only scattered case reports prior to 1978 appeared to describe the same entity. In 1980 a case definition was established by the CDC, and the association of TSS with menses was first recognized (20–22, 36, 110). Seven early and subsequent case-control studies demonstrated that wearing tampons was associated with an increased risk of acquiring TSS (10, 36, 59, 65, 71, 91, 104, 110). The second CDC case-control study, completed in September 1980, reported that the use of Rely brand tampons, which contained carboxymethyl cellulose chips and polyester foam, was associated with a greater relative risk of developing menstrual TSS than were other brands (110). Rely was voluntarily withdrawn from the market by the manufacturer. In 1985, all polyacrylate-containing tampons were removed from the market following a 10-million-dollar lawsuit against one of the manufacturers, in conjunction with a widely publicized in vitro laboratory study (*O'Gilvie v. International Playtex*, no. 83-1845, vol 37 [DC Kan, March 21, 1985] [Post-trial motion and court findings]).

In vitro data have not demonstrated clear, reproducible differences among the different tampon constituents in terms of their ability to induce or enhance production of TSST-1 by *S. aureus* isolates (12). Rather, the epidemiologic studies strongly support the overall absorbency of a tampon as the measure of its relative risk in terms of being associated with TSS (10, 91).

Tampon absorbency is standardized by the syngyna test based on in vitro salt water absorbency and expressed in grams on a scale of 0 to 20 (82). In the CDC case-control study of 285 tampon-associated menstrual TSS cases, the odds ratio, a measure of the relative risk of a given tampon brand to cause TSS, correlated best with the absorbency. Within each category of tampon composition, the risk of illness increased with absorbency; e.g., Tampax Regular had an absorbency of 6.32 g and an odds ratio of 4.7, whereas Playtex Super Plus had an absorbency of 17.23 and an odds ratio of 40.3, compared with non-tampon users with an odds ratio of 1 (10). Standardized absorbency labels are now included on all tampon boxes, indicating the relative absorbency of that particular brand (143). Superabsorbent tampons are no longer available, and the incidence of TSS has dropped dramatically since the first reports in 1978 (24).

Why more-absorbent tampons increase the risk for TSS is unclear. As the vagina is normally an anaerobic environment, it may be that tampons introduce oxygen, which is required for TSST-1 production (45, 133). Although many other potential theories about how tampons act to increase the risk of TSS have been proposed and studied, the answer is as yet unclear.

In addition to tampon use, the risk of acquiring menstrual TSS is related to both cervicovaginal colonization with TSST-1-producing strains of *S. aureus* and the absence of antibody to TSST-1. The prevalence of *S. aureus* in genital cultures was evaluated prospectively in a group of 600 women being followed for routine pregnancy-related or problem-associated visits (81). Of 175 individuals seen for a routine visit, 20 (7%) had a positive labial or vaginal culture for *S. aureus*, and 9 (3%) had a positive vaginal culture only. Three of the 20 isolates produced TSST-1. Thus, overall, approximately 1% of women of childbearing age have cervicovaginal colonization with TSST-1-producing strains of *S. aureus*. The highest *S. aureus* colonization rates were found in postpartum women; 14 of 81 (17%) postpartum women had positive genital cultures, compared with 41 of 519 (8%) other women. The reasons for this increase in postpartum colonization are not clear.

Absence of antibody to TSST-1 is uncommon in women of childbearing age. In one study, 85 of 95 (91%) of patients with TSS had no antibody at disease onset, as determined by radioimmunoassay testing (8, 120). In the general population in the same state, antibody to TSST-1 was found in 70% of individuals by age 10 years, 88% by age 20 years, and 96% by ages 30 and 50 years (131). Thus, absence of antibody appears to be a risk factor for menstrual TSS.

TSS Toxin

S. aureus strains isolated from patients with menstrual TSS produce an exoprotein with a molecular weight of 22,000, TSST-1 (8, 105). More than 90% of menstrual isolates produce TSST-1, compared with 30% of non-TSS *S. aureus* strains. This protein has now been well characterized, and the structural gene for its production, a 10.6-kb unit, has been cloned in *E. coli* (76).

TSST-1 appears to be an important marker for menstrual *S. aureus* isolates, and in the rabbit model it produces many of the manifestations of TSS (98). *S. aureus* isolates from nonmenstrual cases of TSS produce TSST-1 less often. In one study, only 20 of 32 (62.5%) such strains isolated in pure culture from normally sterile *S. aureus*-infected sites in TSS produced TSST-1 (50). Thus, it appears that other substances produced by *S. aureus* may also lead to TSS. Other known toxins produced by

S. aureus that have been suggested as possible causes of TSS are the enterotoxins, in particular, enterotoxin B (27, 57). Additional, as yet unidentified, toxins may play a role.

Clinical Manifestations

The way in which TSST-1 acts in rabbits or humans to produce the manifestations of TSS is unclear but may be related to its role as a superantigen, able to simultaneously and rapidly induce production of both monokines and lymphokines (27, 30, 57).

Multisystem organ damage and massive capillary vasodilation with intravascular fluid loss constitute the apparent toxin-mediated damage of TSS (20, 26, 27). Prolonged hypotension following the loss of intravascular volume may result in ischemic organ damage that further compounds the damage. The onset of illness is abrupt, with symptoms and signs of moderate to severe disease including fever, chills, malaise, headache, sore throat, myalgias, muscle tenderness, fatigue, vomiting, diarrhea, abdominal pain, and orthostatic dizziness or syncope.

Over the next 24 to 48 h, diffuse erythema, severe watery diarrhea (often with incontinence), decreased urine output, cyanosis, and edema of the extremities may be noted. Cerebral ischemia, edema, or a toxin-mediated effect on the central nervous system rapidly results in somnolence, confusion, irritability, agitation, and (occasionally) hallucinations.

Histopathology

The histopathologic findings found at autopsy support the concept that TSS is triggered by a toxin and/or an endogenous mediator (79, 93). Typically, there is a total absence of tissue invasion by bacteria and minimal evidence of an inflammatory reaction in most organs. Cervicovaginal ulcerations are the only characteristic lesions noted in the genital tract in fatal cases. These ulcerations have been noted on postmortem examination of a patient with menstrual TSS who had never used tampons (79). The ulcerations are superficial; capillary vasodilation and thrombosis with inflammation of the mucosa are present, but no deep tissue bacterial invasion is seen. The layer of vacuolization and separation in the ulcers occurs beneath the basal layer. The same type of ulcer has also been found in the bladder and esophagus, suggesting that these ulcerations may be due to the toxin(s) and not to tampon use.

SUTURES AND OTHER FOREIGN BODIES

TSS has occurred following many different gynecologic procedures (47, 94). As for many other postoperative cases of TSS, most of these cases may have been secondary to wound infections. Whether the wound infection is a result of the well-recognized propensity of *S. aureus* to colonize foreign bodies such as sutures is unclear. The increased risk of TSS for women postpartum suggests that sutures in the episiotomy and/or the repair of the cervical lacerations may provide the nidus for the initial *S. aureus* replication and toxin production (15, 27, 47).

SUMMARY

The importance of population control and the convenience of both IUD and tampon use suggest that healthy women worldwide will continue to use both IUDs and tampons. Removal of the Dalkon Shield and Rely and polyacrylate tampons from the market has significantly reduced the incidence of complications associated with their use. Adverse publicity in the early 1970s regarding a possible association between IUDs and PID was most closely related to the peak of sexually transmitted diseases in 1973 and use of the Dalkon Shield. This publicity resulted in a significant decrease in the use of IUDs in the United States. Recent reassessments of IUD use suggest that there is no increase in the incidence of IUD-associated PID for women who are married and monogamous, except for the 20 to 30 days following insertion. The incidence of PID for other women using IUDs is similar to PID estimates in sexually active women in industrial countries.

Continued epidemiologic and basic research are needed to evaluate the remaining products on the market and to create new and safer products. The future will be enriched by continued research into such areas as incorporation of materials to prevent IUD bacterial colonization and glycocalyx formation and making safer tampons.

REFERENCES

1. **Avonts, D., M. Sercu, P. Heyerick, I. Vandermeeven, A. Meheus, and P. Piot.** 1990. Incidence of uncomplicated genital infections in women using oral contraception or an intrauterine device: a prospective study. *Sex. Transm. Dis.* **17:**23–29.
2. **Bank, H. L., and H. O. Williamson.** 1983. Scanning electron microscopy of Dalkon Shield tails. *Fertil. Steril.* **40:**334–339.
3. **Bank, H. L., H. O. Williamson, and K. Manning.** 1975. Scanning electron microscopy of copper containing intrauterine devices: long-term changes in utero. *Fertil. Steril.* **26:**503–508.
4. **Barrett, K. F., S. Bledsoe, B. E. Greet, and W. Droegemueller.** 1977. Tampon-induced vaginal or cervical ulceration. *Am. J. Obstet. Gynecol.* **127:**332–333.
5. **Batar, I., L. G. Lampe, and H. Allonen.** 1991. Clinical experience with intrauterine devices inserted with and without tail. *Int. J. Gynaecol. Obstet.* **36:**137–40.
6. **Beerthuizen, R. J., J. A. Van Wijck, T. K. Eskes, A. H. Vermeulen, and G. P. Vooijs.**

1982. IUD and salpingitis: a prospective study of the pathomorphological changes in the oviducts in IUD users. *Eur. J. Obstet. Gynecol. Reprod. Biol.* **13**:31–41.

7. **Bergdoll, M. S., and P. J. Chesney.** 1991. *Toxic Shock Syndrome.* CRC Press, Inc., Boca Raton, Fla.

8. **Bergdoll, M. S., B. A. Crass, R. F. Reiser, R. N. Robbins, and J. P. Davis.** 1981. A new staphylococcal enterotoxin, enterotoxin F, associated with toxic-shock syndrome *Staphylococcus aureus* isolates. *Lancet* **i**:1017–1021.

9. **Berkeley, A. S., J. P. Micha, K. S. Freedman, and J. C. Hirsch.** 1985. The potential of digitally inserted tampons to induce vaginal lesions. *Obstet. Gynecol.* **66**:31–35.

10. **Berkley, S. F., A. W. Hightower, C. V. Broome, and A. L. Reingold.** 1987. The relationship of tampon characteristics to menstrual toxic-shock syndrome. *JAMA* **258**:917–920.

11. **Bernstein, G. S., L. H. Kilzer, A. H. Coulson, R. M. Nakamura, G. C. Smith, R. Berstein, R. Frezieres, V. A. Clark, and C. Coan.** 1982. Studies of cervical caps. I. Vaginal lesions associated with use of the Vimule cap. *Contraception* **26**:443–436.

12. **Broome, C. V., P. S. Hayes, G. W. Ajello, J. C. Free, R. J. Gibson, S. L. M. Grave, G. A. Hancock, R. L. Anderson, A. K. Highsmith, D. C. Mackel, N. T. Hargrett, and A. L. Reingold.** 1982. In vitro studies of interactions between tampons and *Staphylococcus aureus. Ann. Intern. Med.* **96**:959–962.

13. **Buchan, H., L. Villard-Mackintosh, M. Vessey, D. Yeates, and K. McPherson.** 1990. Epidemiology of pelvic inflammatory disease in parous women with special reference to intrauterine device use. *Br. J. Obstet. Gynaecol.* **97**:780–788.

14. **Buhler, M., and E. Papiernik.** 1983. Successive pregnancies in women fitted with intrauterine devices who take antiinflammatory drugs. *Lancet* **i**:483–484.

15. **Burkman, R. T.** 1981. Women's Health Study: association between intrauterine device and pelvic inflammatory disease. *Obstet. Gynecol.* **57**:269–276.

16. **Burkman R. T.** 1991. Intrauterine devices. *Curr. Opin. Obstet. Gynecol.* **3**:482–485.

17. **Burkman, R. T., and M. T. Damewood.** 1985. Actinomyces and the intrauterine contraceptive device, p. 427–437. *In* G. I. Zatuchni, A. Goldsmith, and J. J. Sciarra (ed.), *Intrauterine Contraception: Advances and Future Prospects.* J. B. Lippincott Co., Philadelphia.

18. **Burnakis, T. G., and N. B. Hildebrandt.** 1986. Pelvic inflammatory disease: a review with emphasis on antimicrobial therapy. *Rev. Infect. Dis.* **8**:86–94.

19. **Cates, W., Jr., H. W. Ory, R. W. Rochat, and C. W. Tyler, Jr.** 1976. The intrauterine devices and deaths from spontaneous abortion. *N. Engl. J. Med.* **295**:1155–1159.

20. **Centers for Disease Control.** 1980. Toxic-shock syndrome—United States. *Morbid. Mortal. Weekly Rep.* **29**:220–230.

21. **Centers for Disease Control.** 1980. Follow-up on toxic-shock syndrome—United States. *Morbid. Mortal. Weekly Rep.* **29**:297–299.

22. **Centers for Disease Control.** 1980. Follow-up on toxic-shock syndrome. *Morbid. Mortal. Weekly Rep.* **29**:441–445.

23. **Centers for Disease Control.** 1984. Toxic-shock syndrome and the vaginal contraceptive sponge. *Morbid. Mortal. Weekly Rep.* **33**:43–44.

24. **Centers for Disease Control.** 1990. Reduced incidence of toxic-shock syndrome. United States 1980–1990. *Morbid. Mortal. Weekly Rep.* **39**:421–422.

25. **Chain, W., M. Mazor, and A. Wiznitzer.** 1992. The prevalence and clinical significance of intraamniotic infection with Candida species in women with preterm labor. *Arch. Gynecol. Obstet.* **251**:9–15.

26. **Chesney, P. J., B. A. Crass, M. B. Polyak, P. J. Wand, R. F. Warner, J. M. Vergeront, J. P. Davis, R. W. Tofte, R. W. Chesney, and M. S. Bergoll.** 1982. Toxic-shock syndrome: management and long-term sequelae. *Ann. Intern. Med.* **96**:847–851.

27. **Chesney, P. J., and J. P. Davis.** 1992. Toxic shock syndrome, p. 1277–1295. *In* R. D. Feigin and J. D. Cherry (ed.), *Textbook of Pediatric Infectious Disease*, 3rd ed. The W.B. Saunders Co., Philadelphia.

28. **Cleghorn, A. G., and R. G. Wilkinson.** 1981. The IUCD-associated incidence of Actinomyces israelii in the female genital tract. *Aust. N. Z. J. Obstet. Gynaecol.* **29:** 445–449.

29. **Cramer, D. W., I. Schiff, S. C. Schoenbaum, M. Gibson, S. Belisle, B. Albrecht, R. J. Stillman, M. J. Berger, E. Wilson, B. V. Stadel, and M. Scibel.** 1985. Tubal infertility and the intrauterine device. *N. Engl. J. Med.* **312:**941–947.

30. **Crass, B. A., and M. S. Bergdoll.** 1986. Involvement of staphylococcal enterotoxins in nonmenstrual toxic shock syndrome. *J. Clin. Microbiol.* **23:**1138–1139.

31. **Culliton, B. J., and D. S. Knopman.** 1974. Dalkon Shield affair: a bad lesson in science and decision making. *Science* **185:**839–842.

32. **Curtis, E. M., and L. Pine.** 1981. Actinomyces in the vaginas of women with and without intrauterine contraceptive devices. *Am. J. Obstet. Gynecol.* **140:**880–884.

33. **Daling, J. R., N. S. Weiss, B. J. Metch, W. H. Chow, R. M. Soderstrom, D. E. Moore, L. R. Spadoni, and B. V. Stadel.** 1985. Primary tubal infertility in relation to the use of intrauterine device. *N. Engl. J. Med.* **312:**937–941.

34. **Danielson, R. W.** 1983. Vaginal ulcers caused by tampons. *Am. J. Obstet. Gynecol.* **146:**547–549.

35. **Dart, R. C., and M. A. Levitt.** 1985. Toxic-shock syndrome associated with the use of the vaginal contraceptive sponge. *JAMA* **253:**1877.

36. **Davis, J. P., P. J. Chesney, P. J. Wand, and the Investigation and Laboratory Team.** 1980. Toxic-shock syndrome. Epidemiologic features, recurrences, risk factors, and prevention. *N. Engl. J. Med.* **303:**1429–1455.

37. **Donders, G. G., P. Moerman, J. Caudron, and F. A. Van Assche.** 1991. Intra-uterine Candida infection: a report of four infected fetuses from two mothers. *Eur. J. Obstet. Gynecol. Reprod. Biol.* **38:**233–238.

38. **Edelman, D. A., G. S. Berger, and L. Keith.** 1982. The use of IUD's and their relationship to pelvic inflammatory disease: a review of epidemiologic and clinical studies. *Curr. Probl. Obstet. Gynecol.* **6**(3):33–34.

39. **Eschenbach, D. A.** 1980. Epidemiology and diagnosis of acute pelvic inflammatory disease. *Obstet. Gynecol.* **55**(5)(Suppl.):142S-152S.

40. **Eschenbach, D. A., J. P. Harnisch, and K. L. Homes.** 1977. Pathogenesis of acute pelvic inflammatory disease: role of contraception and other risk factors. *Am. J. Obstet. Gynecol.* **128:**838–850.

41. **Eschenbach, D. A., and R. M. Soderstrom.** 1980. IUD and salpingitis, p. 140–158. *In* E. S. E. Hafez (ed.), *IUD Pathology and Management.* International Medical Publishers, Lancaster, England.

42. **Evans, D. T.** 1993. Actinomyces israelii in the female genital tract: a review. *Genitourin. Med.* **69:**54–59.

43. **Faich, G., K. Pearson, D. Fleming, S. Sobel, and C. Anello.** 1986. Toxic-shock syndrome and the vaginal contraceptive sponge. *JAMA* **255:**216–218.

44. **Farley, T. M. M., M. J. Rosenberg, P. J. Rowe, J. H. Chen, and O. Meirik.** 1992. Intrauterine devices and pelvic inflammatory disease: an international prospective. *Lancet* **339:**785–788.

45. **Fischetti, V. A., F. Chapman, R. Kakani, J. James, E. Grun, and J. B. Zabriskie.** 1989. Role of air in growth and production of toxic shock syndrome toxin 1 by *Staphylococcus aureus* in experimental cotton and rayon tampons. *Rev. Infect. Dis.* **11**(Suppl. 1):S176.

46. Flesh, G., J. M. Weiner, R. C. Corlett, Jr., C. Boice, D. R. Mishell, Jr., and R. M. Wolf. 1979. The intrauterine contraceptive device and acute salpingitis: a multifactor analysis. *Am. J. Obstet. Gynecol.* **135**:402–408.

47. Friedell, S., and L. J. Mercer. 1986. Non-menstrual toxic-shock syndrome. *Obstet. Gynecol. Surv.* **41**:336–341.

48. Friedrich, E. G., Jr., and K. A. Siegesmund. 1980. Tampon-associated vaginal ulcerations. *Obstet. Gynecol.* **55**:149–156.

49. Galvez, R. S., L. Galich, A. M. Guirola, L. P. Cole, and C. Waszak. 1989. A comparative study of the T Cu 200 B with and without strings. *Adv. Contracept. Deliv. Syst.* **6**:107–112.

50. Garbe, P. L., R. J. Arko, A. L. Reingold, L. M. Graves, P. S. Hayes, A. W. Hightower, F. W. Chandler, and C. V. Broome. 1985. Staphylococcus aureus isolates from patients with nonmenstrual toxic shock syndrome. *JAMA* **253**:2538–2542.

51. Gard, P. R., J. S. Malhi, and G. W. Haulon. 1993. Uterine contamination in the guinea pig following transcervical uterine monofilament insertion. *Gynecol. Obstet. Invest.* **35**:49–52.

52. Ghosh, K., I. Gupta, and S. K. Gupta. 1989. Asymptomatic salpingitis in intrauterine contraceptive device users. *Asia Oceania J. Obstet.* **15**:37–40.

53. Goldacre, M. J., B. Watt, N. London, L. J. Milne, J. D. Loudon, and M. P. Vessey. 1979. Vaginal microbial flora in normal young women. *Br. Med. J.* **1**:1450–1454.

54. Gonzalez, E. R. 1981. Calcium deposits on IUD's may play a role in infections. *JAMA* **245**:1625–1626.

55. Gosden, C., A. Ross, and N. B. Loudon. 1977. Intrauterine deposition of calcium on copper-bearing intrauterine contraceptive devices. *Br. Med. J.* **1**:202–206.

56. Gupta, P. K., D. H. Hollandu, and J. K. Frost. 1976. Actinomycetes in cervico vaginal smears: an association with IUD usage. *Acta Cytol.* **20**:2945–2947.

57. Hackett, S. P., and D. L. Stevens. 1993. Superantigens associated with staphylococcal and streptococcal toxic-shock-syndrome are potent inducers of tumor necrosis factor-b synthesis. *J. Infect. Dis.* **168**:232–235.

58. Haukkamaa, M. P. Stranden, H. Jousimies-Somer, and A. Siitonen. 1986. Bacterial flora of the cervix in women using different methods of contraception. *Am. J. Obstet. Gynecol.* **154**:520–524.

59. Helgerson, S. D., and L. R. Foster. 1982. Toxic shock syndrome in Oregon. Epidemiologic findings. *Ann. Intern. Med.* **96**:909–911.

60. Hill, B. G. 1991. *Eubacterium nodatum* mimics actinomyces in intrauterine device-associated infections and other settings within the female genital tract. *Obstet. Gynecol.* **79**:534–538.

61. Hill, J. A., E. Talledo, and J. Steele. 1986. Quantitative transcervical uterine cultures in asymptomatic women using an intrauterine contraceptive device. *Obstet. Gynecol.* **68**:700–703.

62. Holmes, K. K., D. A. Eschenbach, and J. S. Knapp. 1980. Salpingitis: overview of etiology and epidemiology. *Ann. J. Obstet. Gynecol.* **138**:893–900.

62a. Hooton, T. A., S. D. Fihn, C. Johnson, P. L. Roberts, and W. E. Stamm. 1989. Association between bacterial vaginosis and acute cystitis in women using diaphragms. *Arch. Intern. Med.* **149**:1932–1936.

63. **Indian Council of Medical Research, Task Force on IUD.** 1989. Randomized clinical trial with intrauterine devices (levonorgestrel intrauterine device (LNG) CUT, 380 Ag. CUT 220C, and CUT 200B) *Contraception* **39**:37–52.

64. Ishihama, A. 1959. Clinical study on intrauterine rings, especially the present state of contraception in Japan and the experiences in the use of intrauterine rings. *Yokohama Med. Bull.* **10**:89–105.

65. **Jacobson, J. A., C. R. Nicholas, and E. M. Kasworm.** 1985. Toxic-shock syndrome in Utah. 1976–1983. *West. J. Med.* **43**:337–341.

66. **Jimerson, S. D., and J. D. Becker.** 1980. Vaginal ulcers associated with tampon usage. *Obstet. Gynecol.* **56**:97–99.

67. **Kafka, D., and R. B. Gold.** 1983. Food and Drug Administration approves vaginal sponge. *Fam. Plann. Perspect.* **15**:146–147.

68. **Kahn, H. S., and C. W. Tyler.** 1976. An association between the Dalkon Shield and complicated pregnancies among women hospitalized for intrauterine contraceptive device related disorders. *Am. J. Obstet. Gynecol.* **125**:83–86.

69. **Kapiga, S., D. S. Hunter, J. F. Shae, G. Lwihula, J. Mtui, and E. Mbena.** 1992. Contraceptive practice and HIV-1 infection among family planning clients in Dar-es-Salaam, Tanzania. *Int. Conf. AIDS* **8**(2):C302 (#PoC4343).

70. **Kaufman, D. W., J. Watson, L. Rosenberg, S. P. Helmrich, D. R. Miller, O. Miettinen, P. D. Stolley, and S. Shapiro.** 1983. The effects of different types of intrauterine devices on the risk of pelvic inflammatory disease. *JAMA* **250**:759–762.

71. **Kehrberg, M. W., R. H. Latham, B. T. Haslam, A. Hightower, M. Tanner, J. A. Jacobson, A. G. Barbour, V. Nobel, and C. B. Smith.** 1981. Risk factors for staphylococcal toxic-shock syndrome. *Am. J. Epidemiol.* **114**:873–879.

72. **Keith, L. G., R. Bailey, and M. Method.** 1986. Ljubljana IUD's: further observations on surface morphology. *Adv. Contracept.* **2**:37–54.

73. **Keith, L. G., and G. S. Berger.** 1985. The pathogenic mechanisms of pelvic infection, p. 450–471. *In* G. I. Zatuchni, A. Golsmith, and J. J. Sciarra (ed.), *Intrauterine Contraception: Advances and Future Prospects.* J. B. Lippincott Co., Philadelphia.

74. **Kessel, E.** 1989. Pelvic inflammatory disease with intrauterine device use: a reassessment. *Fertil. Steril.* **51**:1–11.

75. **Khan, S. R., and E. J. Wilkinson.** 1985. Scanning electron microscopy as an analytical tool for the study of calcified intrauterine contraceptive devices. *Scanning Electron Microsc.* **3**:1247–1251.

76. **Kreiswirth, B. N., J. P. Handley, P. M. Schlievert, and R. P. Novick.** 1987. Cloning and expression of streptococcal pyrogenic exotoxin A and staphylococcal toxic shock syndrome toxin-1 in Bacillus subtilis. *Mol. Gen. Genet.* **208**:84–87.

77. **Ladipo, O. A., G. Farr, E. Otolorin, J. C. Konje, K. Sturgen, P. Cox, and C. B. Champion.** 1991. Prevention of IUD-related pelvic infection: the efficacy of prophylactic doxycycline at IUD insertion. *Adv. Contracept.* **7**:43–54.

78. **Lanes, S. F., C. Pook, N. A. Dryer, and L. Lanza.** 1986. Toxic-shock syndrome, contraceptive methods and vaginitis. *Am. J. Obstet. Gynecol.* **154**:989–991.

79. **Larkin, S. M., D. N. Williams, M. T. Osterholm, R. W. Tofte, and Z. Posalaky.** 1982. Toxic shock syndrome: clinical, laboratory, and pathologic findings in nine fatal cases. *Ann. Intern. Med.* **96**:858–864.

80. **Lee, N. C., G. Rubin, H. W. Ory, and R. T. Burkman.** 1983. Type of intrauterine device and the risk of pelvic inflammatory disease. *Obstet. Gynecol.* **62**:1–6.

81. **Linneman, C. C., Jr., J. L. Staneck, S. Hornstein, T. P. Barden, J. L. Rauth, P. F. Bonventre, C. R. Buncher, and A. Beiting.** 1981. The epidemiology of genital colonization with *Staphylococcus aureus. Ann. Intern. Med.* **96**:940–944.

82. **Marlow, D. E., R. M. Weigle, and R. S. Stauffenbert.** 1981. *Measurement of Tampon Absorbency: Evaluation of Tampon Brands.* Bureau of Medical Devices, Food and Drug Administration, Rockville, Md.

83. **Marrie, T. J., and J. W. Costerton.** 1983. A scanning and transmission electron microscopic study of the surfaces of intrauterine contraceptive devices. *Am. J. Obstet. Gynecol.* **146**:384–394.

84. **Mishell, D. R., Jr.** 1985. Current status of intrauterine devices. *N. Engl. J. Med.* **312:** 984–985.
85. **Mishell, D. R., Jr., J. H. Bell, R. G. Good, and D. L. Moyer.** 1966. The intrauterine device: a bacteriologic study of the endometrial cavity. *Am. J. Obstet. Gynecol.* **96:** 119–126.
86. **Mueller, B. A., M. Luz-Jimenez, J. R. Daling, D. E. Moore, B. McKnight, N. S. Weiss.** 1992. Risk factors for tubal infertility. Influence of history of prior pelvic inflammation disease. *Sex. Transm. Dis.* **19:**28–34.
87. **Mumford, S. D., and E. Kessel.** 1991. Was the Dalkon Shield a safe and effective intrauterine device? The contact between case-control and clinical trial study findings. *Fertil. Steril.* **57:**1151–1175.
88. **Murray, S., J. B. Hickey, and E. Houang.** 1987. Significant bacteremia associated with replacement of intrauterine contraceptive device. *Am. J. Obstet. Gynecol.* **156:** 698–700.
89. **Myatt, L., M. A. Bray, D. Gordon, and J. Morley.** 1975. Macrophages on intrauterine contraceptive devices produce prostaglandins. *Nature* (London) **257:**227–228.
90. **Newton, J. R., and D. Tacchi.** 1990. Long-term use of IUD's. *Lancet* **335:**1322–1323.
91. **Osterholm, M. T., J. P. Davis, R. W. Gibson, J. S. Mandel, L. A. Wintermeyer, C. M. Helms, J. C. Forfang, J. Rondeau, and J. M. Vergeront.** 1982. Tri-state toxic-shock syndrome study. I. Epidemiologic findings. *J. Infect. Dis.* **145:**431–440.
92. **Pap-Åkeson, M., F. Solheim, G. Thorbert, and M. Åkerlund.** 1992. Genital tract infections associated with the intrauterine contraceptive device can be reduced by inserting the threads into the uterine cavity. *Br. J. Obset. Gynaecol.* **99:**676–679.
93. **Paris, L. A., L. A. Herwaldt, D. Blum, G. P. Schmid, K. N. Shands, and C. V. Broome.** 1982. Pathologic findings in twelve fatal cases of toxic shock syndrome. *Ann. Intern. Med.* **96:**852–857.
94. **Petitti, D. B., D. Yamamoto, and N. N. Morgenstern.** 1983. Factors associated with actinomyces-like organisms on Papanicolaou smears in users of intrauterine contraceptive devices. *Am. J. Obstet. Gynecol.* **145:**338–341.
95. **Population Information Program.** 1984. New developments in vaginal contraception: barrier methods. *Popul. Rep.* **XII**(1)(seriesH[7]):H157–H190.
96. **Pritchard, J. A., P. C. MacDonald, and N. F. Gant (ed.).** 1985. Intrauterine contraceptive devices, p. 811–835. *In Williams Obstetrics,* 17th ed. Appleton & Lange, Norwalk, Conn.
97. **Purrier, B. G. A., R. A. Sparks, P. M. Watt, and M. Elstein.** 1979. In vitro study of the possible role of the intrauterine contraceptive device tail in ascending infection of the genital tract. *Br. J. Obstet. Gynaecol.* **86:**374–378.
98. **Rasheed, J. K., R. J. Arko, J. C. Feeley, F. W. Chandler, C. Thornsberry, R. J. Gibson, M. L. Cohen, C. D. Jeffries, and C. V. Broome.** 1985. Acquired ability of *Staphylococcus aureus* to produce toxic shock-associated protein and resulting illness in a rabbit model. *Infect. Immun.* **47:**598–604.
99. **Reingold, A. L.** 1986. Toxic-shock syndrome and the contraceptive sponge. *JAMA* **255:**242–243.
100. **Reingold, A. L., N. T. Hargrett, B. B. Dan, K. N. Shands, B. Y. Strickland, and C. V. Broome.** 1982. Nonmenstrual toxic-shock syndrome. *Ann. Intern. Med.* **96:**871–876.
101. **Rossing, M. A., and N. S. Weiss.** 1992. MD's and pelvic inflammatory disease. *Lancet* **340:**248–249.
102. **Roy, S.** 1991. Nonbarrier contraceptives and vaginitis and vaginosis. *Am. J. Obstet. Gynecol.* **165:**1240–1244.
103. **Sagiroglu, N., and E. Sagrioglu.** 1970. Biologic mode of action of the Lippes loop in intrauterine contraception. *Am. J. Obstet. Gynecol.* **106:**506–515.

104. **Schlech, W. F., III, K. N. Shands, A. L. Reingold, B. B. Dan, G. P. Schmid, N. T. Hargrett, A. Hightower, L. A. Herwalt, M. A. Neill, J. D. Band, and J. V. Bennett.** 1982. Risk factors for development of toxic shock syndrome: association with a tampon brand. *JAMA* **7**:835–839.
105. **Schlievert, P. M., K. N. Shands, B. B. Dan, G. P. Schmid, and R. D. Nishimura.** 1981. Identification and characterization of an exotoxin from *Staphylococcus aureus* associated with toxic-shock syndrome. *J. Infect. Dis.* **143**:509–516.
106. **Schmidt, W. A.** 1982. IUD's, inflammation, and infection: assessment after two decades of IUD use. *Hum. Pathol.* **13**:878–881.
107. **Schmidt, W. A., C. W. M. Bedrossian, V. Ali, J. A. Webb, and F. O. Bastian.** 1980. Actinomycosis and intrauterine contraceptive devices—the clinicopathologic entity. *Diagn. Gynecol. Obstet.* **2**:165–167.
108. **Schmidt, W. A., and K. L. Schmidt.** 1986. Intrauterine device associated pathology: a review of pathogenic mechanisms. *Scanning Electron Micros.* **2**:735–756.
109. **Schwartz, B., S. Gaventa, C. V. Broome, A. L. Reingold, A. W. Hightower, J. A. Perlman, P. H. Wolf, and the Toxic Shock Syndrome Study Group.** 1989. Nonmenstrual toxic shock syndrome associated with barrier contraceptives: report of a case-control study. *Rev. Infect. Dis.* **11**(Suppl. 1):S43.
110. **Shands, K. N., G. P. Schmid, B. B. Dan, D. Blum, R. J. Guidotti, N. T. Hargrett, R. L. Anderson, D. L. Hill, C. V. Broome, J. D. Band, and D. W. Fraser.** 1980. Toxic-shock syndrome in menstruating women. Association with tampon use and *Staphylococcus aureus* and clinical features in 52 cases. *N. Engl. J. Med.* **303**:1436–1442.
111. **Shaw, S. T., Jr.,** 1985. Endometrial histopathology and ultrastructural changes with IUD use, p. 276–296. *In* G. I. Zatuchni, A. Goldsmith, and J. J. Sciarra (ed.), *Intrauterine Contraception: Advances and Future Prospects.* J. B. Lippincott Co., Philadelphia.
112. **Sheppard, B. L., and J. Bonnar.** 1982. Scanning and transmission electron microscopy of material adherent to intrauterine contraceptive devices. *Br. J. Obstet. Gynaecol.* **106**:506–515.
113. **Sinei, S. A., K. F. Schultz, P. R. Lamptey, D. A. Grimes, J. G. Mati, S. M. Rosenthal, M. J. Rosenber, G. Riara, P. N. Njage, V. B. Vhullar, and H. V. Ogembo.** 1990. Preventing IUCD-related pelvic infection: the efficacy of prophylactic doxycycline at insertion. *Br. J. Obstet. Gynaecol.* **97**:412–419.
114. **Sivin, I., S. Elmahgoub, T. McCarthy, et al.** 1990. Long-term contraception with the Levonorgestrel 20 mcg/day (LNg 20) and the Copper T 380 Ag intrauterine devices: a five year randomized study. *Contraception* **42**:361–378.
115. **Skangalis, M., C. S. Mahoney, and W. M. O'Leary.** 1982. Microbial presence in the uterine cavity as detected by varieties of intrauterine contraceptive devices. *Fertil. Steril.* **37**:263–269.
116. **Smith, M. R., and R. Soderstrom.** 1976. Salpingitis: a frequent response to intrauterine contraception. *J. Reprod. Med.* **16**:159–165.
117. **Sparks, R. A., B. G. A. Purrier, P. J. Watt, and M. Elstein.** 1981. Bacteriological colonization of the uterine cavity: role of tailed intrauterine contraceptive devices. *Br. Med. J.* **282**:1189–1191.
118. **Spence, M. R., D. R. Stutz, and W. Paniom.** 1975. Effect of a copper-containing intrauterine contraceptive device on *Neisseria gonorrhoeae* in vitro. *Am. J. Obstet. Gynecol.* **122**:783–784.
119. **Stadel, B. V., and S. Schlesselman.** 1984. Extent of surgery for pelvic inflammatory disease in relation to duration of intra-uterine device use. *Obstet. Gynecol.* **63**:171–177.
120. **Stolz, S. J., J. Davis, J. M. Vergeront, B. A. Crass, P. J. Chesney, P. Wand, and M. S. Bergdoll.** 1985. Development of serum antibody to toxic shock toxin among individuals with toxic shock in Wisconsin. *J. Infect. Dis.* **151**:883–889.

121. **Strithers, B. J.** 1991. Copper IUD's, PID and fertility in nulliparous women. *Adv. Contracept.* **7:**211–230.

122. **Tatum, H. J., and E. B. Connell-Tatum.** 1981. Barrier-contraception: a comprehensive review. *Fertil. Steril.* **36:**1–12.

123. **Tatum, H., F. H. Schmidt, D. Phillips, M. McCarty, and W. M. O'Leary.** 1975. The Dalkon shield controversy: structural and bacteriological studies of IUD tails. *JAMA* **231:**711–717.

124. **Tatum, H. J., F. H. Schmidt, and D. M. Phillips.** 1975. Morphological studies of Dalkon Shield tails removed from patients. *Contraception* **11:**465–468.

125. **Todd, J. K., M. Fishaut, F. Kaptral, and T. Welch.** 1978. Toxic-shock syndrome associated with phage-group-1 staphylococci. *Lancet* **ii:**1116–1118.

126. **Toivonen, J.** 1993. Intrauterine contraceptive device and pelvic inflammatory disease. *Ann. Med.* (Finland) **25:**171–173.

127. **Toivonen, J., T. Luukkainen, and H. Allonen.** 1991. Protective effect of intrauterine release of levonorgestrel on pelvic infection: three years comparative experience of levonorgestrel- and copper-releasing intrauterine devices. *Obstet. Gynecol.* **77:**261–264.

128. **Toye, B., C. Laferriere, P. Claman, P. Jessamine, and R. Peeling.** 1993. Association between antibody to the chlamydial heat-shock protein and tubal infertility. *J. Infect. Dis.* **168:**1236–1240.

129. **Trebichavsky, I., and O. Nylkicek.** 1979. Description of the population and ultra-structure of cells on IUD's. *Acta Cytol.* **23:**366–369.

130. **U.S. Food and Drug Administration.** 1974. FDA investigating IUD's after deaths reported. *FDA Drug Bull.* **4:**19.

131. **Vergeront, J. M., S. J. Stolz, B. A. Crass, D. B. Nelson, J. P. Davis, and M. S. Bergdol.** 1983. Prevalence of serum antibody to staphylococcal enterotoxin F among Wisconsin residents: implications for toxic-shock syndrome. *J. Infect. Dis.* **148:**692–698.

132. **Vessey, M., R. Doll, and R. Peto.** 1976. A longterm followup study of women using different methods of contraception. An interim report. *J. Biosoc. Sci.* **8:**373–378.

133. **Wagner, G., L. Bohr, P. Wagner, and L. N. Petersen.** 1984. Tampon-induced changes in vaginal oxygen and carbon dioxide tensions. *Am. J. Obstet. Gynecol.* **148:**147–150.

134. **Wagner, H., M. Pfautsch, and F. K. Beller.** 1976. Investigation of the Dalkon Shield by scanning and transmission electron microscopy and bacteriologic studies. *Arch. Gynecol.* **221:**17–20.

135. **Weissberg, S. M., and M. G. Dodson.** 1983. Recurrent vaginal and cervical ulcers associated with tampon use. *JAMA* **25:**1430–1431.

136. **Westrom, L.** 1980. Incidence, prevalence, and trends of acute pelvic inflammatory disease and its consequences in industrialized countries. *Am. J. Obstet. Gynecol.* **138:**880–892.

137. **Westrom, L., L. P. Bengtsson, and P. A. Mardh.** 1976. The risk of pelvic inflammatory disease in women using intrauterine contraceptive devices compared to nonusers. *Lancet* **ii:**221–225.

138. **WHO Task Force Report.** 1990. The T Cu 380A, Multiload 250 and Nova T IUD's at 3, 5, and 7 years of use. *Contraception* **42:**142–158.

139. **Wilkins, K. M., G. W. Hanlon, G. P. Martin, and C. Marriott.** 1989. The migration of bacteria through gels in the presence of IUCD monofilament tails. *Contraception* **39:**205–216.

140. **Willson, J. R.** 1987. Family planning, p. 192–209. *In* W. J. Ledger, R. K. Laros, Jr., S. H. Mattox, J. R. Willson, and E. R. Carrington (ed.), *Obstetrics and Gynecology,* 8th ed. The C. V. Mosby Co., St. Louis.

141. **Winkler, B., and R. M. Richart.** 1985. Cervical/uterine pathologic considerations in pelvic infection, p. 438–449. *In* G. I. Zatuchni, A. Goldsmith, and J. J. Sciarra (ed.), *Intrauterine Contraception: Advances and Future Prospects.* J. B. Lippincott Co., Philadelphia.

142. **Wolf, A. S., and D. Krieger.** 1986. Bacterial colonization of intrauterine devices (IUD's). *Arch. Gynecol.* **239:**31–37.

143. **Wolfe, S. M.** 1987. Dangerous delays in tampon absorbency warnings. *JAMA* **258:** 949–951.

144. **Wolner-Hanssen, P.** 1991. Pelvic inflammatory disease. *Curr. Opin. Obstet. Gynecol.* **3:**687–691.

145. **Zatuchni, G. I., A. Goldsmith, and J. B. Sciarra (ed.).** 1985. *Intrauterine Contraception: Advances and Future Prospects.* J. B. Lippincott Co., Philadelphia.

146. **Zighelboim, I., W. Szczedrin, and O. Zambrano.** 1990. Management of IUD users with non-visible threads. *Adv. Contracept.* **6(2):**91–104.

147. **Zipper, J., M. Medel, and R. Prager.** 1969. Supression of fertility by intrauterine copper and zinc in rabbits: a new approach to intrauterine contraception. *Am. J. Obstet. Gynecol.* **105:**529–534.

Infections Associated with Indwelling Medical Devices, 2nd ed.
Edited by Alan L. Bisno and Francis A. Waldvogel
© 1994 American Society for Microbiology, Washington, DC 20005

Chapter 15

Antimicrobial Prophylaxis of Infections Associated with Foreign Bodies

David W. Haas and Allen B. Kaiser

The administration of antimicrobial agents prophylactically during the perioperative period has become standard practice for surgical procedures involving the implantation of prosthetic material, and most authorities in the field of surgical wound prophylaxis have endorsed this practice (3, 26, 34, 42, 46, 53). With few exceptions, however, placebo-controlled clinical trials have failed to clearly demonstrate the efficacy of antimicrobial agents in preventing infection of implanted foreign bodies. As outlined in Table 1, numerous attempts to verify the utility of prophylactic antimicrobial agents in this setting have been published. Only two controlled studies have documented an unequivocal benefit of prophylaxis: Ericson et al. (hip arthroplasty) and Bennion et al. (placement of vascular access grafts) (4, 19). A third study, by Blomstedt, demonstrated the efficacy of prophylaxis in ventricular shunt placement (5), but four other similar studies of antimicrobial prophylaxis in ventricular shunt placement have not corroborated these results (40, 50, 58, 62). A prospective study of 8,052 patients undergoing total knee or hip arthroplasty also suggested that prophylactic antibiotics significantly decreased the rate of joint sepsis and that this effect was multiplicative with the use of ultraclean air (41). Unfortunately, the use of ultraclean air rather than antibiotics was randomized in this study.

In general, placebo-controlled studies of antimicrobial prophylaxis

David W. Haas and Allen B. Kaiser • Department of Medicine, Vanderbilt University School of Medicine, Nashville, Tennessee 37232.

Table 1. Prospective placebo-controlled trials of antimicrobial prophylaxis of foreign device infections

Surgical specialty[a]	Reference	Procedure	Results (no. of infections/total no. of patients) and comment[b]
Cardiac	Goodman et al. (25)	Cardiac valve replacement[c]	Placebo control terminated when pneumococcal endocarditis developed in two placebo recipients
	Muers et al. (44)	Pacemaker placement	Cloxacillin (1/50) vs placebo (7/50) $(0.05 < P < 0.1)$
	Jacobson et al. (29)	Pacemaker placement	Penicillin and cloxacillin (2/234) vs placebo (7/197) $(0.05 < P < 0.1)$
Orthopedic	Ericson et al. (19)	Hip repair[d]	Cloxacillin (0/83) vs placebo (4/76) $(0.05 < P < 0.1)$; early (<2 wk) onset of infection
	Carlsson et al. (10)	Hip repair	Cloxacillin (3/60) vs placebo (21/58) $(P < 0.001, \chi^2)$; follow-up of late (1–6 yr) infections from above study
	Boyd et al. (6)	Hip repair	Reported significant differences between nafcillin and placebo infection rates, but the site of infection (i.e., prosthesis vs wound) was not differentiated
	Hill et al. (28)	Hip repair	Reported significant differences between cefazolin and placebo infection rates, but the site of infection (i.e., prosthesis vs wound) was not differentiated
Neuro-	Lambert et al. (40)	Ventricular shunt placement	Gentamicin (1/24) vs placebo (4/20) $(P > 0.1)$
	Wang et al. (58)	Ventriculoperitoneal shunt placement	Sulfamethoxazole-trimethoprim (4/55) vs placebo (5/65) $(P > 0.1)$
	Blomstedt (5)	Ventricular shunt placement	Sulfamethoxazole-trimethoprim (14/60) vs placebo (4/60) $(P < 0.05, \chi^2)$
	Yogev (62)	Ventriculoperitoneal shunt placement	Nafcillin with or without rifampin (2/106) vs placebo (6/84) $(P > 0.1)$
	Schmidt et al. (50)	Ventricular shunt placement	Methicillin (7/79) vs placebo (4/73) $(P > 0.5, \chi^2)$

Continued on following page

Table 1. *Continued.*

Surgical specialty[a]	Reference	Procedure	Results (no. of infections/total no. of patients) and comment[b]
Vascular	Kaiser et al. (35)	Arterial reconstruction	Cefazolin (0/225) vs placebo (4/237) ($P > 0.1$)
	Salzmann (49)	Arterial reconstruction	Cefuroxime or cefotaxime (1/134) vs placebo (4/166) ($P > 0.1$)
	Hasselgren et al. (27)	Arterial reconstruction	Cefuroxime (0/66) vs placebo (1/44) ($P > 0.1$)
	Jensen et al. (31)	Arterial reconstruction	Vancomycin (0/101) vs placebo (3/99) ($P > 0.1$)
	Bennion et al. (4)	Vascular access placement	Cefamandole (1/19) vs placebo (8/19) ($P < 0.02$)

[a] Ophthalmologic, no placebo-controlled studies in lens implantation have been published; urologic, no placebo-controlled studies in penile prosthesis surgery have been published.
[b] Unless otherwise noted, all statistical analyses were performed by using the two-tailed Fisher exact test.
[c] No other placebo-controlled studies in valve surgery have been published.
[d] Four additional studies (9, 24, 47, 55) of infection prevention in hip repair noted a significant improvement of antibiotic regimens over the placebo, but direct infectious involvement of prosthetic devices was not reported.

of implant infection have either ended prematurely because of the devastating consequences of implant infections among placebo recipients or have yielded inconclusive results. For example, in 1968 Goodman et al. abandoned the placebo arm of a prospective trial of antimicrobial prophylaxis in prosthetic valve surgery when pneumococcal endocarditis developed in two placebo recipients (25). Similarly, Kaiser et al. terminated their study of prophylactic cefazolin in vascular surgery after four graft infections had occurred in the placebo group versus none in the cefazolin group (35). Although the differences in rates of infection of implanted material did not achieve statistical significance ($P > 0.1$), high mortality and morbidity (two deaths and two leg amputations) in the infected patients persuaded the authors to conclude their study. The inconclusive results of many other studies have been related to the large number of patients required to achieve statistical significance, especially when infection of the implanted device itself is the end point. For example, in a 2-year study involving 128 patients undergoing arterial surgery, Jensen et al. documented significantly fewer total wound infections (superficial and deep) in vancomycin recipients than in placebo recipients (31). However, infections that directly involved the implanted grafts (deep infections) occurred in only three patients (all placebo recipients), too few to convincingly demonstrate the efficacy of vancomycin in preventing this much more serious infection. The authors estimated that an 800-patient study would be required to obtain significant results. At their previous rate of patient enrollment, a study of this size would span 12 years! In view of the problems of conducting suitable clinical trials and the dire consequences associated with infection of most prosthetic devices, prophylactic antibiotics have become the standard of care in implantation surgery and will likely remain so, despite the fact that proof of efficacy is, for the most part, lacking.

While clinical studies verifying that perioperative antibiotics significantly reduce implant infection rates are not available for the majority of such procedures, significant benefits frequently have been demonstrated when infections within any part of the surgical incision, not just the prosthetic device, are included in the evaluation. For example, six prospective, randomized, and placebo-controlled studies of vascular surgery concluded that antimicrobial prophylaxis significantly reduced surgical wound infections (27, 31, 35, 48, 49, 60). The incidence of infection of the prosthetic material itself was not shown to be significantly reduced in any of these studies. Nevertheless, clinicians have frequently extrapolated from the results of such studies to assume that prophylaxis will also lower rates of infections that directly involve implanted prostheses. In general, such extrapolation appears to be justified because soft tissue infections may be separated by only a few millimeters from the implanted vascular prosthesis and because the pathogens in the soft tissue and vascular graft infections are similar. On the other hand, the predominant pathogen causing infection in newly implanted prosthetic heart valves (i.e., coagulase-negative staphylococci) differs substantially from the predominant pathogen causing infection in the sternal incisions (i.e., *Staphylococcus aureus*). Yet another pathogen, the alpha-hemolytic streptococcus, is a major cause of prosthetic valve endocarditis developing during the late (i.e., >6 months) postoperative period. These data suggest that the epidemiology and pathophysiology of implanted-device infections may differ in important, but as yet mostly unidentified, ways from infections involving host tissues. Given the difficulty in convincingly demonstrating a benefit of antibiotics over placebo in most controlled studies, it is not surprising that data that directly address the efficacy or choice of individual antibiotic regimens in prophylaxis of prosthetic device infection are simply not available. No prospective study has demonstrated a clear benefit of one antimicrobial regimen over another in this situation.

Understandably, given the paucity of definitive information, there is widespread disagreement concerning the details of prophylactic antimicrobial administration. Penicillins, cephalosporins, vancomycin, and aminoglycosides are used in various combinations in surgical centers across the United States, with marked variations in the dose of antibiotic(s) and duration of administration. In addition, the considerable variation in pathogen spectrum and infection rates has made it virtually impossible to combine or compare data from different institutions. For example, in settings where methicillin-resistant *S. aureus* or methicillin-resistant coagulase-negative staphylococci are frequently encountered following implantation surgery, surgeons have routinely substituted vancomycin for cephalosporins. Such an agent would be totally inappropriate in settings where these pathogens are rarely encountered.

Until recently, cefazolin has been the mainstay of prophylaxis. Its relatively long half-life and excellent in vitro activity against *S. aureus*, methicillin-sensitive coagulase-negative staphylococci, and common gram-negative rods established this antimicrobial agent as the workhorse of prophylactic agents in clean surgery, including those procedures involving implanted material. However, a low but persistent rate of infection of implanted material despite the use of cefazolin and the emergence of methicillin-resistant *S. aureus* and methicillin-resistant coagulase-negative staphylococci as significant pathogens in this setting have prompted clinicians to look elsewhere for routine prophylactic coverage. Findings from controlled studies in cardiac surgery suggest that cefazolin may be inferior to either cefuroxime or cefamandole in preventing sternal infection due to methicillin-sensitive staphylococci (32, 52). Experimental evidence strongly suggests that enhanced susceptibility of cefazolin to hydrolysis by *S. aureus* type A β-lactamase, an enzyme expressed by some but not all clinical isolates, may explain this observation (38). Cephalosporins such as cefamandole and cefuroxime are much more resistant to hydrolysis by staphylococcal β-lactamase than is cefazolin. However, two prospective, randomized studies failed to demonstrate a benefit of cefamandole over cefazolin prophylaxis in total joint arthroplasty (7, 21). Similarly, neither cefamandole nor cefuroxime proved superior to cefazolin in two prospective randomized studies of wound infection in vascular surgery (17, 18). Conversely, Doebbeling et al. found cefuroxime to be significantly less effective than cefazolin in preventing infections following cardiac surgery (15). Although the failure to provide intraoperative redosing of cefamandole and cefuroxime (which have relatively short half-lives compared with cefazolin) may account for some of these differences (36), the relative efficacy of the various cephalosporins in prophylaxis remains undefined, even when dosed optimally. Lacking any consensus regarding the best prophylactic agent, and faced with a persistent albeit low rate of prosthetic material infection, other cephalosporins and other antimicrobial agents, such as vancomycin and gentamicin, are being used with increasing frequency. The role of newer antimicrobial agents, including the quinolones, for prophylaxis during prosthetic device implantation is uncertain. It appears unlikely that the issue of the choice of the most appropriate prophylactic antimicrobial agent in implantation surgery will be settled in the near future. Clinicians will be forced to carefully collect information on infecting pathogens in their respective institutions and, working with microbiologists and infectious disease specialists, choose an antibiotic regimen that offers a reasonable balance of spectrum of activity, cost, and side effects.

One of the more controversial issues in prophylaxis of implantation device infection relates to the duration of prophylaxis in the postoperative period. Disagreement exists on the role of prophylactic antibiotics both in the immediate postoperative and in the late or postdischarge period. Many authorities forcefully condemn the practice of extending prophylaxis beyond the immediate perioperative period (1, 14). However, in a randomized study of cefuroxime prophylaxis in 2,651 arthroplasties, joint sepsis occurred in approximately half as many patients who received three doses every 8 h as in those who received a single preoperative dose (11 versus 6, respectively). Although these differences did not achieve statistical significance because of the paucity of infections observed in either group, the authors advocated the three-dose regimen pending more definitive data (61). In the prophylaxis of infection in implantation devices, particularly those positioned within the intravascular space, concern has been expressed over the possibility of hematogenous seeding of such devices during the immediate (<72 h) postoperative period (12, 39). The demonstration of coagulase-negative staphylococci as a common pathogen in early prosthetic valve endocarditis lends some support to this concept. Coagulase-negative staphylococci are dominant pathogens in intravascular catheter infection. Although the presence of numerous intravascular catheters during the early postoperative period following prosthetic valve implantation seems more than coincidental, a causal relationship has not been proven. Equally important, the efficacy of prolonged postoperative antibiotics in preventing such hematogenous seeding has never been adequately evaluated. Furthermore, the potential for mucocutaneous colonization by resistant bacterial populations during antibiotic administration argues against indiscriminant prolonged antimicrobial courses. A number of studies of infection following clean elective surgery have compared infection rates of patients receiving short (usually <24 h) and those receiving long (≥72 h) postoperative prophylaxis (14). Without exception, no difference in wound infection rates has been observed. Equally important, however, all of these studies have involved relatively small numbers of patients, and true differences in infection rates would have been missed. This is an area in which an ambitious prospective clinical study or an appropriately designed animal model might offer useful information. In the absence of such data, definitive conclusions regarding the optimal duration of perioperative antimicrobial prophylaxis in implantation surgery are not possible.

Equally difficult is the question of antimicrobial prophylaxis for the prevention of infection in the remote posthospitalization period during subsequent procedures that may be associated with a risk of transient bacteremia (e.g., dental procedures). Once again, definitive data are lacking. In prophylaxis of prosthetic valve endocarditis, however, anecdotal associations between episodes of transient bacteremia and endocarditis have led to an almost universal recommendation for aggressive antimicrobial prophylaxis for patients with prosthetic valves who undergo dental procedures, surgery, etc. (13, 20). However, for patients with other types of implantation devices, the association between bacteremia and infections is much less clear. A case has been made for antibiotic prophylaxis in arthroplasty patients during dental procedures, using oral penicillin V, cephalexin, erythromycin, or clindamycin (11, 30, 45). The occurrence of late-onset (>6 months) infections in such prostheses has prompted these recommendations. However, few well-documented cases of late hematogenous prosthetic joint infection that followed dental manipulation and that were caused by oral flora have been described. Sullivan et al. reported a patient who presented with acute prosthetic hip infection due to peptostreptococci 3 days after undergoing dental surgery for a fractured molar (54). However, the infecting pathogen in most cases of late prosthetic joint infection is *S. aureus* or coagulase-negative staphylococci, organisms not commonly detected in the bacteremia associated with dental procedures. The source of staphylococci in late hip infections is unknown, but at least some of these infections are related to contamination that occurred, occasionally years earlier, at the time of surgery (10). In support of this concept, perioperative prophylaxis with cefazolin was shown in a large, multicenter study not only to decrease the incidence of hip abscess, septicemia, or lethal infection significantly during the first year following prosthetic hip placement (28) but also to prevent "late" hip infections (i.e., those infections first diagnosed >3 years postoperatively). Indeed, among 2,137 patients initially randomized, 14 such infections occurred in the prophylaxis group versus none in placebo recipients (16). On the basis of these considerations, we agree with the Working Party of the British Society for Antimicrobial Chemotherapy that more information is needed before the routine use of prophylactic antibiotics can be recommended for all patients with

Table 2. Guidelines for antimicrobial prophylaxis of implant device infections

Surgical specialty/ procedure	Predominant pathogen(s)	Prophylactic regimen[a]
Cardiac surgery/valve replacement (13, 34)	Early-onset postoperative infection—CNS,[b] S. aureus, and gram-negative rods	Cefuroxime (1.5 g i.v. at the induction of anesthesia followed by 750 mg q4h during surgery or cefamandole, 2 g i.v. at the induction of anesthesia followed by 1 g q2h during surgery)[c,d,e,f]
	Late-onset infection—alpha-streptococci and enterococci	As recommended by the American Heart Association for patients undergoing dental and surgical procedures
Vascular surgery/arterial reconstruction (34)	S. aureus	Cefazolin (1 g i.v. at induction of anesthesia followed by 1 g q6h for 3 doses)[c,d,e]
Vascular surgery/ vascular access placement (4)	S. aureus and CNS	Cefazolin (1 g i.v. at induction of anesthesia followed by 1 g q6h for 3 doses)[c,d,e]
Neurosurgery/ ventricular shunt placement (34)	CNS, S. aureus, and gram-negative rods	Prophylactic antimicrobial agents are not recommended in institutions with low infection rates (<10%); trimethoprim (160 mg) + sulfamethoxazole (800 mg) i.v. preoperatively and q12h (3 doses) postoperatively may be beneficial in institutions with high infection rates

Continued on following page

prosthetic joints who undergo procedures known to produce transient bacteremia (51). Providing antimicrobial prophylaxis for selected patients with prosthetic joints and particularly severe periodontal disease, however, may be reasonable pending more data. There is currently little support for posthospitalization prophylaxis of other implanted devices, such as vascular grafts and penile prostheses. For further discussion of this issue, the reader should see chapter 11.

A consensus regarding prophylactic antimicrobial agent use is not currently available for any of the various procedures involving the surgical implantation of prosthetic material. A reasonable approach to the choice of a prophylactic agent is presented in Table 2. Intraoperative dosing of the prophylactic antimicrobial agent(s) should be scheduled

Table 2. *Continued.*

Surgical specialty/ procedure	Predominant pathogen(s)	Prophylactic regimen[a]
Orthopedic/hip repair (and placement of prosthetic material in other joint repair procedures) (33, 34)	Early-onset postoperative infection—*S. aureus* and CNS	Cefazolin (1 g i.v. at the induction of anesthesia, followed by 1 g q6h for 3 doses)[c,d,e]; gentamicin incorporated into bone cement may prove valuable as a substitute for or supplement to systemic antimicrobial prophylaxis
	Late-onset infection—CNS	Antimicrobial prophylaxis during outpatient dental procedures or other invasive procedures is not routinely recommended; may be considered for oral surgery associated with dental sepsis or a major breach of oral mucosa (see late-onset cardiac valve prophylaxis above)
Urology/penile prosthesis (43)	CNS, *S. aureus*, and gram-negative rods	Cefazolin (1 g i.v. at induction of anesthesia followed by 1 g q6h for 3 doses)[c,d,e]

[a] In the absence of definitive studies, the choice of prophylactic regimen is based primarily on the predominant pathogen(s), antibiotic spectrum, and pharmacology of the prophylactic antimicrobial agent(s). i.v., intravenously; q2h, q4h, q6h, and q12h, every 2, 4, 6, and 12 h, respectively.
[b] CNS, coagulase-negative staphylococci.
[c] If methicillin-susceptible *S. aureus* infections continue to occur, consider substituting cefuroxime (1,500 mg intravenously at the induction of anesthesia and 750 mg every 4 h throughout the procedure) or cefamandole (2 g at induction of anesthesia and 1 g every 2 h throughout the operative procedure) (37, 52).
[d] If methicillin-susceptible coagulase-negative staphylococcal infections continue to occur despite cefazolin or cefuroxime prophylaxis, consider using cefamandole (2 g at the induction of anesthesia and 1 g every 2 h throughout the operative procedure) (59).
[e] If methicillin-resistant staphylococcal infections become frequent, vancomycin (15 mg/kg preoperatively and 10 mg/kg every 8 h during surgery thereafter) should be considered (22).
[f] Postoperative dosing (every 4 to 6 h) of prophylactic antimicrobial agents for up to 72 h should be considered if intravascular lines are in place.

so that adequte serum and tissue levels are maintained throughout the operative procedure. Importantly, if a tourniquet is used for hemostasis, antibiotics should be administered before tourniquet application, to ensure adequate antibiotics in the tissues at the time of bacterial contamination (2, 32). To this end, a review of the pharmacokinetics of cefazolin, cefamandole, cefuroxime, and vancomycin suggests that these agents should be redosed during the operative period at 6, 2, 4, and 8 h, respectively (8, 22, 37). The duration of postoperative prophylaxis should, in general, be as short as possible, although the role of prolonged prophylaxis in procedures involving the implantation of intravascular devices remains to be defined.

The most important approach to prophylactic management may be to develop a program that systematically evaluates trends in prophylaxis failure. Occasional failures of prophylactic antimicrobial agents may be inevitable, but recurrent pathogens demand aggressive evaluation. Moreover, as the incidence of resistant pathogens such as methicillin-resistant *S. aureus* and methicillin-resistant coagulase-negative staphylococci continues to increase, the need to compare prophylactic regimens will escalate. The choice of antimicrobial regimen and the duration of use remain matters of great confusion. When recurrent pathogens are encountered, a systematic evaluation of new prophylactic regimens, possibly in the form of ongoing randomized trials, may provide a data base for a rational approach to infection prevention in implantation surgery.

In surgical centers where active surveillance shows methicillin-resistant *S. aureus* or methicillin-resistant coagulase-negative staphylococci to be common causes of device-related infections, consideration should be given to prophylaxis with vancomycin. Although randomized studies demonstrating a benefit of vancomycin in this setting are not available, this drug should provide effective prophylaxis against methicillin-resistant staphylococcal infections. However, two words of caution are in order. First, unlike cephalosporins, vancomycin is not active against gram-negative bacteria. While such organisms cause only a minority of device-related infections, the possibility that decreased staphylococcal infections will be offset by increased gram-negative infections should be carefully weighed. Second, widespread use of vancomycin in surgical prophylaxis may, over time, encourage the emergence of gram-positive bacteria in the community which are resistant to vancomycin (especially enterococci and staphylococci). Deep-seated infections caused by these organisms may be extremely difficult to cure with currently available antibiotics.

For prophylaxis to be optimally effective, the first antibiotic dose should ideally be given intravenously a few minutes prior to the first skin incision (often coinciding with the induction of anesthesia); repeated doses should be administered during the procedure, based upon the pharmacokinetics of the individual agents (Table 2). Maintaining adequate tissue levels throughout surgery may be essential to success (37). Unfortunately, in the sometimes hectic environment of the operating room, the focus on more emergent demands may cause the operative team to overlook the need to provide intraoperative redosing of prophylactic antibiotics. For this reason, each surgical center should establish an ongoing system for ensuring that antibiotic prophylaxis is consistently administered in a timely fashion, as well as periodic review to ensure continued success of the system.

As the prevalence of bacteria that are resistant to traditional antimicrobial agents continues to increase in both the community and the hospital, so will the need to develop new ways to prevent prosthetic device infection. Strategies that may be used in the future (based upon very preliminary in vitro and in vivo studies) include specifically blocking the attachment of bacteria to host proteins such as fibrin or fibronectin (23, 57), locally administering cytokines at the time of implantation (56), and immunizing the patient against selected pathogens. The prevention of implanted foreign body infection poses a continuing challenge to surgeons, infectious diseases specialists, and microbiologists for the forseeable future.

REFERENCES

1. **Austin, T. W., J. C. Coles, R. Burnett, and M. Goldbach.** 1980. Aortocoronary bypass procedures and sternotomy infections: a study of antistaphylococcal prophylaxis. *Can. J. Surg.* **23:**483–485.
2. **Bannister, G. C., J. M. Auchincloss, D. P. Johnson, and J. H. Newman.** 1988. The timing of tourniquet application in relation to prophylactic antibiotic administration. *J. Bone Jt. Surg. Br. Vol.* **70B:**322–324.
3. **Beam, T. R., Jr.** 1985. Perioperative prevention of infection in cardiac surgery. *Antibiot. Chemother.* **33:**114–139.
4. **Bennion, R. S., J. R. Hiatt, R. A. Williams, and S. E. Wilson.** 1985. A randomized, prospective study of perioperative antimicrobial prophylaxis for vascular access surgery. *J. Cardiovasc. Surg.* **26:**270–274.
5. **Blomstedt, G. C.** 1985. Results of trimethoprim-sulfamethoxazole prophylaxis in ventriculostomy and shunting procedures: a double-blind randomized trial. *J. Neurosurg.* **62:**694–697.
6. **Boyd, R. J., J. F. Burke, and T. Colton.** 1973. A double-blind clinical trial of prophylactic antibiotics in hip fractures. *J. Bone Jt. Surg. Am. Vol.* **55A:**1251–1258.
7. **Bryan, C. S., S. L. Morgan, R. J. Caton, and E. M. Lunceford, Jr.** 1988. Cefazolin versus cefamandole for prophylaxis during total joint arthroplasty. *Clin. Orthop. Relat. Res.* **223:**117–122.
8. **Bundtzen, R. W., R. D. Toothaker, O. S. Nielson, P. O. Madsen, P. G. Welling, and W. A. Craig.** 1981. Pharmacokinetics of cefuroxime in normal and impaired renal function: comparison of high-pressure liquid chromatography and microbiological assays. *Antimicrob. Agents Chemother.* **19:**443–449.
9. **Burnett, J. W., R. B. Gustilo, D. N. Williams, and A. C. Kind.** 1980. Prophylactic antibiotics in hip fractures. *J. Bone Jt. Surg. Am. Vol.* **62A:**457–462.
10. **Carlsson, A. S., L. Lidgren, and L. Lindberg.** 1977. Prophylactic antibiotics against early and late deep infections after total hip replacements. *Acta Orthop. Scand.* **48:**405–410.
11. **Cioffi, G. A., G. T. Terezhalmy, and G. M. Taybos.** 1988. Total joint replacement:

a consideration for antimicrobial prophylaxis. *Oral Surg. Oral Med. Oral Pathol.* **66:** 124–129.

12. **Culbertson, W. R., W. A. Altemeier, L. L. Gonzalez, and E. O. Hill.** 1961. Studies on the epidemiology of postoperative infection of clean operative wounds. *Ann. Surg.* **154:**599–610.

13. **Dajani, A. S., A. L. Bisno, K. J. Chung, D. T. Durack, M. Freed, M. A. Gerber, A. W. Karchmer, H. D. Millard, S. Rahimtoola, S. T. Shulman, C. Watanakunakorn, and K. A. Taubert.** 1990. Prevention of bacterial endocarditis: recommendations by the American Heart Association. *JAMA* **264:**2919–2922.

14. **DiPiro, J. T., R. P. F. Cheung, T. A. Bowden, Jr., and J. A. Mansberger.** 1986. Single dose systemic antibiotic prophylaxis of surgical wound infections. *Am. J. Surg.* **152:** 552–559.

15. **Doebbeling, B. N., M. A. Pfaller, K. R. Kuhns, R. M. Massanari, D. M. Behrendt, and R. P. Wenzel.** 1990. Cardiovascular surgery prophylaxis: a randomized, controlled comparison of cefazolin and cefuroxime. *J. Thorac. Cardiovasc. Surg.* **99:**981–989.

16. **Doyon, F., J. Evrard, F. Mazas, and C. Hill.** 1987. Long-term results of prophylactic cefazolin versus placebo in total hip replacement. *Lancet* **i:**860.

17. **Edwards, W. H., Jr., A. B. Kaiser, D. S. Kernodle, T. C. Appleby, W. H. Edwards, Sr., R. S. Martin, J. L. Mulherin, and C. A. Wood, Jr.** 1992. Cefuroxime versus cefazolin as prophylaxis in vascular surgery. *J. Vasc. Surg.* **15:**35–42.

18. **Edwards, W. H., Jr., A. B. Kaiser, S. Tapper, W. H. Edwards, Sr., R. S. Martin III, J. L. Mulherin, Jr., J. Jenkins, and A. Roach.** 1993. Cefamandole versus cefazolin in vascular surgical wound infection prophylaxis: cost effectiveness and risk factors. *J. Vasc. Dis.* **18:**470–475.

19. **Ericson, C., L. Lidgren, and L. Lindberg.** 1973. Cloxacillin in the prophylaxis of postoperative infections of the hip. *J. Bone Jt. Surg. Am. Vol.* **55A:**808–843.

20. **Everett, E. D., and J. V. Hirschmann.** 1977. Transient bacteremia and endocarditis prophylaxis: a review. *Medicine* **56:**61–77.

21. **Evrard, J., F. Doyan, J. F. Acar, J. C. Mazas, and R. Flanant.** 1988. Two-day cefamandole versus five-day cephazolin prophylaxis in 965 total hip replacements. *Int. Orthop.* **12:**69–73.

22. **Farber, B. F., A. W. Karchmer, M. J. Buckley, and R. C. Moellering.** 1983. Vancomycin prophylaxis in cardiac operations: determination of an optimal dosage regimen. *J. Thorac. Cardiovasc. Surg.* **85:**933–940.

23. **Froman, G., L. M. Switalski, P. Speziale, and M. Hook.** 1987. Isolation and characterization of a fibronectin receptor from Staphylococcus aureus. *J. Biol. Chem.* **262:** 6564–6571.

24. **Gatell, J. M., J. Riba, M. L. Lozano, J. Mana, R. Ramon, and J. G. SanMiguel.** 1984. Prophylactic cefamandole in orthopaedic surgery. *J. Bone Jt. Surg. Am. Vol.* **66:** 1219–1222.

25. **Goodman, J. S., W. Schaffner, H. A. Collins, E. J. Battersby, and M. G. Koenig.** 1968. Infection after cardiovascular surgery: clinical study including examination of antimicrobial prophylaxis. *N. Engl. J. Med.* **278:**117–123.

26. **Guglielmo, B. J., D. C. Hohn, P. J. Koo, T. K. Hunt, R. L. Sweet, and J. E. Conte, Jr.** 1983. Antibiotic prophylaxis in surgical procedures: a critical review of the literature. *Arch. Surg.* **118:**943–955.

27. **Hasselgren, P., L. Ivarsson, B. Risberg, and T. Seeman.** 1984. Effects of prophylactic antibiotics in vascular surgery. *Ann. Surg.* **200:**86–92.

28. **Hill, C., R. Flamant, F. Mazas, and J. Evrard.** 1981. Prophylactic cefazolin versus placebo in total hip replacement. *Lancet* **i:**795–797.

29. Jacobson, B., G. Bluhm, I. Julander, and C. E. Nord. 1983. Coagulase-negative staphylococci and cloxacillin prophylaxis in pacemaker surgery. *Acta Pathol. Microbiol. Immunol. Scand.* **91:**97–99.
30. Jacobson, P. L., and W. Murray. 1980. Prophylactic coverage of dental patients with artificial joints: a retrospective analysis of thirty-three infections in hip prostheses. *Oral Surg.* **50:**130–133.
31. Jensen, L. J., M. T. Aagaard, and S. Schifter. 1985. Prophylactic vancomycin versus placebo in arterial prosthetic reconstructions. *Thorac. Cardiovasc. Surgeon* **33:**300–303.
32. Johnson, D. P. 1987. Antibiotic prophylaxis with cefuroxime in arthroplasty of the knee. *J. Bone Jt. Surg. Br. Vol.* **69B:**787–789.
33. Josefsson, G., L. Lindberg, and B. Wiklander. 1981. Systemic antibiotics and gentamicin-containing bone cement in the prophylaxis of postoperative infections in total hip arthroplasty. *Clin. Orthop. Relat. Res.* **159:**194–200.
34. Kaiser, A. B. 1986. Antimicrobial prophylaxis in surgery. *N. Engl. J. Med.* **315:** 1129–1138.
35. Kaiser, A. B., K. R. Clayson, J. L. Mulherin, Jr., A. C. Roach, T. R. Allen, W. H. Edwards, and W. A. Dale. 1978. Antibiotic prophylaxis in vascular surgery. *Ann. Surg.* **188:**283–289.
36. Kaiser, A. B., and D. S. Kernodle. 1992. Inappropriate dosing of cefuroxime in cardiac surgery. *J. Thorac. Cardiovasc. Surg.* **103:**167–68.
37. Kaiser, A. B., M. R. Petracek, J. W. Lea IV, D. S. Kernodle, A. C. Roach, W. C. Alford, Jr., G. R. Burrus, D. M. Glassford, Jr., C. S. Thomas, Jr., and W. S. Stoney. 1987. Efficacy of cefazolin, cefamandole, and gentamicin as prophylactic agents in cardiac surgery: results of a prospective, randomized, double-blind trial in 1030 patients. *Ann. Surg.* **206:**791–797.
38. Kernodle, D. S., D. C. Classen, J. P. Burke, and A. B. Kaiser. 1990. Failure of cephalosporins to prevent *Staphylococcus aureus* surgical wound infections. *JAMA* **263:**961–966.
39. Krieger, J. N., D. L. Kaiser, and R. P. Wenzel. 1983. Nosocomial urinary tract infections cause wound infections postoperatively in surgical patients. *Surg. Gynecol. Obstet.* **156:**313–318.
40. Lambert, M., A. E. MacKinnon, and A. Vaishnav. 1984. Comparison of two methods of prophylaxis against CSF shunt infection. *Z. Kinderchir.* **39:**109–110.
41. Lidwell, O. M., R. A. Elson, E. J. L. Lowbury, W. Whyte, R. Blowers, S. J. Stanley, and D. Lowe. 1987. Ultraclean air and antibiotics for prevention of postoperative infection. *Acta Orthop. Scand.* **58:**4–13.
42. Lidwell, O. M., E. J. L. Lowbury, W. Whyte, R. Blowers, S. J. Stanley, and D. Lowe. 1982. Effect of ultraclean air in operating rooms on deep sepsis in the joint after total hip or knee replacement: a randomized study. *Br. Med. J.* **285:**10–14.
43. Montague, D. K. 1987. Periprosthetic infections. *J. Urol.* **138:**68–69.
44. Muers, M. F., A. G. Arnold, and P. Sleight. 1981. Prophylactic antibiotics for cardiac pacemaker implantation: a prospective trial. *Br. Heart J.* **46:**539–544.
45. Nelson, J. P., R. H. Fitzgerald, Jr., M. T. Jaspers, and J. W. Little. 1990. Prophylactic antimicrobial coverage in arthroplasty patients. *J. Bone Jt. Surg. Am. Vol.* **72A:**1.
46. Norden, C. W. 1991. Antibiotic prophylaxis in orthopedic surgery. *Rev. Infect. Dis.* **13:** S842–846.
47. Pavel, A., R. L. Smith, A. Ballard, and I. J. Larson. 1977. Prophylactic antibiotics in elective orthopedic surgery: a prospective study of 1,591 cases. *South. Med. J.* **70:**50–55.
48. Pitt, H. A., R. G. Postier, W. A. L. MacGowan, L. W. Frank, A. J. Surmak, J. V. Sitzman, and D. Bouchier-Hayes. 1980. Prophylactic antibiotics in vascular surgery. Topical, systemic, or both? *Ann. Surg.* **192:**356–364.

49. **Salzmann, G.** 1983. Perioperative infection prophylaxis in vascular surgery—a randomized prospective study. *Thorac. Cardiovasc. Surgeon* **31**:239–242.

50. **Schmidt, K., F. Gjerris, O. Osgaard, E. F. Hvidberg, J. E. Kristiansen, B. Dahlerup, and C. Kruse-Larsen.** 1985. Antibiotic prophylaxis in cerebrospinal fluid shunting: a prospective randomized trial in 152 hydrocephalic patients. *Neurosurgery* **17**:1–5.

51. **Simmons, N. A., A. P. Ball, R. A. Cawson, S. J. Eykyn, S. P. F. Hughes, D. A. McGowan, and D. C. Shanson.** 1992. Case against antibiotic prophylaxis for dental treatment of patients with joint prostheses. *Lancet* **339**:301.

52. **Slama, T. G., S. J. Sklar, J. Misinski, and S. W. Fess.** 1986. Randomized comparison of cefamandole, cefazolin, and cefuroxime prophylaxis in open-heart surgery. *Antimicrob. Agents Chemother.* **29**:744–747.

53. **Strachan, C.** 1982. Antibiotic prophylaxis in "clean" surgical procedures. *World J. Surg.* **6**:273–280.

54. **Sullivan, P. M., R. C. Johnston, and S. S. Kelley.** 1990. Late infection after total hip replacement caused by an oral organism after dental manipulation. *J. Bone Jt. Surg. Am. Vol.* **72A**:121–123.

55. **Tengve, B., and J. Kjellander.** 1978. Antibiotic prophylaxis in operations on trochanteric femoral fractures. *J. Bone Jt. Surg. Am. Vol.* **60A**:97–99.

56. **Vaudaux, P., G. E. Grau, E. Huggler, F. Schumacher-Perdreau, F. Fiedler, F. A. Waldvogel, and D. P. Lew.** 1992. Contribution of tumor necrosis factor to host defense against staphylococci in a guinea pig model of foreign body infections. *J. Infect. Dis.* **166**:58–64.

57. **Vaudaux, P., D. Pittet, A. Haeberli, E. Huggler, U. E. Nydegger, D. P. Lew, and F. A. Waldvogel.** 1989. Host factors selectively increase staphylococcal adherence on inserted catheters: a role for fibronectin and fibrinogen or fibrin. *J. Infect. Dis.* **160**:865–875.

58. **Wang, E. E. L., C. G. Prober, B. E. Hendrick, H. J. Hoffman, and R. P. Humphreys.** 1984. Prophylactic sulfamethoxazole and trimethoprim in ventriculoperitoneal shunt surgery: a double-blind, randomized, placebo-controlled trial. *JAMA* **251**:1174–1177.

59. **Woods, G. L., C. C. Knapp, and J. A. Washington II.** 1987. Relationship between cefamandole and cefuroxime activity against oxacillin-resistant *Staphylococcus epidermidis* and oxacillin resistance phenotype. *Antimicrob. Agents Chemother.* **31**:1332–1337.

60. **Worning, A. M., N. Frimodt-Moller, P. Ostri, T. Nilsson, K. Hojholdt, and C. Frimodt-Moller.** 1986. Antibiotic prophylaxis in vascular reconstructive surgery: a double-blind placebo-controlled study. *J. Antimicrob. Chemother.* **17**:105–113.

61. **Wymenga, A., J. van Horn, A. Theeuwes, H. Muytjens, and T. Slooff.** 1988. Cefuroxime for prevention of postoperative coxitis. *Acta Orthop. Scand.* **63**:19–24.

62. **Yogev, A. M.** 1985. Cerebrospinal fluid shunt infections: a personal view. *Pediatr. Infect. Dis. J.* **4**:113–118.

Index